KT-131-736

'Good Health at Low Cost'
25 years on

What makes a successful health system?

'GOOD HEALTH AT LOW COST' 25 YEARS ON

WHAT MAKES A SUCCESSFUL HEALTH SYSTEM?

Editors: Dina Balabanova, Martin McKee and Anne Mills

© **The London School of Hygiene & Tropical Medicine 2011**

This study was funded by the Rockefeller Foundation.

The opinions expressed in this publication do not necessarily reflect the policies of the London School of Hygiene & Tropical Medicine or the Rockefeller Foundation.

This publication may be reviewed, abstracted or reproduced in part when fully referenced, but may not be sold or used for commercial purposes.

Cover design by: Nexus Design and Print in partnership with Pamoja Consulting Ltd, Sensor House, 10–12 Lewes Road, Brighton BN2 3HP, United Kingdom www.pamojaconsulting.co.uk

Book design by: Sarah Moncrieff, Westminster European, 23 Charlwood Street London SW1V 2EA, United Kingdom

Printed and bound by: Charlesworth Press, Flanshaw Way, Flanshaw Lane, Wakefield WF2 9LP, United Kingdom. www.charlesworth.com

Citation:

Balabanova D, McKee M and Mills A (eds). *'Good health at low cost' 25 years on. What makes a successful health system?* London: London School of Hygiene & Tropical Medicine, 2011.

The London School of Hygiene & Tropical Medicine
Department of Global Health & Development,
15–17 Tavistock Place, London WC1H 9SH
United Kingdom
Website: www.healthsystems.lshtm.ac.uk

ISBN 978-0-902657-84-7

FRONT COVER IMAGES

Top left *Kyrgyzstan*
Credit: © 2006 Anara Doolotova, Courtesy of Photoshare
Caption: An IMCI-trained visiting nurse examines an infant in Bazarkorgondistrict, Jalalabat province, Kyrgyzstan, as part of Project HOPE's Child Survival program.

Top right *Thailand*
Credit: © 2010 Patrick Brown, Panos Pictures
Caption: A woman brings her 4 month old child to a doctor.

Bottom right *Bangladesh*
Credit: © 2002 Shehzad Noorani, Courtesy of World Bank
Caption: A Non Formal Primary Education (NFPE) school. Girls writing on slate board.

Bottom left *Ethiopia*
Credit: © 2007 Bonnie Gillespie, Courtesy of Photoshare
Caption: A community health worker in rural Ethiopia tests a boy for malaria.

BACK COVER IMAGES

Top left *Tamil Nadu*
Credit: © 2005 Chris Stowers, Panos Pictures
Caption: At start of the Pongal Harvest Festival, celebrating the beginning of the Tamil New Year, a mother and her child stir a pot of sweet Pongal, the rice dish after which the festival is named.

Top, second from left *Ethiopia*
Credit: © 2005 Virginia Lamprecht, Courtesy of Photoshare
Caption: A local man of the village and a community-based distribution agent are engaged in a spirited conversation about family planning.

Top, second from right *Bishkek, Kyrgyzstan*
Credit: © 2006 Dmitry Shevkun/IFES, Courtesy of Photoshare
Caption: Thousands gather in Bishkek's Alatoo Square in Kyrgyzstan on November 3, 2006 to protest the slow pace of economic and political reforms since the country's 2005 Tulip revolution.

Top right *Khuda Lahora, India*
Credit: © 2007 Pradeep Tewari, Courtesy of Photoshare
Caption: A health worker educates rural women on sexually transmitted diseases and reproductive and sexual health at a health awareness camp organized by the Sports and Welfare Club and the Teen Club of Khuda Lahora village, India. The clubs are affiliated with Nehru Yuvak Kender (Ministry of Youth, Welfare, and Sports) in Chandigarh.

Bottom *Thailand*
Credit: © 2011 Philippe Huguen, AFP/Getty Images
Caption: Mother and child from mountain region near Chiang Mai.

CONTENTS

FOREWORD

It is now all too apparent that the presence of well-functioning health systems is a prerequisite for progress in global health. Yet, while we may know what we need to achieve in creating such systems, we know much less about how to do so. Health systems are complex, dynamic systems existing in a world characterized by limited resources and changing demands. They are designed by humans, with all their strengths and weaknesses, and are easily thrown off course by events that may be entirely unpredictable. Think, for a minute, of the transformation of health care delivery that has resulted from the emergence of AIDS.

In this book, an international team of authors have sought to understand how five countries have made progress towards the ultimate goal of *Good health at low cost* in recent decades (and what has happened to others that were viewed as successes 25 years ago). They take a holistic approach, demonstrating the strengths of collaboration across disciplines and continents. In doing so, they provide important lessons for other countries seeking to emulate success.

Although each of the health systems they study is unique, it is possible to discern some common factors, such as political vision and the ability to mobilize all those who can contribute to better health care and, ultimately, health. Faced with a shortage of financial and human resources, these health systems embrace innovation. They are responsive to the changing needs of their populations while maintaining continuity over time. They combine resilience with flexibility and have developed mechanisms that allow them to learn from the past and anticipate the future. Yet health systems are, essentially, collections of people. This book contains examples of individuals who have been able to seize opportunities and implement solutions to seemingly intractable problems, adapting them to the national context.

This book provides many immediate lessons for those seeking to strengthen health systems, but it also provides an agenda for future research. There is still much that we do not understand. It also provides a rich resource for teaching, which will support the development of the next generation of health policy analysts and practitioners that the world so needs. I am delighted that the London School of Hygiene & Tropical Medicine and its network of collaborators in many countries has had the opportunity to be associated with this exercise and I look forward to following its impact over the next 25 years.

Peter Piot
Director LSHTM

In a 1975 article on 'The changing relation between mortality and level of economic development', Samuel Preston described the characteristic log-liner curve in which at lower levels of income, relatively small increases in income are associated with larger gains in life expectancy than at greater levels of development. The relation held for data in the 1900s, 1930s and the 1960s. It further noted an upward shift over time, which suggested factors other than income accounted for 80% plus of the gains. The 'Preston curves' have held subsequently always showing a number of countries doing even better than expected.

With this work in mind, the Rockefeller Foundation brought together a team in 1985 including a new generation of health policy experts to ask how some countries were able to achieve much better health outcomes than would be expected given their limited resources. The 'positive deviants' at this time were China, Costa Rica, Cuba, the Indian state of Kerala, and Sri Lanka. The result was a seminal report entitled *Good health at low cost*. This iconic report highlighted the importance of political commitment to health, sustained investment, the pursuit of equity, community engagement and action on the wider determinants of health.

Twenty-five years on, as the Foundation developed its Transforming Health Systems initiative, it decided that it was time to revisit these issues on the comparative performance of different health systems. How had the countries included in the original study fared since the original study? How well had the lessons been learned? Are the lessons learned years ago still relevant in the new era of global health? What new lessons could be drawn from countries that had made more recent progress towards *Good health at low cost*?

This book provides many of the answers to these questions. An international team of authors, including a new generation of health policy experts, has assembled a detailed set of studies that brings us up to date on the original countries and adds five more. Based on a practical conceptual framework linking health systems to health, they confirm the enduring importance of the issues identified in the original report. However, looking across time reveals there are many distinct pathways to *Good health at low cost*. Each of the pathways is shaped by individuals, institutions, events and national context. These broad perspectives remind us of the importance of looking beyond the health sector itself, both to understand the wider determinants of health and the influences that shape health system design.

The Rockefeller Foundation is pleased to have supported this work. It is extremely timely, appearing just when many countries are facing years of economic austerity. We hope that it will stimulate a vigorous debate among academics, policy-makers, and practitioners from which will emerge innovative thinking on the most appropriate and cost-effective ways to improve health outcomes for those most in need.

Ariel Pablos-Méndez
The Rockefeller Foundation

ACKNOWLEDGEMENTS

This project would not have been possible without the intellectual and methodological contributions of all the partners, each of whom provided valuable insights and ideas but also contributed time and effort to enable an understanding of what was happening in situations where data were often scarce. We are particularly grateful to the Thai team for their quantitative work that underpinned the initial discussions.

We are indebted to the Steering Committee for their generous and continuous support, challenging our emerging ideas and contributing their detailed knowledge and interpretations to the country chapters. In addition, Lucy Gilson was instrumental in helping us to identify research priorities, frame research questions, and identify appropriate study designs. Gill Walt provided many thoughtful comments and injected a degree of helpful pragmatism at all stages of the project.

The project was instigated and funded by the Rockefeller Foundation, who identified the importance of conducting research on aspects of health systems that are hotly debated but often poorly documented. We would particularly like to thank Ariel Pablos-Mendes, Stefan Nachuk, Lily Dorment and Mushtak Chowdhury for their continual support and stimulating ideas. Miriam Rabkin from Columbia University contributed to the initial formulation of research questions and approach. We look forward to continuing to work with them in the future.

External participants in our meeting in Bellagio in August 2010 included Scott Halstead, who led the original *Good health at low cost* report published in 1985, Joe Kutzin, Abraham Mengistu and Margaret Whitehead, all of whom helped us to strengthen the analytical rigour of the project and to distil its key messages within the framework established by the original report.

Simon Cousens, Mushtak Khan, Kent Ranson, Carine Ronsmans and Nicola Watt all provided valuable comments on specific draft chapters.

Our technical editors, Joanne McManus, Wendy Wisbaum, Jane Ward and Elizabeth Hoile, have made a huge contribution to clarifying the messages in the book. Sarah Moncrieff went well beyond the duties expected of a designer and we benefited greatly from her wealth of expertise.

Administrative support was provided by the LSHTM team headed by Nicola Lord, Programmes Co-ordinator in the Department of Global Health and Development; we also benefited from the wisdom of Jonathan North with the production process and from the energy of Loveday Penn-Kekana and Benjamin Palafox in helping to pull together the final product. We are grateful to the Thai team who organized an analytical workshop in Bangkok in March 2010, which brought all the partners together and helped to identify cross-cutting themes emerging from the research.

We are also grateful to many former MSc students at LSHTM, especially Jenny Maisoneuve, Adele Fox, Julia Rahman, Hamsadvani Kuganantham, Sidney Sunwoo and Aftab Mukhi, who undertook MSc dissertations on topics related to the project. Interactions with them helped us to explore alternative approaches and flesh out research areas that were beyond the scope of the book, but are important in individual country settings.

Dina Balabanova, Martin McKee and Anne Mills
July 2011, London

CONTRIBUTORS

Partners

The London School of Hygiene & Tropical Medicine

The London School of Hygiene & Tropical Medicine (LSHTM) is a renowned research-led postgraduate institution of public health and global health. Its mission is to improve health in the UK and worldwide through the pursuit of excellence in research, postgraduate teaching and advanced training in national and international public health and tropical medicine, and through informing policy and practice in these areas. Part of the University of London, the School is the largest institution of its kind in Europe with a remarkable depth and breadth of expertise encompassing many disciplines associated with public health.

Dina Balabanova, PhD, Senior Lecturer in Health Systems/Policy, Department of Global Health and Development, LSHTM

Lesong Conteh, PhD, Senior Lecturer in Health Economics, Centre for Health Policy, Institute of Global Health Innovation, Imperial College London (formerly Department of Global Health and Development, LSHTM)

Lucy Gilson, PhD, Professor of Health Policy and Systems, Department of Global Health and Development, LSHTM, and School of Public Health and Family Medicine, University of Cape Town

Ulla Griffiths, MSc, Lecturer in Health Economics, Department of Global Health and Development, LSHTM

Andrew Harmer, PhD, Research Fellow, Department of Global Health and Development, LSHTM

Martin McKee, MD, Professor of European Public Health, Department of Health Services Research and Policy, LSHTM

Anne Mills, PhD, Professor of Health Economics and Policy, Department of Global Health and Development, LSHTM

Benjamin Palafox, MSc, Research Fellow in Pharmaceutical Policy & Economics, Department of Global Health and Development, LSHTM

Loveday Penn-Kekana, MA, Research Fellow, Department of Global Health and Development, LSHTM

Tim Powell-Jackson, PhD, Lecturer in Health Economics, Department of Global Health and Development, LSHTM

Bangladesh

ICDDR,B is an international health research organization dedicated to solving critical public health problems facing the people of Bangladesh and beyond – especially those who are most vulnerable – by generating knowledge and translating it into policy and practice. Located in Dhaka, Bangladesh, with nine rural and urban field sites around the country, ICDDR,B also provides vital humanitarian services to some of Bangladesh's poorest people. Its research activity is funded by competitive grants and its work in general is supported by over 50 donor countries and organizations, including: the Government of Bangladesh, UN agencies, foundations, universities, and private sector companies.

Tracey Pérez Koehlmoos, PhD, MHA, Health Systems Scientist, Centre for Equity & Health Systems, ICDDR,B

Ziaul Islam, MSc, MBBS, Associate Scientist, Centre for Equity & Health Systems, ICDDR,B

Shahela Anwar, MPH, Research Investigator, Centre for Equity & Health Systems, ICDDR,B

Rukhsana Gazi, MSc, MBBS, Associate Scientist, Centre for Equity & Health Systems, ICDDR,B

Shaikh A. Shahed Hossain, MSc, MBBS, Associate Scientist, Centre for Equity & Health Systems, ICDDR,B

Peter Kim Streatfield, MSc, PhD, Director, Centre for Population, Urbanisation & Climate Change, ICDDR,B

Abbas Bhuiya, PhD, Deputy Executive Director, ICDDR,B and Centre for Equity & Health Systems.

Ethiopia

The Miz-Hasab Research Center is an Addis Ababa-based independent institution established in 1996 to conduct reproductive health research, focusing on infectious diseases, family planning and nutrition, in Ethiopia. Resources available to the Center include a devoted, well-trained and disciplined full-time staff of 16 (including senior and junior researchers); data collection and entry personnel; demographic and statistical software (including CSPro, SPSS, ATLASti and NUDIST); 12 desktop, laptop networked computers, with Internet connections; a documentation center; and a vehicle.

The Center has worked (directly or indirectly) with several reputable local and international universities (Addis Ababa University, Johns Hopkins University, London School of Hygiene & Tropical Medicine), NGOs (ICRW, PATH, Pathfinder, Engenderhealth), international development organizations (USAID, DIFID, World Bank, UNDP) as well as private research companies (Abt Associates, Macro International) . In addition, our Center is proud and privileged to have hosted and shared knowledge with several interns and graduate students from various local and international schools; and conducted dissemination workshops to share its findings with stakeholders.

Hailom Banteyerga, PhD, Senior Researcher; Principal Investigator of GHLC Ethiopia study, and an Associate Professor of Discourse Analysis and Health Communication in the College of Social Sciences and Humanities, Addis Ababa University

Aklilu Kidanu, PhD, Director; Project Manager of GHLC Ethiopia study

Kyrgyzstan

The Health Policy Analysis Center (HPAC), a public foundation, was established in 2009. The Foundation is a successor of the Health Policy Analysis Project that started in 2000 with support of WHO-Euro and DFID. The main goal of HPAC is to support evidence-based decision making of the Ministry of Health (MOH) and the wider Kyrgyz public sector in order to achieve better health, good access to high-quality medical care, and reasonable financial burden of health care seeking for all Kyrgyz citizens. HPAC carries out research activities in the area of health policy. The MOH identifies the research priorities and topics; so far about 70 studies have already been conducted in such areas as poverty and equity, health financing, public health sector efficiency, health service delivery, human resources and public health. In addition, HPAC actively participated in development of monitoring and evaluation (M&E) packages for both national health programmes (*Manas* and *Manas Taalimi*) in Kyrgyzstan and was involved in the evaluation of both these programmes. In addition, HPAC organizes round-table discussions and seminars on the research findings and important health policy issues to facilitate exchange of information, open debate and consensus building so as to support policy dialogue on current health care problems. HPAC is also actively involved in conducting local and international training courses (mainly Commonwealth of Independent States (CIS)) on health management and health systems including Flagship Courses on Health Systems Development and Sustainable Financing in collaboration with WBI and WHO-Euro. In addition, HPAC team members carrying out consultancy activities in CIS region in the areas mentioned above.

Ainura Ibraimova, MD, PhD, Consultant to WHO Regional Office for Europe until 2011 (currently Deputy Regional Director at the USAID-funded Central Asia Quality Health Care Project)

Baktygul Akkazieva, MBA, MSc, Director of the Health Policy Analysis Center until 2011 (currently Deputy Regional Director for M&E at the USAID-funded Central Asia Quality Health Care Project)

Gulgun Murzalieva, MD, Senior Policy Analyst until 2011 (currently Director of the Health Policy Analysis Center)

Tamil Nadu

The *Indian Institute of Technology, Madras*, established in 1959 by the Government of India, is a leader in tertiary education in engineering, sciences, and humanities and social sciences, in South Asia. The master's and doctoral programmes of the Department of Humanities and Social Sciences at the Indian Institute of Technology (IIT) Madras are among the best offered in Indian Universities. During the past 15 years, the Department of Humanities and Social Sciences has been active in promoting comparative public policy studies with special reference to health sector in India. Their current research work includes health care financing, health systems efficiency, public–private partnership and history of health care in south India. They are also actively involved in the health policy-making processes both state and national level.

VR Muraleedharan, PhD, Professor in the Department of Humanities and Social Sciences, IIT (Madras)

Umakant Dash, PhD, Associate Professor in the Department of Humanities and Social Sciences, IIT (Madras)

Thailand

The *International Health Policy Programme* (IHPP), Thailand is a semi-autonomous programme conducting research on the national health priorities related to health systems and policy. IHPP is a part of the Bureau of Policy and Strategy, Thai Ministry of Public Health (MOPH). It aims to improve the national health systems through generating knowledge and evidence on improving health systems and policy to the public and Thai policy-makers. Another important aim of IHPP is to strengthen the capacity of Thai researchers to conduct policy-relevant research in the areas of health financing; equity monitoring before and after Universal Health Coverage; human resources for health; health policy analysis; and health promotion and disease prevention, including alcohol study. IHPP has focused not only on research but also on policy processes and policy utility of research findings; this required researchers to work closely with related stakeholders in each particular field. IHPP has physical proximity to, but an arm-length relationship with, policy-makers in and outside the Ministry of Public Health in order to maintain policy relevance and scientific integrity and independence.

Walaiporn Patcharanarumol, PhD, Researcher of IHPP, MOPH

Viroj Tangcharoensathien, PhD, Senior Advisor of IHPP, MOPH

Supon Limwattananon, PhD, Associate Professor, Khon Kaen University, Senior Researcher of IHPP, MOPH

Warisa Panichkriangkrai, MPH, Researcher of IHPP, MOPH

Kumaree Pachanee, MA, Research Assistant of IHPP, MOPH

Waraporn Poungkantha, MA, Research Coordinator of IHPP, MOPH

Steering committee

Simon Cousens, MA, DipMathStat, Professor of Epidemiology and Medical Statistics, Department of Infectious Disease Epidemiology, LSHTM

Richard Coker, MD, FFPH, Professor in Public Health, Department of Global Health and Development, LSHTM, and Communicable Diseases Policy Research Group, LSHTM, Bangkok, Thailand

Carine Ronsmans, MD, DrPH, Professor of Epidemiology, Department of Infectious Disease Epidemiology, LSHTM

Gill Walt, PhD, Emeritus Professor of International Health Policy, Department of Global Health and Development, LSHTM

LIST OF ABBREVIATIONS

AIDS	Acquired immunodeficiency syndrome
BRAC	Bangladesh Rural Advancement Committee
CCSS	Costa Rican Social Security Fund
CIS	Commonwealth of Independent States
DANIDA	Danish International Development Agency
DFID	United Kingdom Department for International Development
DOTS	Directly observed treatment, short-course
EBAIS	Equipos Básicos de Atención Integral en Salud, Costa Rica
EPRDF	Ethiopian People's Revolutionary Democratic Front
GAVI	GAVI Alliance (formerly the Global Alliance for Vaccines and Immunisation)
GDI	Gender-related development index
GDP	Gross domestic product
GEM	Gender empowerment measure
GHLC	*Good health at low cost*, 1985 report
Gini	Gini coefficient or generalised inequality index Definition: a measure of inequality of income or wealth, where a value of 0 expresses total equality and a value of 1 total inequality
Global Fund	formerly the Global Fund to Fight AIDS, Tuberculosis and Malaria
GNI	Gross national income
HDI	Human Development Index
HIV	Human Immunodeficiency Virus
ICDDR,B	International Centre for Diarrhoeal Disease Research, Bangladesh
IHP	International Health Partnership
IHPP	International Health Policy Programme (Thailand)
IMCI	Integrated management of childhood illness
IMF	International Monetary Fund
Int$	International dollar (Geary-Khamis dollar) Definition: a hypothetical unit of currency that has the same purchasing power that the US dollar had in the United States at a given point in time (e.g. in 2005)

LSHTM	London School of Hygiene & Tropical Medicine
MDG	Millennium Development Goal
MHIF	Mandatory Health Insurance Fund (Kyrgyzstan)
MoHFW	Ministry of Health and Family Welfare (Bangladesh)
MOPH	Ministry of Public Health
MoWCA	Ministry of Women and Children Affairs (Bangladesh)
NESDP	National Economic and Social Development Plans, Thailand
NGO	Nongovernmental organization
NRCMCS	New Rural Cooperative Medical Care System (China)
ORS	Oral rehydration solution
PASDEP	Plan for Accelerated and Sustained Development to End Poverty (Ethiopia)
PEPFAR	President's Emergency Plan for AIDS Relief
RCMCS	Rural Cooperative Medical Care System, China
SGBP	State Guaranteed Benefits Package, Kyrgyzstan
SWAp	Sector-wide approach
TNMSC	Tamil Nadu Medical Services Corporation
UN	United Nations
UNICEF	United Nations International Children's Emergency Fund
USAID	United States Agency for International Development
USSR	Union of Soviet Socialist Republics
WDI	World Development Indicators
WGI	Worldwide Governance Indicators
	Definition: aggregate and individual governance indicators for 213 economies for six dimensions of governance: voice and accountability, political stability and absence of violence, government effectiveness, regulatory quality, rule of law, and control of corruption. The aggregate indicators combine the views of a variety respondents in industrial and developing countries. The individual data sources underlying the aggregate indicators are drawn from a diverse variety of survey institutes, think tanks, NGOs and international organizations
WHO	World Health Organization

LIST OF BOXES, TABLES AND FIGURES

Boxes

Tables

Figures

Chapter 1

INTRODUCTION

Good Health at Low Cost research team

In 1985, the Rockefeller Foundation commissioned a report (published as a compendium of papers and thematic analyses) exploring the question of why some poor countries were able to achieve better health outcomes than others at similar levels of income[1]. The report, entitled *Good health at low cost* (GHLC), identified China, Costa Rica, Kerala State in India and Sri Lanka as such countries[a] and sought to identify factors underpinning their relative success. 'Good health at low cost' was used as a catchy way of referring to success in improving health with relatively limited economic resources.

The original *Good health at low cost* volume reflected a contemporary interest in eliciting the multiple determinants of health and understanding how these are distributed across populations. The report was published in the aftermath of a series of economic difficulties, including the oil crisis of 1973, at a time when structural adjustment programmes advocated by the International Monetary Fund (IMF) and World Bank were being implemented in many low-income countries. It demonstrated a new understanding of the importance of comprehensive and community-oriented primary health care as a key element of the health system, a view expounded a few years previously at the 1978 joint World Health Organization (WHO)/United Nations International Children's Emergency Fund (UNICEF) conference on primary health care at Alma-Ata.

The *Good health at low cost* volume has become an iconic publication, influencing the international debate on health systems, and political and practical strategies to improve health. Its key contribution was to highlight the social determinants of health, now widely accepted but then far from the dominant paradigm. By highlighting the existence of multiple causes of ill health interacting in many complex ways, it was able to show how social, economic and health policies contributed to improvements in health status. The report convincingly dispelled the myth that economic growth is a sufficient driver of development and, with it, better population health. For the first time, it brought together a corpus of empirical evidence to support what had previously been mainly theoretical arguments[2] to show how many low-income countries had achieved vast improvements in a number of measures of health, often reaching levels comparable to those seen in developed countries, even though they had experienced only modest growth in income and, in the case of Sri Lanka, internal conflict.

One important finding was that all the countries studied had achieved above-average investment, in both financial and human terms, in their health systems, and particularly in primary health care. However, the original *Good health at low cost* volume concurred with the view set out at Alma-Ata that primary health care

---

[a] For convenience, "countries" is used as the generic term, although Kerala is a state within India.

was not just a means of delivering a package of interventions, as was then being promoted, among others, by UNICEF. Instead, it was the focal point of the health care system and a platform to address other social issues, such as participation and empowerment. All the countries studied also showed commitment to prevention, as judged by their patterns of expenditure. Crucially, in the view of the report's authors, these policies were underpinned by a commitment to equity both within the health system and beyond. This was seen as ensuring that provision of services was tailored to the needs of the most vulnerable

> **Box 1.1 Factors contributing to good health, from GHLC 1985**
>
> - Political and historical commitment to health as a social goal
> - Strong societal values of equity, political participation and community involvement in health
> - High-level investment in primary health care and other community-based services
> - Widespread education, especially of women
> - Intersectoral linkages for health.

groups in the population, whose status was, simultaneously, being advanced by enhanced engagement and political participation, especially by women (Box 1.1). A second finding was the importance of good governance, seen as a government's commitment to development. In time, this influenced the WHO's health system framework[3], where governance is fundamental to all other aspects of the health system. The factors identified by the report's authors are set out in Table 1.1.

Each country implemented health care strategies that reflected their individual circumstances. In both Kerala and Sri Lanka, there was an emphasis on expansion of primary health care programmes as a means of improving essential care and, in particular, greater utilization of essential maternal and child health services such as immunization, antenatal and postnatal care, skilled birth attendance, and prompt intervention to treat infections. In Kerala, "ancillary nurse midwives" were deployed in underserved rural areas. In contrast, Costa Rica adopted a broader development perspective, recognizing the need to employ a combination of strategies to tackle neonatal mortality (for example, promoting family planning to reduce fertility, extending and improving inpatient services) and post-neonatal mortality (improvements in immunization, clean water and sanitation). In China, the barefoot doctor system was seen as a way of rapidly scaling up the basic provision of care in rural areas, while patriotic health campaigns addressed some of the broader determinants of health, such as sanitation. Such links to broader policies were identified elsewhere too. For example, a malaria control campaign in Sri Lanka was an integral component of land reform and the social development agenda during the 1950s and 1960s. The reform was designed not only to tackle historical inequities but also to enhance

Table 1.1 Social and political factors supporting 'good health at low cost'

Political and historical commitment to health as a social goal	Legislation
	Government expenditure on health
	Establishment of health facilities
	Historical and cultural influences
Social welfare orientation to development	Preventive orientation
	Support for basic necessities
	Educational programmes
	Land reform
Participation in the political process	Universal franchise and political engagement
	Extent of decentralization
	Community involvement
Equity-oriented services	Health, education and nutrition status of women, minorities, etc.
	Urban–rural coverage
	Income–asset distribution
Intersectoral linkages for health	Mechanisms to ensure linkage
	Incentives to ensure linkage
	Recognition that health is socially determined

Source: Adapted from reference 4

agricultural productivity and thus improve income and food security, as well as to reduce the transmission of malaria. Many other health policies also benefited from it indirectly; associated improvements in transportation infrastructure benefited economic growth but also improved physical access to health facilities.

All of the countries studied provided examples of explicit policies to address inequalities of different types. These included gender equity (promotion of female literacy in Kerala), social exclusion (measures to tackle the inherent inequalities in the caste system in Kerala), urban–rural disparities in coverage (expansion of primary health care in rural areas, particularly maternal and child health services, coupled with universal health insurance in Costa Rica), and disparities in distribution of income and assets (land reform in Sri Lanka and Kerala, trade union friendly policies and action to increase wage levels in Kerala).

The countries studied also demonstrated that access to at least basic health care was seen as a fundamental human right. Strong political commitment to making this happen was manifest in different ways. One was in the creation of structures, as in Costa Rica, where the government had established social security and health insurance systems that were effective in reaching out to the entire population. Another was in the priority given to different types of expenditure. Costa Rica had abolished its armed forces in 1948, spending money instead on social development. Kerala had the highest per capita expenditure on health care (14.5% of total government expenditure in 1981) of any Indian state.

Political factors were important. These included the existence of a universal franchise (although, as in China, not necessarily multi-party elections) and political engagement of communities and grassroots groups. To varying degrees, all of the countries were left wing. Unusual among Indian states, Kerala has had Marxist governments for much of the time since independence, while China remains a communist state. Political engagement by women also emerged as a potentially important factor, facilitated by high levels of female literacy in, for example, Kerala and Sri Lanka; this may have created political pressure to develop services relevant to the needs of women. In China, the largest of the countries studied, decentralization of many administrative functions, although tightly regulated by the centre, was seen as contributing to strong local administrative structures that could manage health care delivery effectively. Cultural factors also played a part. Sri Lanka had a long tradition of public welfare, which the authors of the report linked to both the Ayurvedic system of medicine and the British legacy of free public services; after independence, this tradition was apparent in areas such as food subsidies, land reform and pro-poor pricing policies.

Since the original *Good health at low cost* report was published, coverage of effective health care has increased worldwide. Life expectancy has increased markedly in many countries, with the exception of those countries in Africa and the Caribbean worst affected by the HIV/AIDS epidemic and a few countries suffering from conflict (such as Iraq and Afghanistan) or gross political mismanagement (Democratic People's Republic of Korea). Some of these gains have resulted from "picking the low hanging fruit", for example through vector control to reduce transmission of malaria or Integrated Management of Childhood Illness (IMCI) to prevent death from easily treatable conditions. Yet there is still much to be done and, in many countries, progress towards the health-related Millennium Development Goals (MDGs) is either slow or, in some cases, regressing. Of the 68 countries that account for the vast majority of child and maternal deaths in the world, 49 are unlikely to meet the child health goal[5]. At the same time, many new challenges are emerging.

The first relates to the nature of disease. Acute illnesses from which victims either recovered spontaneously or died have been replaced by complex chronic disorders. These include the increasing prevalence of AIDS, due to a combination of disease spread and enhanced survival, and the growing burden of non-communicable diseases driven by successes in areas such as food security[6], coupled with access to motorized transport and agricultural mechanization that has led to rapid increases in risk factors such as injuries, accidents and obesity. A second development has been the growth in therapeutic capability. The handful of effective medicines in the 1940s has expanded into an enormous armamentarium, with a particularly large increase in drugs that require long-term administration, often for life, as well as monitoring to ensure optimum treatment and avoidance of side-effects. A third development has been the recognition that optimal care often requires the involvement of multi-professional teams working across different levels of care. Two conditions, diabetes and AIDS, exemplify these challenges, requiring long-term management by a range of health workers who handle not just the primary disorder but also, and often more importantly, its complications.

This poses enormous challenges to health systems[7]. To close the gap between what is possible and what is currently available for a large proportion of the world's population, it is necessary to put in place systems that can deliver skilled health workers, reliable supplies of medication, appropriate facilities to treat patients, lifelong learning to ensure that those delivering care are using the latest knowledge, and managerial processes that can make all this happen in a way that is both effective and affordable. Yet it is now very clear that such complex responses do not emerge spontaneously, as is the case in many of the world's poorest nations. Despite economic recession, almost all industrialized countries (with the exception of Italy) have confirmed or even increased their commitments to development assistance, exemplified by their commitment to the eight United Nations (UN) MDGs[8]. These initiatives enshrine the lessons of the original GHLC report, demonstrating increasing acceptance of the principle that social development can be addressed only via comprehensive multisectoral strategies, involving many partners at both national and international level.

At the same time, new global structures have been created to facilitate the flow of assistance. The Global Alliance for Vaccines and Immunisation (GAVI) was established in 2000 and the Global Fund to Fight AIDS, Tuberculosis and Malaria (now Global Fund) followed in 2001. While the resulting massive scaling up of resources has had some success (in the rollout of antiretroviral treatment for example), it has also confronted the limited absorptive ability of many health systems[9]. Progress has also been hampered by the absence of many of the factors identified in the GHLC report, such as political commitment and policies to promote broader social change. As a result, donor and recipient governments are now reassessing their policies.

A key conclusion emerging from this reassessment is the importance of strengthening health systems. Much of the additional funding has been delivered through vertical approaches that, although improving access to specific treatments, have not succeeded in building sustainable capacity within the health system. This goes beyond the longstanding debate about vertical and horizontal approaches to health care delivery; in fact, in many cases, the differences have been overstated, as programmes designed as vertical at the top have horizontal elements at lower levels. For example, centrally designed and donor-funded programmes are often delivered by frontline staff who are actually responsible for a broad range of primary care services[10]. As a consequence, many global organizations are modifying their approach[11,12], devoting an increased share of resources to health system strengthening, now accounting for 30% of the overall budget of GAVI. This increased focus on health systems reflects not only their obvious role in the delivery of care but also their role as an entry point to address wider social problems, including improving the status of women and access to other public services.

Yet the recognition that health systems matter is not being accompanied by an adequate understanding of what health system strengthening actually involves[13]. Current experience suggests a need for investment in expertise within donor organizations and recipient governments to ensure that such funds are spent effectively[14]. In parallel, there is a need for evidence on what works. Recent years have seen a vast range of "health sector reform" initiatives, including cost sharing, decentralization, market-based models and community financing, few of which have been adequately evaluated.

In this new study, we update and extend the original analysis in *Good health at low cost* which looked at the constellation of factors that affect health, tracing the subsequent experience of the four countries in the original report (China, Costa Rica, Kerala and Sri Lanka), asking whether their earlier achievements have been sustained given the extensive political, social and economic changes each country has undergone. However our main focus has been to explore five new countries that have achieved significant success in improving health – in particular maternal and child health – compared with other countries with similar levels of economic resources. This study, conducted through a partnership of research teams in each of the countries and at the London School of Hygiene & Tropical Medicine, includes Bangladesh, Ethiopia, Kyrgyzstan, the Indian state of Tamil Nadu and Thailand.[b] The research process was underpinned by

---

[b] Partners: ICDDR,B, Bangladesh; Miz-Hasab Research Center, Ethiopia; Health Policy Analysis Center, Kyrgyzstan; Indian Institute of Technology (Madras), India; International Health Policy Program, Thailand; LSHTM, United Kingdom.

effective participation and interaction of all partners at every stage of the process through a series of meetings and regular communication. A steering committee provided strategic leadership. All partners met in Bellagio, Italy, to discuss emerging findings and identify cross-cutting themes beyond individual country experience. The research process built on our long-term engagement with each country partner and previous work amassing a critical body of knowledge.

Our major focus is on the role of health systems, which we treat as an entry point to understanding the complex interrelationships among different determinants of health. By employing established frameworks for studying health systems, we seek to identify what factors contribute to their success.

Our starting point is the original *Good health at low cost* report and, in particular, the factors that it identified as important. One was the key role played by the state. A commitment to development was critical and the public sector provided the infrastructure, financing and multisectoral development policies that led to good health; the role of the private sector in health was relatively small. Since 1985, however, the relationship between the public and private sectors has changed significantly; the private sector is expanding rapidly, in different forms (offering extensive services in low- and middle-income countries, including primary care, private insurance, training, cross-border services, etc.). Given the already high and growing inequalities within countries since the 1980s, this situation has major implications for "good health" in the future, especially among the poor or marginalized groups that are often least attractive to private investors.

Another key factor that was identified as leading to good health is primary health care and expanded access to essential services, with developments in both the public and private sectors. However, we recognize that the term "primary health care" has been interpreted in many ways in different places. We ask whether particular aspects of primary care now emerge as especially important. For example, can effective and accessible primary care be attributed to the existence of formal programmes, the availability of health workers, mechanisms to deliver services in outlying and otherwise underserved areas, implementation of packages of basic services, or coordination and institutional support? Clearly, the existence of a formal programme developed by national leaders does not necessarily mean that it is actually operating at district level.

We then seek to identify key drivers for health system performance, considering organization and financing, delivery of services, policy processes and regulation and governance arrangements. We extend the earlier work by taking a whole system approach, seeking to explain why and how changes came about, and to understand what combination of factors explain success in a particular setting.

While the original report listed a broad range of factors, we seek to disentangle the complex interrelationships among these factors. Analysis focuses on the multifaceted interaction among three types of factor: health systems-related factors; public sector provisioning and policy factors; and broader contextual factors (for example, the political system in a country).

In a further extension to the original study, we then identify plausible pathways through which these factors influence health. For example, while factors identified in the original report such as empowerment of women and female literacy have long been known to be associated with improved health outcomes, the ways in which they affect health have been less well understood. It may be that literate, empowered women are more aware of services and can communicate more effectively with providers, or it may be that female empowerment operates through political processes, increasing the likelihood that appropriate services will be made available for all women, regardless of their level of literacy. We also explore the context in which all of these factors operate and interact, seeking to elicit the circumstances under which specific policies and interventions are likely to be successful.

Finally, this is a comparative study, so we take advantage of the similarities and differences among the five new countries and the four original *Good health at low cost* countries. Our countries share a history of success in delivering good health at modest income levels but are in many other ways quite different, with differing burdens of disease, income levels and resources used to deliver health care. Where possible, we extend our comparisons to include countries' neighbours, while also looking at changes over time. These "within and across" country analyses make it possible to generate putative explanations for differences in outcomes.

In Chapter 2 of this book, we describe the purpose, analytical approach and methods employed in conducting the research. In Chapters 3–7, we examine the experience of each of the study countries, while in Chapter 8, we explore the changes in the four original countries since publication of the 1985 report. In Chapters 9 and 10, we discuss cross-cutting themes and features of the health systems and beyond that emerge from the study and have been found to promote good health and access to care in diverse settings. Finally, in the concluding Chapter 11, we offer reflections on the implications of the findings.

REFERENCES

1. Halstead S, Walsh J, Warren K, eds. *Good health at low cost*. Bellagio: Rockefeller Foundation; 1985.

2. Ahmad E et al., eds. *Social security in developing countries*. Oxford: Oxford University Press; 1991.

3. WHO. *The World Health Report 2000. Health systems: improving performance*. Geneva: World Health Organization; 2000.

4. Rosenfield PI. The contribution of social and political factors to good health. In: Halstead S, Walsh J, Warren K, eds. *Good health at low cost*. Bellagio: Rockefeller Foundation; 1985.

5. Aga Khan University et al. *Countdown to 2015: taking stock of maternal, newborn and child survival*. Geneva: WHO and UNICEF; 2010.

6. Beaglehole R et al. Priority actions for the non-communicable disease crisis. *Lancet* 2011; 377(9775):1438–47.

7. McKee M, Nolte E, Figueras J. Strategies for health services. In: *Oxford Textbook of Public Health. 5th ed*. Beaglehole R, et al., eds. Oxford: Oxford University Press; 2009. p. 1668–81.

8. United Nations Millennium Declaration. General Assembly Resolution, 55th session, document A/RES/55/2. 8 September 2000.

9. Subramanian S, Peters D, Willis J. *How are health services, financing and status evaluated? An analysis of implementation completion reports of World Bank assistance in health*. Washington, DC: World Bank; 2006 (HNP Discussion Paper).

10. Oliveira-Cruz V, Kurowski C, Mills A. Delivery of priority health services: searching for synergies within the vertical versus horizontal debate. *Journal of International Development* 2003; 15:67–86.

11. GFATM. Health systems strengthening. In: *7th Policy and Strategy Committee Meeting*. Geneva: Global Fund to fight AIDS Tuberculosis and Malaria; 2007.

12. WHO. *The Global Fund strategic approach to health systems strengthening. Report from WHO to the Global Fund Secretariat*. Geneva: World Health Organization; 2007.

13. Marchal B, Cavalli A, Kegels G. Global health actors claim to support health system strengthening: is this reality or rhetoric? *PLoS Medicine* 2009; 6(4):e1000059.

14. Balabanova D et al. What can global health institutions do to help strengthen health systems in low income countries? *Health Research Policy and Systems* 2010; 8(1):22.

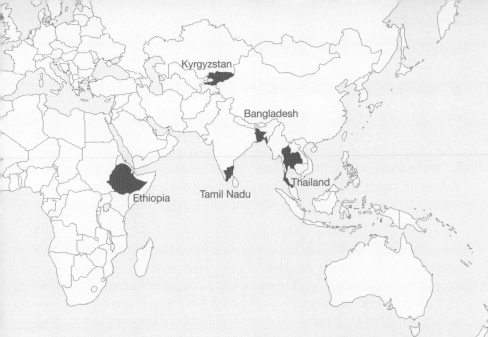

Chapter 2

RESEARCH APPROACH AND METHODS
HIGHLIGHTS FROM STUDY COUNTRIES

Good Health at Low Cost research team

■ Purpose and objectives

As in the original *Good health at low cost* report, we aimed to identify plausible explanations for why some countries have achieved better health outcomes than others in a similar economic position. Since the term 'good health at low cost' has become so iconic, at times we refer to this as our theme, although – as with the original report – we share the interpretation of this as good health relative to income.

We sought to explore these explanations further in five countries that were not included in the original report but were seen as success stories in specific areas of health and health systems development. We were interested in exploring the meaning and value of the 'good health at low cost' concept and also in identifying how the range of determinants of health has changed over the past two decades. This chapter explains the research objectives, framework and methods used. It also presents the rationale behind the selection of the five study countries.

The overall objective of the study was to examine how certain factors – both individually and combined – contribute to improvements in health and in access to key services:

- factors related to the health system (the main focus of the study);

- factors related to living conditions and public services (e.g. policies in other sectors);

- factors related to the institutional environment (e.g. political, economic, social); and

- factors related to the context (e.g. geography, climate).

The study was conducted by a partnership of researchers in the selected countries and within the London School of Hygiene & Tropical Medicine (LSHTM). The formulation of the approach to research and initial proposals involved intensive interactions within the research team. The case studies were conducted by each respective partner drawing on the insight and the intellectual contribution from the rest of the team. A common research framework and research tools were initially created for the purpose of achieving methodological and conceptual consistency and were adapted to countries by each partner institution. In-country research presented a rich context and accentuated country differences. Various combinations of methods and data sources were used in each setting, reflecting national specificities (see Annex). International Health Policy Program, Thailand (IHPP-Thailand) conducted a series of cross-country quantitative analysis on outcomes and their determinants which informed the development of the research.

Further analytical work facilitated through bilateral and multilateral discussions helped to identify common patterns of development within the health systems, other sectors, and contexts. As the research progressed, there was a continuous process of dialogue with national policy-makers and consultations with external experts and peer reviewers, seeking to validate findings and contribute to national policy processes as well as to the international debate.

■ Conceptual framework

We used the widely accepted WHO definition of the health system as consisting of "...all organizations, people and actions whose primary intent is to promote, restore or maintain health. This includes efforts to influence determinants of health as well as more direct health-improving activities"[1]. This is coherent with the aim of the study, whereby we examine the entire range of "organizations, people and actions" contributing to population health. These extend beyond those in the public sector to include a range of private for-profit and not-for-profit organizations and individuals, as well as actions taken by actors both within and outside the health sector. The unifying theme is that all of these have, as their primary intent, the promotion, restoration or maintenance of health. Underlying this definition is the understanding that the health system is not a fixed entity: its boundaries change over time.

To address the complex task of explaining why some countries have been able to improve the health of their populations even at relatively low levels of economic development, the starting point of the analysis was a conceptual framework that sought to represent the myriad determinants of health, acting at different levels, and the ways in which they interacted with each other (Figure 2.1). We began from the premise that the immediate determinants (or causes) of health, such as infectious agents, inadequate diet, or smoking, are well established. The relationships between these risk factors and disease were not the focus of our attention. Instead, we were interested in the "causes of the causes" of disease and their relationship with the health system. The assessment of the strength of a health system can be made on the basis of how it affects the transition from disease to death, disability or recovery, or prevention of disease in the first place. However, countries face different disease burdens, which, in turn, are influenced by living conditions and the broader environment (which includes factors that are malleable, at least in the medium term) and context (which are those factors such as climate or geography that are relatively fixed). A health system in a country that has been spared the AIDS epidemic or where fertility is low will find it easier to achieve good health than one in which AIDS or fertility are higher.

Figure 2.1 Conceptual model: determinants of health

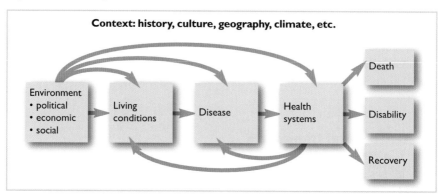

Source: Reference 2.

In this way, we sought to encompass the broader determinants of population health, as well as the more distal political and socioeconomic factors, such as societal inequalities in income and status[3], and the political-economic systems that may or may not favour the accumulation of private wealth over redistribution of power and privilege[4,5]. However, it soon became clear that this framework, while helpful in organizing our thoughts, was unduly ambitious in the settings being studied, due to lack of data. The limited data on outcomes were not matched by data on health determinants or policy responses. The data that were available were often extrapolated from surveys, were episodic and their sources precluded disaggregation. Consequently, it was difficult to establish trends and compare different health outcomes and the changes within health systems and societies that might have been associated with these outcomes.

Given the primary focus on health systems, it was helpful to review how thinking about them has developed in recent years. Historically (and in some quarters, currently) health care is viewed as essentially unproductive, diverting resources from other more productive sectors of the economy. This view has largely given way in the face of evidence[6] that poor health is a drag on economic growth and, conversely, investment in health is, like education, a driver of growth. But health investment decisions are not straightforward. Although there is recognition that, collectively, health care interventions can make a measureable contribution to overall population health, growing evidence demonstrates that health systems do not always achieve their potential. For example, some health systems deliver unduly expensive and inappropriate care to those who need it least while failing to provide effective care to those in most need.

The shift in thinking about the importance of the health system has been matched by changing ideas about how it might be organized. The 1978

Figure 2.2   The WHO health system framework

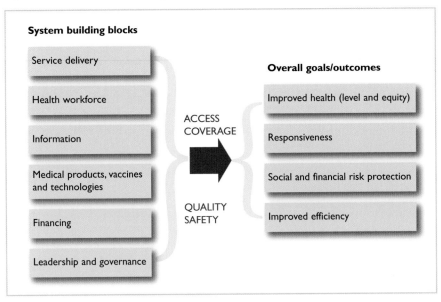

Source: Reproduced from reference 1.

Declaration of Alma-Ata set out a vision of integrated health care, based on a strong primary care component. However, for a variety of reasons, in particular, resource constraints and perceived political feasibility, this was displaced by a focus on targeted delivery of specific interventions, such as the GOBI package (growth monitoring, oral rehydration, breastfeeding, immunization), which helped to create a number of often-isolated vertical systems. These have grown over the years, especially following the creation of a number of specialized global programmes, such as the Global Fund against AIDS, TB and Malaria (Global Fund) and the US President's Emergency Plan for AIDS Relief (PEPFAR).

Over time, the strengths and limitations of the vertical approach have been acknowledged, and some have sought synergies between vertical and integrated approaches, for example by means of what have been termed "diagonal" systems[7]. However, the choice of the most appropriate approach remains the focus of an enduring debate, with different views about what strategy each country should adopt if it is to provide universal access to quality health care on a sustainable basis[8].

Such debates have led to work that has sought to conceptualize the role of a health system in translating inputs into outcomes. The most widely used conceptual model is that developed by the WHO (Figure 2.2)[1], in which a series

Figure 2.3   Conceptual framework: *Good health at low cost* **2011**

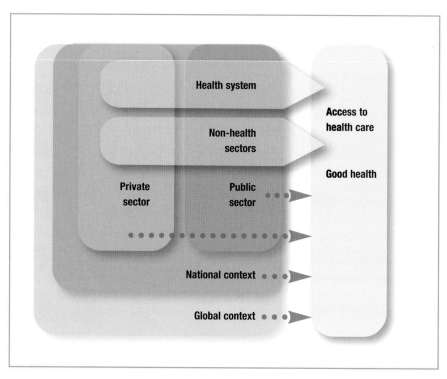

of health system building blocks (such as the health workforce, medical products and leadership) are combined, in a manner that promotes access, coverage, quality and safety, to create better health, greater responsiveness, and protection of individuals from financial risk in an efficient manner.

Other work has examined the mechanisms that are available to ensure the optimal performance of a health system. An example is the Harvard Control Knobs framework, which identifies five 'control knobs' (financing, payment, organization, regulation and behaviour) that can be used by policy-makers to achieve goals such as better health or financial risk protection[9,10]. While the framework has many similarities with the WHO model, and informed its development, it emphasizes that understanding the behaviour of the actors is crucial in translating plans into reality.

Our approach to the research (illustrated in Figure 2.3) draws on these frameworks but goes beyond them in exploring the broader environmental factors – including political, cultural and economic factors – that have influenced the way health systems develop and operate over time and their ability to scale up priority health interventions. These contextual and environmental factors are increasingly seen as influential yet are not easily captured by the WHO framework[11]. They are, however, addressed explicitly in our analyses.

The health system forms the core of our conceptual framework. Our understanding of the role of the health system is as a social institution working with other institutions to promote well-being rather than just providing treatment. In exploring health systems, we pay particular attention not only to structures and resources but also to processes such as communication, integration, collaboration and participation, which are seen as crucial elements of health system performance[12]. In particular, we look at the enabling factors and bottlenecks to achieving effective service provision and good health, as well as the contextual factors that encourage or discourage their development[13–16]. We focus on both private and public sectors, recognizing that in some countries both non-profit and for-profit organizations have significant roles in the health system.

Non-health sectors, however, also influence access to health care and good health. For example, maternal and child survival in poor countries is influenced by education and literacy programmes as well as by access to clean water. If both are made available, outcomes may improve regardless of health system deficiencies. Non-health initiatives may be provided by either the private or the public sector.

The next level of analysis concerns the **national context features** likely to influence health and health systems, as well as other sectors. Achieving good health is likely to be influenced by broad aspects of governance. At its most basic, this entails the presence of a functioning state with viable mechanisms to develop policies and the capacity to implement interventions. Broad norms and approaches to governance in a country obviously influence the governance of the health system, but beyond this, they can promote health, enabling citizens to voice their needs and demand responsive services.

Other important dimensions of national context are economic factors, such as the level and distribution of national income; political factors, such as political freedom, civil liberties, empowerment (especially of women), visionary leadership, and the status of the health ministry within government; and social and cultural factors, such as the level of social, ethnic and religious cohesion. There are also less widely recognized contextual factors which affect health systems. One is geography (for example, whether countries are landlocked); another is population size (for example, the ability to create a critical mass of expertise within government) and yet another is a country's history (for example, attitudes to solidarity or individualism). Elements of national context can affect health status and health systems directly. Thus, a country with a failing economy, where the health ministry is weak and where the government favours military rather than health spending is unlikely to have an effective health care system.

All of these factors are influenced by the **global position of the country**. For example, whether donor funding is important, or what the scope is for migration and brain drain (influenced, for example, by what languages are spoken widely). The global position of a country will have implications for how its health system is shaped and also directly for the health of its population (for example, its openness to trade will affect food security and the prevalence of health-affecting foods and beverages).

■ Approach to the research

Given these considerations relating to the conceptual framework, our approach was driven by several imperatives.

(i) Seeking to capture some of the complexity of the determinants of health and the factors that enable functioning health systems. Determinants of health are inherently complex. Complexities are manifested in the sheer number of pathways involved, the ways in which determinants interact, and the possible time lag between cause and effect. There are many diverse studies of factors associated with improvements in health indicators, particularly maternal and child health. Some have provided periodic country profiles, such as the three Countdown to 2015 Reports tracking factors known to influence maternal and child health[17], while more recent studies have started to explore how the factors interact with each other[18]. We sought to examine hierarchies and interrelationships of factors that affect intermediate and final outcomes.

We also attempted to investigate how different determinants are shaped by context, particularly by social relations, power, trust, politics, cultural norms and values. We drew on the concept of pluralistic health systems as "social contracts between actors, underpinned by shared behavioural norms ... [which] may influence how health systems operate"[19]. Many of these contextual features are likely to influence both health systems and determinants of health outside the health system. Moreover, these factors are likely to influence the behaviour of users and other actors, affecting their preferred means of engagement with the health system[20].

(ii) Taking account of the phenomena of path dependency and dynamic change. Health systems and other social systems are shaped by multiple historical, institutional and political processes, many with origins outside the health sector. The phenomenon of path dependency means that the starting conditions (reflecting

past policies) may constrain the scope for a system to develop in the future[21]. An example is the difficulty that the United States, with the dominance of a private health insurance industry, has faced in implementing a universal health care system. Thus, our analysis is situated within knowledge of the history of political, economic and social change in the country concerned.

At the same time, the health system exists within a wider set of systems, with which it interacts in a dynamic fashion. For instance, while health worker performance is influenced by established professional norms and clinical practices, the political influence and bargaining position of medical associations may affect the status of the particular staff categories and, thus, workers' incentives to deliver good-quality services in the public sector. These interactions are complex, in that they are characterized by non-linear relationships and feedback loops, leading to the presence of unpredictable and unintended consequences[22]. Therefore, our approach seeks to examine examples of factors influencing health and the multiple influences on these factors, historically and currently, and explore what triggers change in established trajectories.

(iii) Tracing pathways by which good health at low cost is achieved. We aim to identify the contribution of multiple factors to good health, while recognizing that attribution of cause and effect must be somewhat speculative. However, we attempt to identify plausible pathways by which health systems might influence health and through which decisions are translated into action, accepting that, in many countries, there is a large gap between the de jure and de facto situations[23].

(iv) Generating propositions through pattern recognition. Our analysis is based on five country studies, which is insufficient for statistical analysis to test hypotheses. However, through an iterative process and drawing on multiple data sources, we aim to identify common patterns among the countries so that propositions about the relationship between health, health systems and social determinants can be generated. Where possible, comparisons are drawn with countries with similar income levels or located in the same geographical regions.

Methods

Country selection

In collaboration with the Rockefeller Foundation, we selected Bangladesh, Ethiopia, Kyrgyzstan, Thailand and the Indian state of Tamil Nadu to be included in the study. Even though Tamil Nadu is a state rather than a country, we refer to them collectively as the five study countries. Countries were chosen as a result of research commissioned by the Rockefeller Foundation, which led to a ranking and ultimately to a shortlist of possible study countries.

Drawing on this list, we identified countries that had undertaken large-scale and innovative system-level reforms, suggesting effective government stewardship, vision and capacity to implement change despite financial constraints. A further criterion was that the sample should include a variety of health system configurations, geographical regions, population sizes and income levels. A third consideration was that the selected countries offered a range of health system configurations and models of governance.

The five study countries have seen considerable improvements in the health of their population or in access to key interventions, beyond what might be expected on the basis of their income level. Many of these positive trends were sustained or accelerated over long periods of time (see Highlights from the study countries, below).

Availability of documented experience from implementing policies and programmes both within the particular country and internationally was also important. Thus, a fourth factor we considered was whether there were well-established research organizations in the countries with expertise and interest in health systems research. Consideration was also given to the scope for policy engagement and the level of international and regional interest likely to be generated through the research.

Finally, we also revisit the original countries included in the 1985 *Good health at low cost* volume: China, Costa Rica, the Indian state of Kerala, and Sri Lanka. At the time of the original report, these four countries had shown dramatic improvements in infant mortality rate and life expectancy, despite severe economic constraints, and their improvements were substantially better than comparable countries.

Mapping data

We began by identifying data on key indicators of maternal and child health, including under-5 mortality, infant mortality, maternal mortality, and life expectancy, as well as intermediate indicators such as the presence of skilled birth attendants and antenatal care. These indicators, while limited as measures of population health, have the benefit of being available over time and of capturing a series of diverse processes within the health system. Thus, effective maternal health care, for instance, requires the presence of a skilled birth attendant and access to emergency care in case of complications; child health requires timely access to antibiotics, immunization, oral rehydration therapy and safe water and sanitation. Each country mapped all data sources available, and identified any discrepancies in definitions and data between national and international sources.

This mapping allowed us to link available data to the framework (Figure 2.3), identifying gaps and duplications and then finding ways to approach these through choice of methods.

Review of literature

We sought to identify country studies that have linked health outcomes with health systems or non-health system factors. We also conducted a desk review of the original countries in the 1985 volume (China, Costa Rica, the state of Kerala, Sri Lanka) to determine whether good health outcomes have been sustained.

The first review, undertaken by researchers at the LSHTM, focused on the published literature. Databases searched included PubMed, MEDLINE, BIDS, HINARI, EconLit, and also media accounts and Google Scholar. The topic did not lend itself to a classic Cochrane-type systematic review that focuses on a single question. Rather, we undertook a scoping review with an iterative search strategy to help to identify key issues[24]. First, country-specific time limits were set, specifying the time period to be considered for each country. Second, papers and texts containing the country name and outcomes of interest (for example, under-5 and child mortality, as well as intermediate outcomes, such as institutional childbirths) were identified, using standard terms in each database. Third, searches were undertaken including the name of the country and major determinants of health related to the health system and other sectors. Fourth, searches were combined to identify papers that considered both outcomes and determinants of health. Finally, abstracts were screened to identify the most relevant papers. This process was guided by key themes emerging from the fieldwork. Since some relevant papers might not have been captured by formal search terms, we supplemented our searches with reference tracing and advice from case study material and key informants.

At country level, the research teams focused on identifying main documents that might have been missed in the first review. These included books, published and unpublished papers, official government or donor reports, research reports, strategy papers and policy documents. Key papers were included on governance, accountability, the country's political structure, decision-making patterns, ideology, gender issues and history, while giving priority to papers that explored the associations of these with health outcomes. The literature sources included both published and grey literature on health policy and systems, but also relevant material from the social sciences. The process was iterative, as data from interviews and the first round of documentary evidence were used to build more refined and focused searches. A large proportion of the data used originated at country level and was found in unpublished sources.

Finally, within each country, trend data were gathered on health-related outcomes, determinants, and inequalities (disaggregated by year, gender, socioeconomic group, urban–rural, important regional divisions and ethnic groups). The main source was the national statistics agency in each country or state. Data were compared with figures from the WHO Statistical Information System, Demographic and Health Surveys, Living Standards Measurement Surveys, World Bank World Development Indicators (WDI) database, World Health Survey, Countdown to 2015 series and UNICEF Multiple Indicator Cluster Surveys.

Data collection and analysis

The case studies were conducted in each study country in late 2009 and the first half of 2010 and involved an in-depth exploration of developments over many years in each country. This historical perspective sought to identify how these developments were affected by institutional, political and cultural factors influencing both government institutions and health systems, as well as the broader context[25]. Recognizing the considerable challenges in attributing causality in complex systems where data are limited, the case studies sought to identify temporal and/or geographical associations among changes in health policies, health determinants (immediate and underlying), and health outcomes.

The case studies triangulated data from multiple sources, drawing on existing quantitative and qualitative data. The approach identified associations and generated and tested plausible explanations of these, drawing on multiple data sources and on the literature, which then generated further propositions. The research process included several stages, each of which built upon each other.

Stage I. Understanding health outcomes and their proximal determinants

The objective of the first stage was to describe how health outcomes, proximal determinants, and other potentially relevant explanatory factors have evolved over time. The trends in under-5 mortality, maternal mortality and other outcome indicators relevant to particular country settings were examined.

In Thailand, determinants of health and mortality that were analysed included the coverage of health interventions and characteristics of individuals and households (for example, wealth and education), and publicly provided infrastructure. The work in the other countries explored and synthesized published literature on determinants of health in their particular settings, particularly factors influencing maternal and child health. This provided the necessary insights into the health problems that each health system faced and pointed to how much health improvements were due to reductions in diseases (for example, vaccine-preventable ones) through a functioning health system. These findings fed into the next stage, where we examined the policy context and the role of health systems.

Quantitative methods included a review of descriptive statistics on mortality, health interventions and health system indicators over time. Much of the analysis drew on standard datasets, in particular Demographic and Health Surveys, Multiple Indicator Cluster Surveys, and other national surveys, as well as time series estimates generated using statistical modelling by the Institute for Health Metrics and Evaluation and WHO. These data were used to generate a set of common country profiles using a range of comparable indicators (related to disease, economic and health system resources) that were compared with global and regional averages. This was complemented with further country-specific reviews of available evidence exploring relevant issues in more depth. These describe how health outcomes, their determinants and other potential explanatory factors have changed over time and how they vary within the population. The latter analyses were informed by knowledge of locally relevant determinants of health inequalities and of disease patterns and their determinants.

Stage II. Analysing the policy context and the health system, including key changes over time

Using our conceptual model described above (Figure 2.3), and drawing on the findings from Stage 1, we now focused on the health system and the wider policy context in which it operates, recognizing the mutual interdependence of all elements of the conceptual model. Drawing on the conceptual framework, the main areas of research were operationalized to specific research questions (Box 2.1).

Health systems. We used WHO's building blocks health systems framework as a basis for our analysis of the country health systems. The focus was not just on which developments took place in public programmes, including the health system, but also how and why these changes were initiated and implemented.

Box 2.1   Steps in the analytical approach

1. Why is the country an example of 'good health at low cost'?

2. What are the key areas of health improvement that have secured 'good health at low cost' over the last few decades (cause-specific health gains in whatever way possible, not only in infant and maternal mortality rates)?
   - How does the country compare with other similar countries?
   - Has the country done it well in all parts of the country and for all groups in the population?

3. How has the country achieved these specific health gains (what diseases/ conditions have been tackled)?
   - What interventions (inside or outside the health sector) have been delivered to address these conditions?
   - Recognize evidence limitations! Plausible arguments.

4. How did the health system and other sectors support the effective delivery of these interventions?
   - What were the key changes over time in the system or other sectors that supported these interventions?

5. How and why were these health system developments and wider policy interventions possible (consider, for example, policy actors, policy processes/ strategies for policy formulation, implementation, institutionalization as well as sociocultural and political influences over these issues)?
   - Key details of sociopolitical context that are relevant.

6. What other sociocultural-political factors may explain health gains through influence over patients/community health behaviours and activities (e.g. employment or gender equity that influence service use and health behaviour)?
   - Key relevant details of sociocultural context that are relevant.

7. Conclusions
   - What lessons can other countries learn from our experience?
   - What are the challenges for the future? Challenges for health and ensuring equitable health systems? Challenges of addressing them?

We also sought to explore the process of *policy change*, with the following key questions:

•   What were the policy changes or reforms in terms of their design, key features and timelines?

•   What were the intended aims and the expected changes in health outcomes and health equity and access (such as maternal mortality), or intermediate outcomes (such as staff retention) of the policy changes or reforms?

•   Were there unintended changes associated with the policy changes?

•   How did the key policy changes take place? What were the main drivers and factors that shaped these policy changes?

•   In what ways have different actors engaged in policy initiation and development, such as setting the agenda, assuming an active role in implementing the policy, or indirectly helping or obstructing it? The range of actors whose roles were explored varied among countries and included politicians, senior civil servants, parliamentarians, health professional groups and lobbies, civil society groups, businesses, the media, professional associations, international organizations and donors.

Policy context. The development and implementation of health and other public policies take place within a national and international context. Our proposition was that health policies that contribute to 'good health at low cost' are more likely to emerge within a supportive social policy and political context. We, therefore, looked for factors such as the constitutional and legislative basis for action; partnerships among stakeholders; economic resources and financial systems; capacity for management, innovation, monitoring and evaluation; attitudes towards gender; the situation regarding human resources (including competing health worker employment, migration); bureaucratic effectiveness; level of solidarity; and the role of civil society. These categories are not, however, exhaustive. The activities of other relevant sectors, such as education, management of natural resources and agriculture, were also considered, as they influence health and the way health systems operate.

Across the five countries, extensive interviews were undertaken with a range of respondents working currently or previously at national, district and local levels, including government representatives, civil servants, donor and civil society representatives and private sector organizations selected to represent a variety of actors in each context (the fieldwork undertaken in each country, along with a description of the settings, data sources and methods, are provided in the

Annex). Key informants were identified through a snowball technique, in order to identify people who had been involved at major stages of health system development, had a good overview of the determinants of health and were knowledgeable about the sequencing of the most important events. These included managers, planners, health practitioners in charge of programmes, and representatives of the private sector and nongovernmental organizations (NGOs) within the health system and beyond. Data were collected using a semi-structured interview guide. To improve consistency and comparability, a generic research guide was developed and adapted to each country. Data collection instruments were translated and tested in each country, and shared among all research teams, while retaining sufficient flexibility to capture unexpected issues. Questions were adapted to the expertise and circumstances of each respondent, but retained an exploratory focus.

Thus, the country case studies adopted an iterative approach with triangulation of both qualitative and quantitative data. The quantitative data were examined critically, given their known weaknesses, with cross-checking of figures from different sources and inspection for discontinuities in time trends as described above. Findings were presented at national workshops and at policy and technical fora; feedback from these, as well as from independent reviewers, was considered. The country case studies are presented in the subsequent chapters.

Stage III. Synthesizing stage: why do some countries achieve 'good health at low cost'?

The final stage of the research integrated the findings from the previous two stages, and sought to explain the health outcomes observed in each country and across countries, with reference to our conceptual model. Some caveats are in order, however. First, it is important to stress that we did not expect to identify a single magic bullet – health outcomes are a consequence of many interacting factors. Second, by focusing on specific outcomes (such as maternal and child health) where we understand the factors that can potentially affect them, we were more likely to be able to determine the possible reasons for observed broad changes in health and health systems. Third, there are huge constraints imposed by what are, in effect, analyses of natural experiments over long time periods, and in situations of limited data. Hence, we did not expect to establish causal associations. Our objective was to draw on relevant evidence, to propose plausible relationships and to identify patterns across countries through comparative analysis.

This study has certain limitations. First, we are focusing on success stories. Ideally, we would have compared the countries included with others that were generally similar but which have failed to improve health outcomes to the same extent. However, this would pose many problems, especially the cost and time required to do in-depth case studies in a large number of countries. In addition, at least some of the other potential countries lack indigenous capacity to undertake the research and have weak data systems. In addition, it may be difficult to identify triggers for implementation of particular programmes and policies. It may be that, especially in political environments where there is considerable insecurity, local policy-makers are reluctant to participate in interviews. We did, however, attempt to compensate for this limitation by making regional comparisons where possible, and including the original four countries in the study to take into account their trajectories and mixed fortunes.

Second, while we can identify potential contributors to 'good health at low cost', we cannot quantify their relative contribution. One promising avenue for investigation could have used subnational longitudinal data on health outcomes and the coverage of health interventions to explore the relative contribution of different determinants on changes over time and to seek associations with policy developments. However, in most cases (with the exception of Thailand), there were severe limitations on the availability of good quality data that precluded such an analysis.

Finally, on a related note, while there were many more data available to us than to the authors of the 1985 *Good health at low cost* report, the quality of data remains variable, often limiting comparisons both nationally and regionally.

▓ Highlights from the study countries

This section introduces the five study countries by comparing their achievements with others in their region and beyond on a number of commonly used metrics. The country chapters provide more detailed information on within-country variations. As the following data demonstrate, each country's performance is generally encouraging.

Achievements in improving health

Figure 2.4 reproduces an updated version of the Preston (1975) curve showing the relationship between life expectancy and gross domestic product (GDP) per capita in current US dollars at purchasing power parity (i.e. as international dollars (Int$)). Average income is strongly associated with improvements in life expectancy for the poorest countries, but at around US$7000, the relationship flattens out. The five study countries have similar or better life expectancy than

Figure 2.4   Life expectancy and GDP per capita, 2005 international dollars

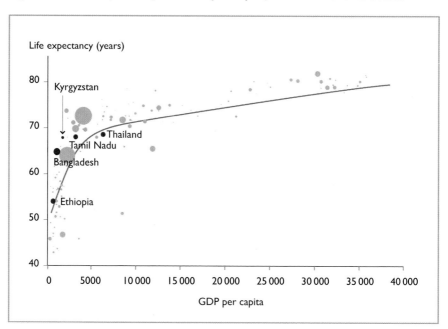

Sources: References 26 and 27.

Note: This is an updated version of the Preston curve[28]. The size of each country data point is proportional to the population size. The line represents a plot of a non-parametric regression. The five study countries are shown in red.

predicted by the regression curve. This static representation, of course, cannot show the trajectories that each country has followed to get to where it is now. Thailand, for example, has seen increases in both income and life expectancy, while Ethiopia's improvements in life expectancy have taken place despite very limited economic growth.

There have been impressive health gains in each of the study countries, although some of these improvements are more recent than others. Figure 2.5 shows trends over time for two health outcomes in each study country and their respective region (or country in the case of Tamil Nadu). Because of the limited availability of data over time, we focus on under-5 mortality and maternal mortality, drawing on recently published estimates[29,30]. We use model estimates for each country, with the exception of Tamil Nadu, where we have vital registration data. In addition, Figure 2.6 shows the proportion of children underweight at two points in time for which good quality data are available.

Figure 2.5 Trends in maternal and child health in the study countries

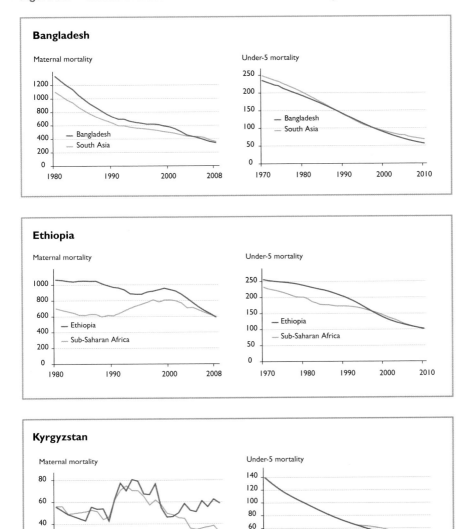

Note to Kyrgyzstan: The reduction in maternal mortality after 2000 may reflect concerted policy efforts to improve maternal and child health in the region (particularly in the Russian Federation), as well as improving standards of living and falling birth rates. However, there are significant concerns with unrecorded births due to out of facility deliveries and underreporting of deaths in countries such as Turkmenistan. In 2004, Kyrgyzstan introduced new WHO live birth criteria while other countries in the region did not, and thus regional comparisons are difficult[31].

Figure 2.5 (continued)

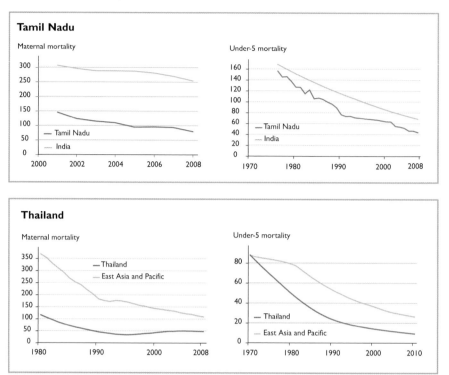

Sources: References 29 and 30.

Notes: The regional trend line uses the median value for the region because the required information to calculate a weighted average across all countries in a region was not available. Maternal mortality per 100 000 live births; under-5 mortality per 1000 live births.

The two health outcomes in the study countries have improved despite significant demographic and geographical challenges, as well as a series of economic and political crises. While undernutrition remains a major problem in three of the countries (Bangladesh, Ethiopia and Tamil Nadu), there have nonetheless been sizeable reductions in all countries. The direction of progress is encouraging.

Although Bangladesh has not outpaced the regional average for maternal and under-5 mortality since independence in 1971, there have been impressive gains. In addition, total fertility fell from 6.1 children per woman in the 1970s to 2.8 in 2010. The country is considered on track to meet Millennium Development Goal number four (MDG4) (reducing child mortality)[17].

Historically, health status in Ethiopia lagged behind other low-income countries in sub-Saharan Africa. In recent years, however, it has caught up and now

Figure 2.6   Improvements in underweight prevalence among children under 5 years of age in the study countries

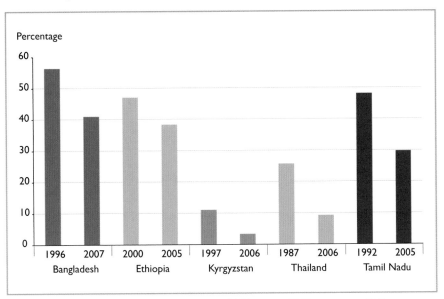

Sources: Bangladesh[32,33]; Ethiopia[34,35]; Kyrgyzstan[36,37]; Thailand[38,39]; Tamil Nadu[40,41].

Notes: Kyrgyzstan data for 1997 is for children under 3 years.

maternal and under-5 mortality are similar to the regional averages. In just five years, between 2000 and 2005, under-5 mortality in Ethiopia fell from 188 to 132 deaths per 1000 live births[34,35]. Over the same period, the proportion of underweight children decreased from 42% to 33% and total fertility rates decreased from 5.9 to 5.4 births per woman.

Kyrgyzstan has achieved improvements in child health outcomes over time, although maternal mortality has stagnated. Despite economic and political challenges, life expectancy (shown in the country chapter) is higher than in many wealthier countries in the former Soviet Union, such as Russia and Kazakhstan. Kyrgyzstan has implemented rigorous vital registration systems that have masked the improvements in mortality rates compared with its neighbours, because previous mortality rates were underestimated. Access to health care is greater than in neighbouring countries due to improved primary care coverage and financial protection for many population groups. Almost all women give birth in a health facility, despite high out-of-pocket payments, in contrast to Tajikistan, where only about 60% of women deliver in a health facility.

Thailand has attracted international attention because of its remarkable health and health system achievements. Maternal and under-5 mortality have both fallen rapidly, far outpacing other countries in the region. By 1990, mortality had already reached very low levels, providing scope for only marginal improvements over the following two decades. This progress not only puts the country on track to achieve MDG4, but has also been accompanied by a narrowing of the rich–poor gap[42]. In addition, Thailand has achieved universal coverage of essential services and substantial protection from the risk of catastrophic health expenditure[43]. Use of public health services, especially primary and secondary care, has increased substantially, with most benefit seen by the poor.

In health terms, Tamil Nadu has long outperformed most other states in India. In 2006, Tamil Nadu had the third lowest rate of under-5 mortality in India (9.2 versus 17 deaths per 1000 live births for all of India), and in 2001–2003, the state was second lowest in terms of maternal mortality (134 per 100 000 lives births versus 301 average for India)[44]. Total fertility, most recently estimated at 1.6 births per woman, compares favourably with the Indian average of 2.7. Although there is variation among districts, the state's population as a whole has relatively good access to public health care facilities.

Coverage of health interventions

The literature points to a wide number of health interventions that are key to improving maternal, neonatal and child health (sometimes referred to as intermediate health outcomes). Coverage indicators for a selection of health interventions mainly related to maternal and child health are presented in Table 2.1. There is wide variation among countries and across interventions. Three of the study countries have almost achieved universal coverage on skilled birth attendance (regarded a good proxy for access to primary health care), while Bangladesh and Ethiopia have a long way to go. As shown by the data, when coverage of skilled birth attendance is low, there is more scope for large inequalities in access. With the exception of Ethiopia, immunization rates are high in the study countries. As will be illustrated in the country chapters, there are dramatic improvements in access to essential interventions over time, leading to health improvements.

Health system inputs

With the exception of Thailand, the GDP per capita of the study countries is substantially less than Int$5000 and all countries spend under Int$500 per capita on health (Figure 2.7). The resource challenges these countries are facing are illustrated in Table 2.2. The five study countries have achieved health gains despite spending (in absolute terms) no more on health than countries that are

Table 2.1   Coverage of key health interventions, most recent year available

Coverage indicators	Bangladesh	Ethiopia	Kyrgyzstan	Tamil Nadu	Thailand
% of births with skilled attendant at delivery	18	6	98	91	97
Skilled attendance at delivery, ratio richest to poorest	11	38	1	1	1
% of births with antenatal care (1 or more visit)	60	28	98	99	99
% of children (12–24 months) vaccinated with DPT	91	32	92[a]	96	94
% of children (12–24 months) vaccinated against measles	83	35	97[a]	93	96
% of currently married women (or in union) using modern contraceptive method	48	14	46	60	70
% of children under 5 years with suspected pneumonia taken to health provider	37	19	62	75	84
% of children under 5 years with diarrhoea receiving appropriate treatment[b]	68	37	22	47	46

Sources: Bangladesh[33]; Ethiopia[35]; Kyrgyzstan[37,45]; Tamil Nadu[41]; Thailand[39].

Notes: DTP: Three doses of combined diphtheria, pertussis, tetanus; [a] Values are for 1 year olds; [b] Appropriate treatment is defined as having received oral rehydration therapy or increased fluids, and continued feeding; value for Ethiopia is only for received oral rehydration therapy or increased fluids.

otherwise comparable in economic development. The usual explanation is that these countries may be spending a greater share of their resources on health. However, as Figure 2.7 shows, per capita health spending in most countries is similar to the level expected on the basis of their national income. If anything, Thailand spends less than would be predicted by its GDP per capita. Thus, the study countries appear to be no different from other countries at similar levels of national income in terms of their health spending.

Figure 2.7 Total health expenditure and GDP per capita, 2005 international dollars

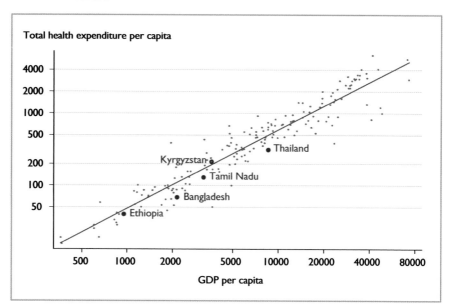

Sources: References 27, 46–48.

These countries have disproved the hypothesis that better outcomes are a result of a larger proportion of GDP per capita spent on health. A related hypothesis is that the governments in the five study countries spend more on health as a proportion of their GDP than other countries with similar levels of national income (that is, that the public share of health expenditure is higher). Figure 2.8 shows that as countries become richer, they tend to spend more on health as a proportion of their GDP. Nevertheless, the evidence suggests that the governments in the five study countries are not unusually generous investors in the health sector and, if anything, spend less as a proportion of GDP than predicted by the linear regression line.

The strong relationship between health workers and health outcomes is well established[56]. Figure 2.9 illustrates this relationship between maternal mortality and the density of nurses and midwives. The relationship between under-5 mortality and density of physicians is almost identical. In countries with scarce human resources, increases in the availability of health workers are strongly associated with reductions in child and maternal mortality. The density of physicians varies quite considerably across the five study countries, with Ethiopia at one end of the scale and Kyrgyzstan at the other. None of the study countries are outliers

Table 2.2   Health system inputs, 2009

	Bangladesh	Ethiopia	Kyrgyzstan	Tamil Nadu[a]	Thailand
Health system capacity[49]					
Density of physicians, nurses and midwives per 10000[b]	6	2–3	80	12[c]	17
Hospital beds per 10000 population[b]	4	2	51	10[50]	22
Health system financing[51]					
Health expenditure, total (% of GDP)	3.4	4.3	6.8	4.0[d,e]	4.3
Health expenditure per capita (current US$)	18.8	14.7	57.1	27.9[d,f]	167.7
Health expenditure per capita (constant 2005 Int$)	48.5	39.9	151.7	–	344.7
Health expenditure, general government (% of total health expenditure)	32.9	47.6	50.9	17.7[d]	75.9
Out-of-pocket health expenditure (% of total health expenditure)	64.8	42.0	39.9	82.0[d]	16.5
Out-of-pocket health expenditure (% of private health expenditure)	96.5	80.1	81.3	100.0[e]	68.1
Private insurance expenditure on health (% of total health expenditure)	0.2	0.8	–	0.2[d,g]	5.9
Formal population coverage (% covered by insurance or tax-based arrangements)	0.4[h]	–	100.0[i]	100.0[j]	97.7[h]

Sources: As indicated in the table and below.

Notes: [a] Data for Tamil Nadu from reference 47 unless otherwise stated; [b] Values are for 2000–2009; [c] Value is for 2008, data from reference 52; [d] Values are for 2004–2005; [e] Estimated value; [f] Exchange rate of US$ 1 = Rs 45; [g] Values is the all-India figure; [h] Values are for 2008, data from reference 53; [i] Depth of coverage varies, data from reference 54; [j] Nominal figure, data from reference 55.

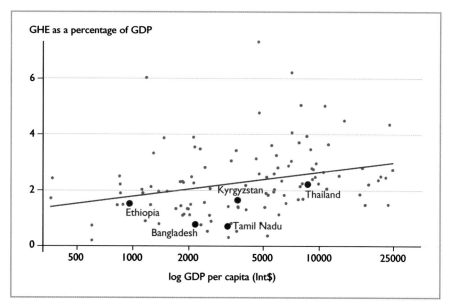

Figure 2.8 Government health expenditure (GHE) as proportion of GDP versus GDP per capita, 2005 international dollars

Sources: References 27, 46–48.

in the relationship between these measures, except Kyrgyzstan, where under-5 mortality is higher than would be expected given its historical density of physicians, an issue that will be discussed in the country chapter. Figure 2.9 exhibits a similar pattern for maternal health, although here, Kyrgyzstan is no longer an outlier.

Other public sector inputs

Sectors outside of health are known to be important for health outcomes. Non-health factors are too numerous to mention; this section focuses on just two – education and sanitation – that are regarded as being particularly influential. Education is a key determinant of health and there is an enormous literature devoted to the study of this relationship. Education may have a direct effect on health through its influence on health-related behaviours or indirectly as a driver of higher income. Figure 2.10 shows the cross-country relationship between under-5 mortality and adult female literacy, with the five study countries highlighted. The first thing to note is that the female literacy rates differ enormously between the five study countries. Second, higher female literacy is associated with lower under-5 mortality. The majority of the five study countries fall below

Figure 2.9 Maternal mortality and nurse/midwife density, latest year

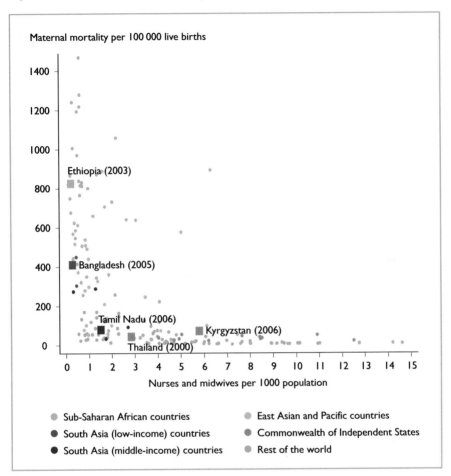

Sources: References 26 and 29.

the linear regression line, suggesting that, on average, they achieve better health outcomes than other countries with similar female literacy rates.

Sanitation is another developmental indicator outside the health system that is regarded as a strong predictor of good health[57] (Figure 2.11). The plot confirms that countries with greater access to sanitation tend to have lower under-5 mortality. As with the previous indicators, there are wide differences in access to sanitation across the five study countries. With the exception of Tamil Nadu, the study countries show levels of mortality that are similar to other countries with the same access to sanitation.

Figure 2.10 Under-5 mortality and adult female literacy, latest year

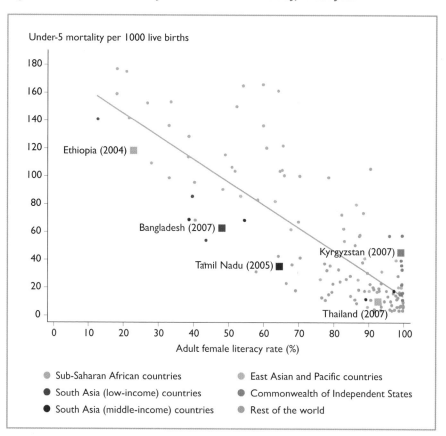

Sources: References 26 and 30.

Innovation and large-scale investment in health sector reforms

All the countries included met the criterion of having undergone large-scale reform in their health sectors, either alone or as part of broader public sector reform. Improvements in maternal and child health in Bangladesh since the 1980s have been linked to the prioritization by government of population control and emergency obstetric care. Since independence, the government and donors invested heavily in a network of community clinics offering curative and preventive services. The large non-state sector developed sophisticated micro-finance schemes that contributed to health and employment.

The government of Ethiopia implemented a series of innovative reforms from 2000 onwards, seeking to achieve universal access to primary health care by

Figure 2.11 Under-5 mortality and access to improved sanitation, 2005

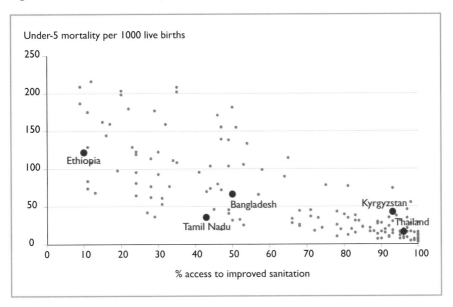

Sources: References 26 and 41.

2017. Its Health Extension Programme, introduced in 2003, has sought to provide two trained health workers in every village health post in the country.

Soon after independence from the USSR in 1991, Kyrgyzstan launched a radical reform plan (MANAS) that has provided a coherent framework for donor investment in the health sector under government leadership. The country represents a unique example of sustained and concerted action in the region. Reforms led to a shift from specialist-oriented care to family practice, implementation of a basic benefits package, hospital rationalization, introduction of contracting, creation of a single payer system, and liberalization of the pharmaceutical market.

The government of Tamil Nadu has implemented extensive health system reforms since the 1970s, most recently within the framework of the 2005 National Rural Health Mission of the Government of India. This study focuses on reforms up until 2005, due to the fact that it is still too early to assess the impact of the Health Mission. Nevertheless, the new reform is addressing fundamental weaknesses of the public health system, including the provision of substantial increases in financing and managerial autonomy. These have been associated with marked increases in the uptake of services in rural areas and unprecedented health improvements, particularly in maternal and child health.

The available evidence indicates that the increased public spending on primary care (particularly preventive care and health promotion) is largely pro-poor (Vaidyanathan G et al. *Do the poor benefit from public spending on healthcare in India? Results from benefit (utilization) incidence analysis in Tamil Nadu and Orissa.* Draft report, May 2010). Tamil Nadu is a good example of a mixed health system, which, despite a growing private sector, has safeguarded key public services (immunization, deliveries, etc.) in the public sector.

Thailand has implemented a range of far-reaching and ambitious reforms over many decades. Coverage was increased step-by-step by expanding insurance schemes for particular income groups. Successive improvements in financial protection through user fee exemption and community and formal sector insurance schemes were consolidated in 2002 to establish a system of universal health care. This has been accompanied by capacity building in public and private sectors, growth of infrastructure and human resources, and extension of primary care, all with only modest increases in total health expenditure.

Although the countries have been selected as success stories, they still face significant challenges, as will be discussed in the chapters that follow. Kyrgyzstan has experienced three coups since independence. In Bangladesh and India, there are persistent concerns about how to regulate the large and complex private sector. There are still high out-of-pocket payments in Bangladesh, Kyrgyzstan and India, placing substantial burdens on households. In addition, considerable income and health inequalities exist in all countries, across population groups and across geographical areas. Most countries face workforce shortages. Despite abundant donor funding in Ethiopia, there are concerns about its capacity to use donor and government funds effectively[58]. Our study explores how the countries are improving health, while managing these challenges and preparing for the future.

Much can be gained by understanding the five countries' achievements and successes. Countries such as Thailand and the state of Tamil Nadu have done well over long periods of time; others, like Ethiopia, Kyrgyzstan and Bangladesh, have demonstrated faster improvements in recent years compared with countries with comparable economic resources. All have implemented ambitious and far-reaching reforms. The following chapters provide individual country case studies to chart how these measurable improvements have developed. This is with a view to providing lessons on how other, less successful countries – at similar stages in their economic development – might follow in their footsteps. A separate chapter analyses the experience of those countries studied in the original *Good health at low cost* report 25 years later.

ACKNOWLEDGEMENTS

The Thai team and, in particular, Supon Limwattananon, produced the multi-country analyses on the determinants of health outcomes for the chapter, which informed the development of its content. Tim Powell-Jackson produced Figures 2.5, 2.6, 2.7, 2.8 and 2.11, and provided accompanying text. Benjamin Palafox produced Tables 2.1 and 2.2.

All GHLC team members and Steering Committee members contributed to the development of the initial ideas, framework for analysis and methodologies.

REFERENCES

1. WHO. *Everybody's business: Strengthening health systems to improve health outcomes. WHO's framework for action.* Geneva: World Health Organization; 2007.

2. Lalonde M. *A new perspective on the health of Canadians. A working document.* Ottawa: Government of Canada; 1974.

3. Marmot M et al. Closing the gap in a generation: health equity through action on the social determinants of health. *Lancet* 2008; 372(9650):1661–9.

4. Birn A-E. Making it politic(al): closing the gap in a generation: health equity through action on the social determinants of health. *Social Medicine* 2009; 4(3): 166–82.

5. Krieger N et al. Who, and what, causes health inequities? Reflections on emerging debates from an exploratory Latin American/North American workshop. *Journal of Epidemiology and Community Health* 2010; 64(9):747–9.

6. WHO. *Macroeconomics and health: investing in health for economic development. Report of the Commission on Macroeconomics and Health.* Geneva: World Health Organization; 2001.

7. Sepúlveda J. Foreword. In: Jamison DT et al., eds. *Disease control priorities in developing countries,* 2nd edn. Washington, DC: Oxford University Press; 2006:xiii–xv.

8. Mills A, Rasheed F, Tollman S. Strengthening health systems. In: D. Jamison et al., eds. *Disease control priorities in developing countries,* 2nd edn. Washington, DC: Oxford University Press; 2006:87–102.

9. Hsiao W. *What is a health system? Why should we care?* Cambridge, MA: Harvard School of Public Health; 2003.

10. Roberts MJ, et al. *Getting health reform right: A guide to improving performance and equity.* New York: Oxford University Press; 2004.

11. Shakarishvili G et al. Converging health systems frameworks: towards a concepts-to-actions roadmap for health systems strengthening in low and middle income countries. *Global Health Governance* 2010; 3(2).

12. Atun R et al. Integration of targeted health interventions into health systems: a conceptual framework for analysis. *Health Policy and Planning* 2010; 25(2):104–11.

13. Atun RA et al. Barriers to sustainable tuberculosis control in the Russian Federation health system. *Bulletin of the World Health Organization* 2005; 83(3):217–23.

14. GAVI/NORAD. *Alleviating system wide barriers to immunization. Issues and conclusions from the Second GAVI Consultation with Country Representatives and Global Partners.* Oslo: Global Fund; 2004.

15. Hanvoravongchai P et al. Pandemic influenza preparedness and health systems challenges in Asia: results from rapid analyses in 6 Asian countries. *BMC Public Health* 2010; 10:322.

16. Travis P et al. Overcoming health-systems constraints to achieve the Millennium Development Goals. *Lancet* 2004; 364(9437):900–6.

17. WHO/UNICEF. *Countdown to 2015 decade report (2000–2010). Taking stock of maternal, newborn and child survival.* Geneva: World Health Organization; 2010.

18. Croghan TW, Beatty A, Ron A. Routes to better health for children in four developing countries. *Milbank Quarterly* 2006; 84(2):333–58.

19. Bloom G, Standing H, Lloyd R. Markets, information asymmetry and health care: towards new social contracts. *Social Science & Medicine* 2008; 66(10):2076–87.

20. WHO Commission on the Social Determinants of Health. *Challenging inequity through health systems. Final report, Knowledge Network on Health Systems.* Geneva: World Health Organization; 2007.

21. Tissot L, Veyrassat BA, eds. *Technological trajectories, markets, institutions: industrialized countries, 19th–20th centuries* [in English and French]. Bern: Peter Lang; 2002.

22. Atun R, Menabde N. Health systems and systems thinking. In: Coker R, Atun R, McKee M, eds. *Health systems and the challenge of communicable disease. Experiences from Europe and Latin America.* Buckingham, UK: Open University Press; 2005:121–140.

23. McPake B, Blaauw D, Sheaff R. *Recognising patterns: health systems research beyond controlled trials.* London: Department for International Development; 2006. (http://www.dfid.gov.uk/r4d/PDF/Outputs/HealthSysDev_KP/recognising_patterns_web_version.pdf, accessed 5 September 2011) (HSD working paper HSD/WP/10?06).

24. Arksey H, O'Malley L. Scoping studies: towards a methodological framework. *International Journal of Social Research Methodology* 2005; 8(1):19–32.

25. Yin RK. *Case study research: design and methods.* Thousand Oaks, CA: Sage; 2003.

26. World Bank. *World development indicators* [online database]. Washington, DC: World Bank; 2011 (http://data.worldbank.org/indicator, accessed March 2011).

27. Heston A, Summers R, Aten B. *Penn world table version 6.3.* Philadelphia, PA: Center for International Comparisons of Production, Income and Prices at University of Pennsylvania; 2009.

28. Preston SH. The changing relationship between mortality and level of economic development. *Population Studies* 1975; 29(2):281.

29. Hogan MC et al. Maternal mortality for 181 countries, 1980–2008: a systematic analysis of progress towards Millennium Development Goal 5. *Lancet* 2010; 375(9726):1609–23.

30. Rajaratnam JK et al. Neonatal, postneonatal, childhood, and under-5 mortality for 187 countries, 1970–2010: a systematic analysis of progress towards Millennium Development Goal 4. *Lancet* 2010; 375(9730):1988–2008.

31. Rechel B, McKee M. The effects of dictatorship on health: the case of Turkmenistan. *BMC Medicine* 2007; 5:21.

32. NIPORT, Mitra and Associates and ORC Macro. *Bangladesh demographic and health survey 1999–2000.* Calverton, MD: National Institute of Population Research and Training, Mitra and Associates, and ORC Macro; 2001.

33. NIPORT, Mitra and Associates, and Macro International. *Bangladesh demographic and health survey 2007.* Calverton, MD: National Institute of Population Research and Training, Mitra and Associates, and Macro International; 2009.

34. Central Statistical Authority, MEASURE DHS and ORC Macro. *Ethiopia demographic and health survey 2000.* Addis Ababa: Central Statistical Authority, MEASURE DHS and ORC Macro; May 2001.

35. Central Statistical Authority, MEASURE DHS and ORC Macro. *Ethiopia demographic and health survey 2005.* Addis Ababa: Central Statistical Authority, MEASURE DHS and ORC Macro; 2005.

36. Research Institute of Obstetrics and Pediatrics, Kyrgyzstan, and Macro International. *Kyrgyz Republic demographic and health survey, 1997*. Bishkek: Research Institute of Obstetrics and Pediatrics, Kyrgyzstan Ministry of Health and Macro International; 1998.

37. National Statistical Committee of the Kyrgyz Republic and UNICEF. *Multiple Indicator Cluster Survey (MICS) Kyrgyz Republic, 2006: Monitoring the situation of children and women*. Bishkek, Kyrgyzstan: National Statistical Committee/United Nations Children's Fund; 2007.

38. Chayovan C, Kamnuansilpa P, Knodel J. *Thailand demographic and health survey 1987*. Bangkok: Institute of Population Studies, Chulalongkorn University and Institute for Resource Development/Westinghouse; 1988.

39. Thailand National Statistical Office. *Thailand multiple indicator cluster survey December 2005–February 2006, final report*. Bangkok: National Statistical Office; 2006.

40. International Institute for Population Sciences. *National family health survey (MCH and family planning), India, 1992–93*. Bombay: International Institute for Population Sciences; 1995.

41. International Institute for Population Sciences and Macro International. *National Family health survey (NFHS-3), India, 2005–06: Tamil Nadu*. Mumbai: International Institute for Population Sciences; 2008.

42. Vapattanawong P et al. Reductions in child mortality levels and inequalities in Thailand: analysis of two censuses. *Lancet* 2007; 369(9564):850–5.

43. Limwattananon S, Tangcharoensathien V, Prakongsai P, *Equity in financing healthcare: impact of universal access to healthcare in Thailand*. Rotterdam: EQUITAP; 2005. (EQUITAP Project Working Paper 16).

44. Datanet India. *Indiastat.com* [online database]. New Delhi: Datanet India; 2011 (http://www.indiastat.com/default.aspx, accessed March 2011).

45. WHO. *World health statistics 2008*. Geneva: World Health Organization; 2008.

46. WHO. *Statistical information system* (WHOSIS), Geneva: World Health Organization (http://www.who.int/whosis/en/, accessed March 2011).

47. Government of India. *National health accounts, India 2004–05*. New Delhi: Government of India; 2009.

48. Government of Tamil Nadu. *Statistical hand book 2010*. Chennai: Department of Economics and Statistics; 2010.

49. WHO. *World health statistics 2010*. Geneva: World Health Organization; 2010.

50. Government of Tamil Nadu. *Statistical hand book 2011, Tamil Nadu.* Chennai: Department of Economics and Statistics; 2011.

51. WHO. *National health accounts, country health information.* Geneva: World Health Organization; 2011 (http://www.who.int/nha/country/en/, accessed 17 June 2011).

52. Rao KD et al. *India's health workforce size, composition and distribution.* New Delhi: Public Health Foundation of India & World Bank; 2008 (HRH technical report 1).

53. International Labour Office, Social Security Department. *Social health protection. An ILO strategy towards universal access to health care.* Geneva: International Labour Organization; 2008 (Social Security Policy Briefing 1).

54. Ibraimova A et al. Kyrgyzstan: Health system review. *Health Systems in Transition* 2011; 13(3):1–152.

55. Government of Tamil Nadu. *Annual policy notes.* Chennai: Department of Health and Family Welfare; 1990–2005.

56. Anand S, Barnighausen T. Human resources and health outcomes: cross-country econometric study. *Lancet* 2004; 364(9445):1603–9.

57. Gakidou E et al. Improving child survival through environmental and nutritional interventions: the importance of targeting interventions toward the poor. *Journal of the American Medical Association* 2007; 298(16):1876–87.

58. Banteyerga H et al. *The system-wide effects of the Global Fund in Ethiopia: baseline study report.* Bethesda, MD: Partners for Health Reform plus Project, Abt Associates; 2005.

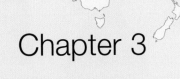

Chapter 3

HEALTH TRANSCENDS POVERTY:
THE BANGLADESH EXPERIENCE

**Tracey Pérez Koehlmoos, Ziaul Islam, Shahela Anwar,
Shaikh A Shahed Hossain, Rukhsana Gazi, Peter Kim Streatfield and
Abbas Uddin Bhuiya**

ICDDR,B, Dhaka, Bangladesh

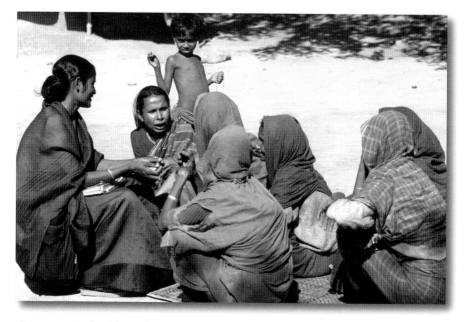

A community health worker gives child nutrition and family planning advice. She also deals with minor medical problem and shows mothers how to mix and administer oral rehydration fluids to treat childhood diarrhoea. Mobarakdi village, Matlab district, Bangladesh

■ Key messages

- Bangladesh became a nation in 1971 under the most difficult circumstances and since then has made huge strides in improving its population's health. A political commitment to health was enshrined in the 1972 Constitution, and policies have transcended political change while constantly adapting to emerging issues.

- Bangladesh was one of the first developing countries to strongly endorse a national family planning programme, resulting in a dramatic reduction in fertility. Bangladesh's basic population and health indicators are on a par with or better than its neighbours, despite having a lower per capita income.

- Bangladesh has continued to be an innovator in health policies and in testing and adapting low cost technologies in the health sector, while maintaining long-term continuity of policies. This is demonstrated by its long history of community and voluntary health workers who bring appropriate technologies to its people.

- Innovation has been facilitated by an environment that has created policy space for the non-state sector. Bangladesh's world renowned non-governmental organisations (NGOs) and initiatives in health have grown and matured alongside public sector activities, often working together to deliver services.

- Bangladesh's health achievements have occurred in the context of improved literacy, economic development and some positive changes in the social fabric of the nation.

■ Introduction

The People's Republic of Bangladesh came into existence in 1971 under the most difficult circumstances. Once part of British India, the region had become East Pakistan at Partition in 1947 but was subjected to oppressive policies by the authorities in the politically dominant West Pakistan. The nine-month War of Liberation in 1971 was among the 20th century's most brutal. An estimated three million Bengalis died and ten million refugees fled into India. Much of the country's infrastructure was destroyed. Mortality rates were high, life expectancy and literacy were low, and poverty was rampant. Other challenges facing the new nation were frequent natural disasters, including seasonal flooding, cyclones and devastating famines such as that of 1974[1,2]. The fledgling government also suffered from widespread inefficiencies[3,4].

During the past 40 years, the country has made enormous advances in life expectancy, child health, literacy and disaster preparedness. The fertility rate has been dramatically reduced and high levels of immunization coverage have been achieved; this, in turn, has led to unprecedented reductions in maternal and child mortality[5]. Bangladesh's basic population and health indicators are on a par with or better than its neighbours, which have higher per capita income. To recognize the great strides the country has made towards good health, in September 2010, Prime Minister Sheikh Hasina accepted a United Nations award on behalf of the people of Bangladesh for outstanding achievements in the reduction of child mortality, one of the eight Millennium Development Goals (MDGs). These achievements have been made with low total health expenditure (3.4% of GDP or US$ 12 per capita in 2007) and even lower health expenditure financed by the public sector (1.1% of GDP or US$ 4 per capita in 2007). The level of total health expenditure is low by regional standards; in contrast, India spends 4.8% and Nepal 5.3% of GDP on health[6].

Although the Bangladeshi economy has grown 5–6% per annum since 1996, it is still one of the poorest nations in the world, with a per capita GDP of US$ 554. In 2007, an estimated 40% of its 160 million people were living on less than US$ 1 a day. Over the past three decades, Bangladesh has experienced one of the highest urban population growth rates in the world[7]. At present, about one quarter of the population lives in urban areas[8], a number that is expected to continue to rise rapidly. The population of Dhaka, the capital city, is expected to reach 22 million by 2025, making it the fourth largest city in the world[9]. An estimated 37% of Dhaka's residents (more than nine million in 2007) live in overcrowded slums, often without access to safe drinking water, adequate nutrition or primary health care services[10,11]. The picture is similar in other major cities and rural areas across the country (Box 3.1).

Box 3.1   **Bangladesh at a glance**

Population   162 million[12]. Among the highest urban population growth rates in the world[7], with 28% urban population (2009)[1] living mainly in poorly serviced slums.

Geography   Most of the country is low lying and subject to frequent floods and cyclones. 20 million people exposed to excessive levels of arsenic in drinking water[13].

Ethnic   Culturally homogeneous; 98% of the population Bengalis.
composition   Minority tribal groups living mainly in hilly regions of country[14].

Government   Gained independence in 1971. Parliamentary democracy since 1990s, except for brief period of military-backed government from 2006 to 2008. Frequent changes in political leadership, but investing in health services is popular politically.

Health   Health expenditure per capita (constant 2005 Int$)[15]: 48.49
system   Density of physicians, nurses and midwives per 10 000[16]: 6
         Pluralistic, relatively decentralized health system, with the state, NGOs, private for-profit sectors all playing a major role. Large numbers of informal and traditional healers. Focus on primary health care and family planning. Coverage of key health interventions varies dependent on intervention (18% of births with skilled attendance at delivery[17], 75% of children under age of 1 year fully immunized nationwide)[18].

Economic,		
demographic GDP per capita (constant 2005 Int$)[12]		1286
and social Economic growth between 2000 and 2005[14]		5.4%
development Population living on less than Int$1.25 a day (2005)[12]		49.6%
Population below the national poverty line[12]		40%
Gini index (2005)[12]		31
Infant mortality rate (2008)[16]		43[a]
Maternal mortality ratio (2010)[19]		194[b]
Adult HIV prevalence[20]		0.1%
Life expectancy (years) (2009)[12]		67
Adult literacy (2009)[21]		55.9%
Ratio girls to boys in education[c] (2008)[12]		108%
Access to improved water source (2008)[12]		80% population

Note: [a] Per 1000 live births; [b] Per 100 000 live births; [c] Primary and secondary education.

This chapter explores the reasons for the country's achievements in health. It shows how these health gains can be attributed to a series of effective health sector strategies and policy processes, and to a strong emphasis on delivery of health and family planning services at the community and household level. It then describes the promotion of low cost and targeted technologies and proven interventions and policies that have played a significant role in improving health

---

Box 3.2 The Government of Bangladesh

The head of state of the People's Republic of Bangladesh is the president, a largely ceremonial post, who is elected every five years by parliament. The legislature is a single-house parliament, consisting of 300 members of parliament, also elected every five years. The executive function resides with the prime minister as the head of government, acting through a Council of Ministers[22]. Implementation of government policies and programmes is vested in Bangladesh's civil service, a corps of trained administrators who form the most influential group of civil servants. The district level is key in policy implementation. The districts are divided into subdistricts, or *upazilas*, and those are further divided into unions, the lowest administrative level.

Democratically elected political parties have led the country since the 1990s, with the exception of a two-year, military-backed caretaker government from 2006 to 2008. Civil society organizations, development partners, the media and human rights groups have continued to lobby for the strengthening of democratic processes. The frequent change in political leadership has implications for turnover among political and administrative staff.

The right to health care is established in the Constitution of Bangladesh, which was adopted on 4 November 1972. The policy-making environment in Bangladesh is a closed one, with a bureaucratic chain of government and top-level officials making all the final decisions. In health, the key policy-makers include the minister of health, the director generals of health services and family planning, and the health secretary. They all have extensive authority and are accountable to the prime minister. However, there is an intensive and institutionalized consultative process involving multiple actors within and outside the government system. Commentators have noted that evidence does inform the decision-making process.

---

outcomes. The chapter concludes by setting Bangladesh's health achievements within a context of economic development and some positive changes in the social fabric of the nation.

Certain common threads weave throughout the chapter. These are the principles of political commitment, leadership, innovation and engagement with the non-state sector, which, taken together, go a long way in explaining why Bangladesh has done so well in comparison to many other low-income countries (Box 3.2).

■ Better health?

Compared with other countries in the region, Bangladesh has among the longest life expectancy for men and women, the lowest total fertility rate and the lowest infant, under-5, and maternal mortality rates (Table 3.1). This section examines the trends in these rates since the mid-1970s (with the exception of maternal mortality, which has only been measured since 2001) (Box 3.3). We will show that population and health gains have not been equitable.

Average life expectancy at birth rose from 58 years in 1994 to 66 in 2008, with women living slightly longer than men (65 years and 64 years, respectively) (Table 3.1).

Bangladesh has experienced dramatic decreases in total fertility among women aged 15–49 years. In the mid-1970s, total fertility was 6.6 births per woman aged 15–49 years; in 1994, it was 3.4; and by 2007, it was 2.7[31,32] (Figure 3.1). The differential in rural–urban fertility has narrowed over the past decade, from 1.3 births in 1997 to 0.4 births in 2007; however, this decline has not been seen across wealth quintiles. The poorest women still have approximately one child more (3.2) than their wealthier counterparts (2.1).

Infant mortality has declined dramatically from 85 deaths per 1000 live births in the late 1980s to 52 deaths per 1000 live births between 2002 and 2006 (Figure 3.2). In recent years, there have been improvements in all wealth

Table 3.1   Comparative health indicators across countries of the region

Countries	GDP PPP per capita (US$)[29]	Total fertility rate[30]	Life expectancy at birth (years)[16] 2008		Mortality rate per 1000 live births[15] 2008		
	2009	2008	Male	Female	Infant	Under-5	Maternal
Bangladesh	1398	2.3	64	65	43	54	380
Bhutan	5312	2.6	61	65	54	81	440
India	2930	2.7	63	66	52	69	450
Myanmar	1156	2.3	59	63	74	103	380
Nepal	1144	2.9	63	64	41	51	830
Pakistan	2624	4.0	63	64	72	89	320

Note: PPP: Purchasing power parity.

Box 3.3 The health system in Bangladesh at a glance

Bangladesh, like most other south Asian countries, has a public system run by the government and a large non-state sector that plays a major role in the delivery of health care services. The latter includes NGOs, private providers of modern and indigenous medicine, and informal providers, such as traditional birth attendants, drug vendors and village doctors.

During the 1970s, the government developed a public health system along the *Health for All* model, with a nationwide network of hospitals, health complexes, family welfare centres, subcentres, and Expanded Programme for Immunization outreach clinics. At the same time, a parallel network of family planning and maternal and child welfare centres was established, in some cases contracting NGOs to provide services[23].

Some 2000 NGOs work in Bangladesh, including some of the largest in the world Bangladesh Rural Advancement Committee ((BRAC), Grameen, ASA and Proshika). NGO activities are mainly concentrated in rural areas, with recent expansion into semi-urban and urban slums.

The traditional medicine practised in Bangladesh includes Unani and Ayurvedic medicine. Formal providers are regulated by a joint governing board, and each has its own network of teaching colleges.

The formal private for-profit sector is large and complex, and since 2000, it has been growing by about 15% per year[24]. For example, in 2000, approximately 682 clinics and hospitals and 838 laboratories and other diagnostic centres were registered with the Ministry of Health and Family Welfare. As of March 2009, those numbers had risen to 2271 and 4735, respectively[23]. In many cities, essential health services are much more widely available in private hospitals than in public hospitals. In the city of Chandpur in 2008, for example, two public hospitals were offering emergency obstetric care, while 24 private hospitals offered the same service.

The non-state sector provides the overwhelming majority of outpatient curative care, while the public sector is used for a larger proportion of hospital deliveries and preventive care. For example, about 90% of care for children with acute respiratory infection or diarrhoea is obtained from the private sector[25,26]. This is partly because of the lack of qualified providers in rural areas[27,28]. It is also because the Essential Services Package does not cover noncommunicable diseases and health workers are not trained to manage these conditions; consequently, for these health issues, people routinely turn to unlicensed providers for treatment.

The total number of private practitioners is estimated to be around 450 000, or 3.6 per 1000 population. Of these, unqualified providers outnumber formally qualified ones by 12 to 1[24].

Figure 3.1 Trends in fertility rate, 1975–2007

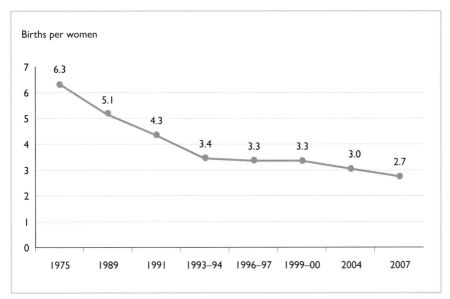

Source: Reference 32.

Figure 3.2 Trends in under-5 and infant mortality rates, 1989–2006

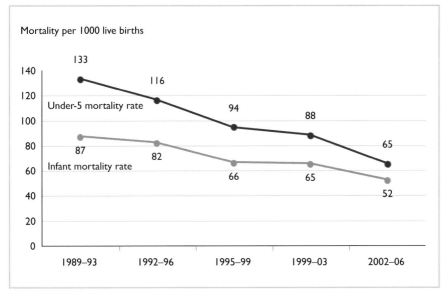

Source: Reference 32.

Figure 3.3   Infant mortality rate by wealth quintile, 2004 and 2007

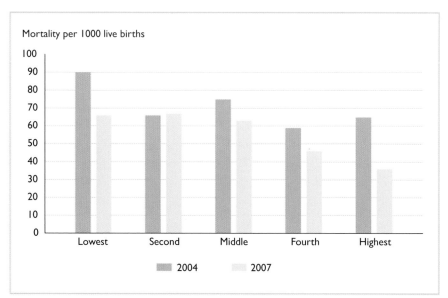

Source: Reference 32.

Figure 3.4   Trends in under-5 mortality rate, urban vs. rural

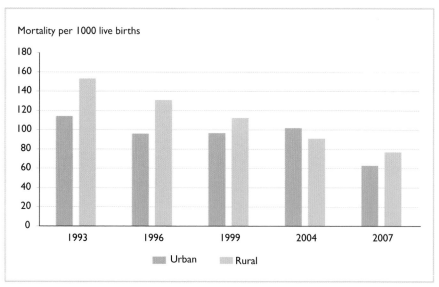

Source: Reference 32.

quintiles (Figure 3.3), but there has been no reduction in inequality and, if anything, disparities between wealth groups have widened. While in 2004 mortality in the richest quintile was 27% lower than in the poorest quintile, this disparity increased to 42% in 2007[32]. However, there have been more equitable advances in infant mortality across the urban–rural divide (Figure 3.4): in 1993, the rate was 81 in urban areas versus 102 in rural areas; by 2007, the difference had fallen to 50 in urban areas versus 59 in rural areas.

Huge improvements in under-5 mortality have taken place: from 202 per 1000 live births in 1979 to 133 in 1989 to 94 in 1995 and to 65 in 2006. As a consequence, Bangladesh is on track to achieve MDG4 to reduce under-5 mortality. Although disparities remain between rural and urban areas (Figure 3.4), child mortality has fallen by at least half in all areas.

There is strong evidence from national and subnational studies that maternal mortality has declined substantially in Bangladesh. Studies conducted in the 1960s suggest that maternal mortality was between 600 and 800 deaths per 100 000 live births at that time[33,34]. A national survey conducted in 2001 reported a decline from 514 deaths per 100 000 live births in the mid-1980s to 322 per 100 000 in the late-1990s[35]. These trends are confirmed by high-quality studies in the Matlab demographic surveillance area[a] in rural Bangladesh: maternal mortality in the Matlab rural area declined from 579 to 247 deaths per 100 000 live births between 1982 and 2005[36]. In order to achieve MDG5 (improve maternal health), maternal mortality must fall to 143 deaths or lower per 100 000 live births by 2015. In fact, a 2010 national survey showed that the maternal mortality ratio had dropped to 194 per 100 000 live births, indicating that Bangladesh is also on track to achieve this goal. However, poor rural women remain disadvantaged[22].

Other health indicators where more progress is needed include low birth weight, malnutrition, and drowning and injuries among children. In addition, an increase in noncommunicable diseases and an ageing population are bringing new challenges to the health system. These are discussed in more detail below.

---

[a] The Matlab Health Research Centre, in rural Bangladesh, is the world's oldest and largest demographic surveillance site in a developing country. Since 1966, researchers at the ICDDR,B have been monitoring population and health indicators for approximately 225 000 residents. Situated 57 km south of Dhaka, it was originally selected for the high incidence of cholera. Now, routine collection is done on births, deaths, nutrition and migration. In recent years, information has been collected regarding risk factors, and morbidity and mortality for noncommunicable diseases. The Health and Demographic Surveillance Site at Matlab is part of the INDEPTH Network.

■ Role of large-scale strategies and policy processes in explaining health gains

The country's leaders have considered the health of the population to be a national priority ever since the drafting of Bangladesh's Constitution in November 1972. This political commitment has transcended political party politics. Under the military rule that lasted from 1975 to 1990, Bangladesh made considerable progress in the health and social development sectors. It is believed that military leaders adopted a set of pro-people programmes to strengthen their popularity, and build the basis for a political platform from which they could subsequently achieve an electoral mandate. In any event, it should be noted that the transition to democracy since the 1990s has served to generate further momentum for the country's overall development.

Figure 3.5 shows the timeframe of major health reforms mapped against outcomes in total fertility and child mortality. In general, political and institutional leadership in the public sector is subject to frequent changes, and depends more on political bent than on specific expertise. Politicians are key actors in the health system. For example, the current political party rose to power on a platform that included the re-establishment of community clinics throughout

Figure 3.5   Health reforms and health gains

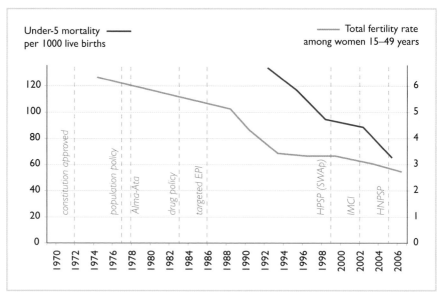

Notes: HPSP: Health and Population Sector Programme; HNPSP: Health, Nutrition and Population Sector Programme.

rural Bangladesh. Despite rapid changes in the political landscape and in key actors, many policies have been sustained for a significant period of time. Individual health professionals, activists, technocrats and civil servants played a critical role in the country s health sector development. There are many examples of individuals who achieved national support for key policies despite the complex political environment. One example from the time of military rule was the promotion and development of Bangladesh's National Drug Policy of 1982 (see below). This innovative policy has survived the transition from military rule to civilian leadership and subsequent changes in governing party.

However, it was the presence of effective civil servants that was essential for implementing complex policies nationwide. The following sections will highlight three policies that had a major impact on the health of the people of Bangladesh: the population policy, the drug policy and the early adoption of the Sector Wide Approach (SWAp). Yet coverage by these policies would not have been as widespread, in terms of geography and their outreach to disadvantaged groups, without the diverse institutions of the voluntary sector. These organizations came into being after the country's independence and grew as the nation was being rebuilt. In many cases, their mandate has been to deliver types of service and reach groups that could not have been reached with existing government capacity. This explains why the voluntary health sector is viewed as an "extender of government". Voluntary organizations have developed strong capacity and often lead the implementation of innovative delivery models and technologies. In reality, they have a considerable scope of freedom of action on the ground. Some of Bangladesh's NGOs have gained worldwide reputations.

The policy environment involves a great deal of flexibility and fluidity between state and non-state sectors. The government has fostered collaboration, working with a series of reputable NGOs on health initiatives that have complemented public sector activities. This has been a two-way exchange, with government providing support but also learning from these organizations[37]:

> NGOs grew and prospered and became the cutting edge for programme improvement. The government, albeit reluctantly, came to accept this and to learn from NGOs.

Population policy and family planning

Population control by means of family planning was a high priority immediately after independence in 1971 and was seen as a main driver of socioeconomic progress and development in an environment with limited resources. It was the main policy goal in the country's first Five Year Plan, 1973–1977[37]. In 1974, the decision was taken to divide the Ministry of Health and Family Welfare

(MoHFW) into separate health services and family planning wings, each with their own director general responsible for supervising and maintaining their respective staff. This separation has been a long standing topic of debate and is frequently challenged, but to date, efforts to unify the two directorates have failed[38]. It is argued that the separation served its purpose at the time, producing benefits in terms of organizational structures that advanced specific policy goals. The MoHFW embodied the government commitment to family planning and helped to safeguard resources and build management capacity in this area.

A population policy was developed in 1976. As part of this, the government decided to implement an innovative, community-based delivery system for family planning services that had been carefully piloted. From the mid-1970s until the 1990s, the family planning programme was largely supply driven and incentive based. The interventions that resulted – namely an aggressive campaign at the community level through household visits with a supply of contraceptive methods – were made possible in large part as a result of the government's impetus.

Drug policy

The pioneering drug policy of 1982 is seen as a major innovation in improving access to drugs in Bangladesh, and it had several components. First, the national policy established a list of mainly generic essential drugs to be procured and used in the public health services. The development of the drug policy under a military government, with key support from the non-state sector, is well documented[39]. Dr Zafrullah Chowdhury[b] of Gonoshasthaya Kendra (GK) played a major role in designing this policy, together with some reputable health professionals and civil servants. WHO worked with government institutions to recommend products to the essential drugs list.

Moreover, the new policy set the stage for establishing in-country production of essential medicines and for a flourishing pharmaceutical sector, facilitating the availability of antibiotics and other medicines for both formal and informal providers throughout the country.

---

[b] Public health activist, freedom fighter, and founder of the NGO Gonoshasthaya Kendra. A UK trained physician, his public health leadership began with the establishment of the first field hospital dedicated to serving other freedom fighters during Bangladesh's War of Liberation. He further served the young nation by championing the Essential Drugs Act, which encouraged national development and discouraged duplication and unsafe practices in the pharmaceutical sector.

Following adoption of this policy, the MoHFW established a drug-production unit (Essential Drugs Company Limited) to ensure an adequate supply of essential drugs in public facilities. Thus, production and distribution facilities exist primarily within the public sector.

The drug policy, the Essential Drugs Company Limited and incentives for the country to produce its own good quality drugs were critical in making essential drugs available to public facilities, filling a previous gap in supply and demand of drugs. By the mid-1990s, the drug policy's positive impact became clear. Not only did drug prices stabilize and medicines became more affordable, but the percentage of essential drugs in all local production increased from 30% (1981) to 80% (mid-1990s). In addition, while only 35% of the country's essential drugs were produced by Bangladeshi companies in the 1980s, this share grew to 60% by the mid-1990s[40]. The reduced dependence on imports and the prioritization of essential drugs are estimated to have saved the country approximately US$ 600 000 million.

In recent years, additional production and distribution facilities have been established within both the public and the private sectors. The pharmaceutical sector in Bangladesh is now thriving, with approximately 224 licensed pharmaceutical factories in the country, six of which are owned by multinational companies[41]. Eighty-five per cent of the raw materials used in the local production of pharmaceuticals are imported, but only 1.1% of locally produced drugs are exported, which has ensured access to drugs that are appropriate to local needs. The pharmaceutical industry lobby is not strong and, in contrast to elsewhere, there has been limited opposition to the essential drug list. This situation may change; in a speech to the parliament of Bangladesh on 11 June 2009, the Minister of Finance, the Honourable Mr Abul Maal Abdul Muhith, recommended the development of export capacity in the pharmaceutical sector as a priority for the economic development of Bangladesh, and this may reduce local availability in the long run.

SWAp

SWAp was introduced in 1998 within the framework of the Health and Population Sector Programme. Although vertical programmes had been successful in reducing overall morbidity, mortality and the total fertility rate, by the late 1990s, it was apparent that duplications and overlap were wasting resources. The SWAp replaced more than 120 separate partner-funded development health projects with 25 integrated annual operational plans, each of them a cost centre whose resources are managed by a single-line director. It is claimed that the SWAp has reduced duplication and financial waste in the health sector and has simplified the process of programme development and implementation. It was carried through the subsequent Health, Nutrition and Population Sector Programme, from 2003 to 2010. The Programme, in place at the time of writing, was extended until 2011 and a new plan called the Health Population Sector Development Programme was under development.

The SWAp is facilitated by the World Bank and the core donor group includes the Governments of Canada, Germany, Japan, the Netherlands, Sweden, the United Kingdom and the United States, as well as the European Union, the Global Fund, GAVI, United Nations Population Fund and UNICEF.

■ Health workers and service delivery at the community level

Strong political commitment has led to investments in human resources and in their innovative use in delivering services, particularly at community and household levels in rural areas, which have made significant contributions to the country's progress in improving population and health outcomes. First of all, household visits by health assistants and family welfare assistants, the public sector's frontline health personnel, have been instrumental in achieving success in health and family planning programmes. Second, alongside the government's drive to increase personnel, NGO participation has been remarkable, training thousands of community health workers and deploying them in rural areas to carry out home visits and raise awareness about good health practices. The large NGOs that deliver health care in Bangladesh began during and in the immediate aftermath of the War of Liberation in the early 1970s, and soon flourished. Third, the many informal providers[c] found in almost every community in Bangladesh have also played an important role. These three distinct groups are described below.

Health assistants and family welfare assistants

Health assistants and family welfare assistants have been particularly instrumental in achieving health improvements in Bangladesh. In the 1960s and early 1970s, there were male smallpox vaccinators and malaria control workers in the

---

[c] Informal providers (also referred to as unlicensed or unqualified practitioners) are predominantly allopathic practitioners such as village doctors and drug sellers, and less commonly, non-allopathic providers such as homeopaths, kabiraj and others. Some of these providers may have received training, but this is not a requirement for them to set up practice; they are not licensed or regulated by public sector authorities.

country. In the mid-1970s, when these two vertical programmes ended, the male field workers were reassigned to the position of health assistants, demonstrating the government's efforts to promote continuity and retain human resources.

In 1976, as part of the new policy to advocate family planning, 13 500 young married women were trained as family welfare assistants, and each was assigned to a population of approximately 5000 people in a rural area. Every two months, these female government employees visited the homes of married women of reproductive age in rural areas, achieving almost universal coverage. Services provided included a wide range of contraceptive methods and education. This was backed by new drug and supply distribution systems and family planning clinics in rural areas, which later started to provide integrated maternal and child health services. Family welfare assistants distributed birth control pills and condoms free of charge and provided information. The initial focus concentrated on birth spacing, but later the family planning programme developed into a comprehensive maternal and child health service aimed to reduce maternal and child mortality. It supplemented the major child and maternal health interventions of the health directorate at that time. Its use of the mass media for education and attitude change was replicated in other countries, such as Kenya and Brazil.

> *Many misconceptions about family planning, childbirth and maternal death have been eliminated from rural society. Nowadays, even "would-be brides" come to us and say they will get married soon, what contraceptive would suit them best? Previously, we did not find such interest in family planning. This change of mindset didn't occur overnight. Sustained campaigning at the doorstep by FWAs, coupled with satellite clinics and facility-based back-up, has resulted in such positive motivation.*
>
> *Family Welfare Assistant (FWA)*

In 1996, the government recruited 4500 women to fill vacancies as health assistants. During home visits, the health assistants carry out health promotion and disease prevention activities, including early detection and reporting of infectious diseases; birth/death registration; distribution of oral rehydration solution (ORS), vitamin A capsules and the supply of medicines for selected diseases; health education campaigns, including motivating men to use condoms and informing them about vasectomy; immunization via Extended Programme of Immunization outreach; and the organization of medical teams during natural disasters. They also make referrals when deemed necessary. The health assistants are assigned to a cluster of 6000 people in the community and they make home visits every two months.

*We clearly inform them about dos and don'ts during pregnancy, delivery
and the postnatal period, through one-to-one contact or group discussion
at their courtyard. We treat minor ailments, vaccinate all babies and
women, educate and motivate them on health, hygiene and family
planning and refer them to the health complex when required. The
community is very familiar to us as we were born and grew up here.*

Health Assistant

Health assistants are recruited by the Directorate General of Health Services,
while family welfare assistants are recruited by the Directorate General of Family
Planning. Both receive basic training followed by periodic refresher courses and
in-service training. The minimum qualification for health assistants and family
welfare assistants is a secondary school certificate[42]. At present, there are 21 000
health assistants, supervised by 4250 assistant health inspectors, and 23 500
family welfare assistants, supervised by 4500 family planning inspectors.

The wide reach and popularity of the family welfare assistant programme can be
explained by its emphasis on home-based contact, which is in response to the
restricted mobility of women due to cultural and geographical factors. Most
importantly, it rejected coercive approaches and responded to real needs at the
time that the programme was conceived[43]. Family planning efforts continue
today, involving health assistants and family welfare assistants, who have broadened their scope to include many different aspects of preventive and, in some
cases, curative health care.

*It is primarily due to our regular home visits over the years that enabled
married women of reproductive age to become aware and users of modern
contraceptive methods, safe delivery practices, child health care and safe
abortion services as well. Nowadays they often call us over cell phones and
seek advice when they need it. This old-time familiarity and intimacy of
FWAs with households has greatly contributed to the reduction of maternal and children's diseases, death and fertility.*

Family Welfare Assistant

Although family welfare assistants, who provide predominantly family planning
services, and health assistants, trained to perform a broader range of tasks, may
operate in the same geographical area and together in the community clinics,
there is little duplication of services, as they cater to the needs of different target
groups.

Bangladesh Rural Advancement Committee and village health workers

In addition to government field workers, NGOs working in the health sector have developed different modalities for using community health workers which have also been extremely effective. Large NGOs have high levels of autonomy and flexibility, and they have been able to play an important role in improving health as well as in reaching populations that have been excluded because of isolation, stigma or lack of resources.

For example, the Bangladesh Rural Advancement Committee (BRAC; originally known as the Bangladesh Rehabilitation Assistance Committee) pioneered the community health volunteer cadre. BRAC was created immediately following the War of Liberation and initially worked on small-scale relief efforts with returning war refugees. By the end of 1972, BRAC had expanded its operation to focus on multisector programmes for the poor and landless, especially women. By the mid-1970s, BRAC's portfolio included microcredit, agriculture, fisheries, vocational training, adult literacy and health and family planning. It had also begun to set up community centres and village organizations to serve as activity hubs.

In 1979, with technical advice from the government and the International Centre for Diarrhoeal Disease Research, Bangladesh (ICDDR,B), BRAC launched its first large-scale nationwide health programme: the Oral Therapy Extension Programme to scale up use of ORS in order to combat the biggest killer of children, diarrhoeal disease. Over a ten-year period, 1200 BRAC employees went door to door in rural Bangladesh and taught 12 million mothers how to prepare and use the life-saving oral saline solution. ORS become popular in the community and BRAC's role in encouraging its use has been seen as a major factor in the significant reduction in infant and child mortality that has been documented. Bangladesh still has the highest ORS use rates in the world. Lessons learned in scaling up were soon translated into youth education programmes and other health programmes.

Since 2006, BRAC has been using trained birth attendants, health workers and volunteers to deliver maternal, neonatal and child health care in urban slums. A newly recruited cadre was created, fully trained and paid for by BRAC, without drawing on public facilities and, thus, did not weaken capacity in the public sector.

Today, BRAC's areas of work include a handicraft business, a dairy and food company, information technology, legal services for the poor, disaster relief services, non-formal primary education, and a university. In collaboration with the government, BRAC delivers directly observed treatment, short-course (DOTS) for tuberculosis. BRAC's 64 000 village health workers touch the lives of more than 110 million people. As the largest NGO in the world, it has more than 120 000 employees, who work in 14 countries, including Afghanistan, Pakistan, the Sudan and Uganda[44,45].

Informal providers

Unlicensed informal practitioners of modern medicine have also played a role in the country's health gains. In addition to selling medicines at affordable rates, they diagnose and treat patients, including children and women, and they provide health education. Although there is no evidence of their effectiveness in providing health services or the value of training them[46], they must be included in any analysis because they provide more health care services than any other cadre of health worker in the country (see Box 3.2). More than 63% of children are cared for by unlicensed providers[26,32]. Informal providers believe that they make good quality, reliable medicines available in rural areas.

> *Besides treating patients, we sell good quality, low-cost antibiotics and other allopath medicines at our chamber cum shop. Medical representatives of various pharmaceutical companies visit us regularly and keep us updated on the use of their products. We've made these modern medicines available to the villagers. Our clients do not need to go far away to buy such medicines. People do rely on our consultation and medicines for they are experienced with our practice for quite a long period of time.*
>
> *A village doctor in a focus group discussion*

During the early 1980s, the national government provided a one-year basic curative training course to approximately 16 000 village doctors, following the Chinese model of the "barefoot doctor". Although this programme did not last beyond 1982, many of its graduates are still working as local practitioners[42,46]. Oversight is sketchy and the effectiveness of investing in the training of informal providers has not been rigorously evaluated; however, their presence in everyday rural life and the access they provide to medical advice and low cost antibiotics and other pharmaceuticals may have played a role in the reduction of childhood mortality and other diseases such as rheumatic heart disease[27,47,48].

In sum, novel approaches to human resources and service delivery have been associated with notable health advances in Bangladesh between 1980 and 2010. Low cost technologies and proven interventions are also credited with playing a large role in explaining these gains. Their role is described in more detail in the next section.

■ What else has Bangladesh done to improve health?

This section addresses the steps that Bangladesh has taken to adopt low cost technologies and adapt proven interventions to the local context. It starts by recognizing the role of grassroots innovation and development and moves on to programmes that have been successfully implemented, such as the Expanded Programme on Immunization, and others that aim to succeed in high-need areas, such as maternal health.

A global leader in developing low cost medical technologies

With a history going back before the War of Liberation, ICDDR,B has become a global leader in population and health research, with a worldwide reputation for developing innovative low cost technologies that have led to improvements in health. ICDDR,B is perhaps best known for its groundbreaking work on ORS, for the treatment of cholera, and for hosting the oldest demographic surveillance sites in a developing country. Zinc for the treatment of childhood diarrhoea is another example of a local innovation that was developed and scaled up in Bangladesh and is now being used in many other developing countries. Delivery kits, *Pustipack* (food supplementation packages), tetanus vaccination for pregnant women, and iodized salt are other important low cost interventions that have spread throughout Bangladesh and to other developing countries. Other innovations, such as a low cost mat that can be used during home deliveries to measure postpartum haemorrhaging, are currently being developed by ICDDR,B.

Implementing proven programme interventions

Long before the emergence of contemporary global health initiatives, the government, the health sector and the population of Bangladesh placed strong emphasis on the importance of childhood immunization as a key mechanism for reducing childhood mortality. The Expanded Programme on Immunization in Bangladesh is considered to be a health system success because of its remarkable progress over the last 20 years. It provides almost universal access to vaccination services, as measured by the percentage of children under 1 year of age who receive BCG (a vaccine against tuberculosis). This increased from 2% in 1985 to 99% in 2009. Coverage for other vaccines has also improved substantially (Figure 3.6).

Although 75% of children aged 12 months nationwide are fully immunized, coverage remains low in some areas[18]. In 22 rural subdistricts, most of which are difficult to access, full immunization coverage ranges between 44% and 64%[32].

Figure 3.6 National vaccination coverage by age 12 months among 12- to 23-month-old children from 1991 to 2009

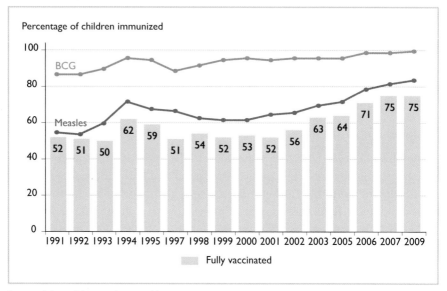

Source: Adapted from reference 18.

Among children living in urban slums, coverage is only 45%[49,50]. The MoHFW, UNICEF and other agencies are actively working to address the needs of these children in hard-to-reach areas.

The Integrated Management of Childhood Illness (IMCI) strategy is also a factor in the country s health gains. Introduced in Bangladesh in 2001, it focuses on effective treatment of diarrhoea, pneumonia, malaria, measles and malnutrition as a means of reducing under-5 mortality. By the end of 2008, 304 out of 508 *upazilas* had implemented IMCI and almost 94% of the health workers in these facilities had been trained in IMCI in the intervention areas where health system support was generally available. A study by Arefin and colleagues has revealed that implementation of IMCI led to improved health worker skills, health system support, and family and community practices, translating into increased care seeking for illnesses from appropriate health care providers. In the IMCI areas, care seeking for sick children from trained providers improved threefold, from about 8% in 2000 to 24% by mid-2007. In IMCI areas, more children under 6 months of age were exclusively breastfed and the prevalence of stunting in children aged 24–59 months decreased more rapidly than in non-IMCI areas. However, the study also found that IMCI implementation had no effect on mortality within the timeframe of the assessment[51].

Piloting initiatives to improve maternal health outcomes

In recent years, the MoHFW has been investing in training skilled birth attendants and posting them to rural areas as a means of improving maternal health.
Since the 1990s, doctors, nurses and paramedics have been trained as part of
comprehensive emergency obstetric care available at district and subdistrict
levels, and basic emergency obstetric care available at most *upazila* health
complexes[32]. However, this led to a massive growth of the private sector, with
providers either engaging in dual practice or leaving the public sector to run
their own private maternity hospitals. The majority of births in Bangladesh still
occur at home and most facility-based deliveries take place in the private sector.
Between 2004 and 2007, the percentage of live births in public facilities
remained at 6.1% and 7.1%, respectively, while the percentage of live births in
private health facilities increased from 3.2% to 7.6% during the same time
period. Skilled birth attendance remains low, at 18%, and the number of trained
attendants at home-based deliveries has held steady at around 4% between 1996
and 2007[32].

Overall, however, more women have access to emergency obstetric care.
Nevertheless, 68% of caesarean sections (a proxy indicator of women's access to
skilled care for complicated deliveries) take place in the private sector[31]. The
delivery rate of caesarean sections for the poorest two quintiles is under 2%, so
clearly there is unmet need for emergency obstetric care. It should be noted that
achieving better outcomes may have been hampered by poor quality of services;
a study that audited 191 comprehensive emergency obstetric care facilities found
that one third of facilities were unable to manage complications of labour
because there were no available qualified providers (obstetricians and anaes-
thetists)[52].

More research is needed to understand why women do not make use of public
sector facilities for normal deliveries[32]. There are indications that the main
reasons are cultural preferences and the tradition of delivering at home, often
with the help of a local or traditional health worker familiar to the family.
However, cost may play an important role, especially for the poorest groups. The
government has recently responded with a series of innovative policies seeking
to reduce home delivery rates. In an effort to create incentives for behaviour
change, a major initiative to reduce maternal mortality is currently underway.
This is the maternal voucher scheme, pilot tested in 33 *upazilas* since 2007[23],
which offers a set of services to encourage use of antenatal, safe-delivery and
postnatal care, as well as a cash incentive for skilled birth attendance. The vouch-
ers can be used with multilevel providers in the public sector and at approved
organizations in the non-state sector. Provider incentives include a half face

value of the coupon for public providers (with the other half retained for facility improvement) and full-value reimbursement for non-state providers, with the intention of encouraging facility births. The higher rate of reimbursement for caesarean sections than for normal deliveries has, predictably, led to an increase in the provision of this service. Although there has not yet been an impact evaluation of the voucher scheme on maternal mortality, it has been enthusiastically received by health providers (including health assistants) and by beneficiaries[53].

■ Role of factors outside the health system in explaining health gains

Broader poverty reduction initiatives have positively impacted on life expectancy and child mortality in Bangladesh. For example, participation in microcredit programmes has been associated with better child survival[54,55]. The expansion of roads and electricity has facilitated the country's huge improvement in childhood immunization, particularly measles control. This section elaborates on three factors outside the health system that are deemed to have had the most significant impact on health gains to date: education, women's empowerment and disaster preparedness.

Education

One non-health system factor – better education – seems to have a direct relationship with health, earning potential and the ability of individuals and families to deal with the consequences of complex health conditions[56]. Bangladesh increased its net primary education enrolment from 74% in 1991 to 87% in 2005. A larger percentage of girls and women aged 15–19 have completed primary education (77.9%) than men and boys (68.6%) in the same age group.

Literacy rates for men increased from 38.9% in 1980 to 61% in 2008, and for women from 15% in 1980 to 54% in 2008 (Figure 3.7). Although the improvement is significant, especially for women, literacy in Bangladesh remains much lower than in other south Asian countries, including India, Nepal and Pakistan[58]. In addition, there is disparity between urban and rural literacy: the rural combined rate for men and women is 46.4%, versus 56.9% for urban areas.

A mass education campaign beginning in the mid-1980s aimed to enroll all girls in primary schools. It is believed to have contributed to women's empowerment as well as to higher literacy rates, contributing to the uptake and success of

Figure 3.7   Adult literacy rate

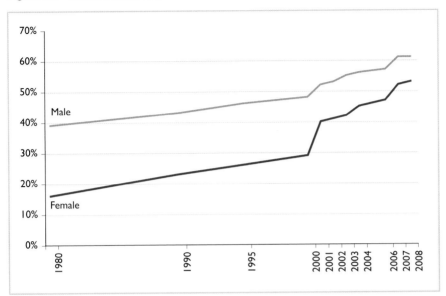

Sources: References 21 and 57.

microcredit programmes. BRAC has been instrumental in the provision of education, especially to girls, and they can also attend government-run primary and secondary schools for free, where they also receive textbooks and a stipend. All the people interviewed agreed that these efforts have encouraged parents to send their daughters to school.

Women's empowerment

Women's empowerment, a major agenda item for the past three decades in Bangladesh, is believed to have had a positive impact on health. Many studies describe the positive associations between work, marriage and education[36] and the contribution of work to maternal and child health in Bangladesh. Women who work are more likely to use contraception and are more likely to seek health services for their children[59].

In the context of growing international and national advocacy for equal rights and opportunities for women, in 1978 the Government of Bangladesh established the Ministry of Women and Children Affairs (MoWCA). The Ministry has been actively engaged in promoting quotas for women in the civil service, the police and defence forces and other services, and provisions have been made for reserved seats for women in the national parliament[60]. The MoWCA works in partnership with the MoHFW, Ministries of Home Affairs, Law and Social Welfare and many NGOs on a number of collaborative programmes. For example, the MoWCA, together with the MoHFW and the Ministry of Home Affairs, has created and operates crisis management centres in larger hospitals that provide medical and legal support to women who are victims of rape, acid burns and other violent acts. The enactment of a law to severely punish those who throw acid at women has been credited with a dramatic reduction in this once common heinous act. However, a 2007 World Bank paper reported that Bangladesh had the second highest incidence of violence against women in the world and that such violent acts were widely accepted: 50% of women interviewed thought that it was a husband's right to beat his wife; 85% felt that it was his right to hit his wife if she was disobedient[61].

The changing employment and social status of women has influenced their position within families and has contributed to lower fertility and better access to key services. Cultural traditions and preferences (for example, for large families) have changed in line with a shift from agriculture and exposure to mass media. For example, women have been further empowered outside of their homes through employment in the garment industry and through the opportunity to access microcredit. However, each of these major societal changes has yet to fully empower women or impact decisively on health outcomes or on health care decision-making for all women[54].

Many women living in rural villages are still not making health-related decisions for themselves or for their families. Only 33% of currently married women decide independently on daily household purchases, and only 8–19% make independent decisions on matters such as major household purchases (8.5%), their own health care (13.8%) or a child's health care (18.8%)[32]. Despite these alarming statistics, grassroots organizations postulate that improvements are occurring and that the long-term impact of women's economic and social empowerment may only be seen 10 to 20 years from now.

Women's empowerment – through education and income-generating activities, improved communication and connectivity (for example, mobile phones), involvement in microcredit programmes, older age at marriage, exposure to media and so on – is seen as essential for reducing the number of maternal deaths. However, cultural norms continue to serve as speed bumps on the road to progress, including the traditional preference to deliver at home, the slow growth of women's decision-making for health care, and women's general inability to determine the use of funds within the household.

Disaster preparedness

Bangladesh's geography and climate make it especially susceptible to natural disasters, with profound consequences for health. Droughts, cyclones and floods present a seemingly endless cycle of challenges. Yet, since the 1980s Bangladesh has become a global example of successful disaster preparedness and response. The building of storm shelters, embankments and barricades, preparing the population to respond, and establishing effective procedures for early warning and coordination of responses have served to mitigate the impact of the unavoidable.

This can be illustrated by comparing Bangladesh's relative success in saving lives after Cyclone Sidr in November 2007 with the devastation (more than 138 000 deaths) and delays in distributing aid in neighbouring Myanmar after Cyclone Nargis in May 2008.

Disaster preparedness is an example of the country's ability to coordinate plans and implement effective action, demonstrating good governance across many public sectors. This shows that incentives to coordinate plans and mount effective action have not been unique to the health sector, and reflect good governance across many public sectors.

■ Lessons learned and future challenges

This chapter describes how Bangladesh has made tremendous progress in improving population health since 1971, an achievement made all the more impressive because the country came into being as one of the poorest nations in the world.

Like many other low-income countries, Bangladesh is in the midst of a demographic and epidemiological transition. Notable successes have been achieved in reducing fertility, and improving access to vaccinations and other basic interventions, often delivered by NGOs. Yet while these programmes were effective responses to the formidable challenges of the past, some of them may have already run their course. New approaches that incorporate innovation while responding to cultural and socioeconomic realities must be developed in response to changing threats. This is because the population is ageing and approximately 51% of deaths are now due to noncommunicable diseases and other chronic health conditions[18] (Figure 3.8). While efforts to lower maternal, newborn and child mortality need to continue in order to attain the health MDGs, the health system must expand further in order to meet the needs of the population, particularly the poor. At the moment, treatment for noncommunicable diseases

Figure 3.8   Causes of mortality in rural Bangladesh (Matlab), 1986–2009

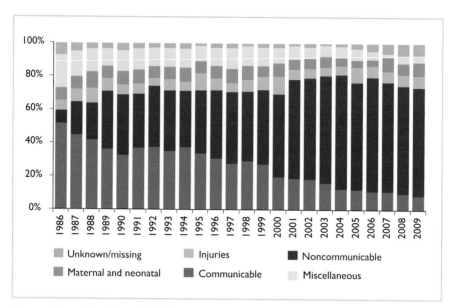

Source: Adapted from Streatfield PK, personal communication, Matlab data.

in the public health system is neither free nor subsidized at the point of service, despite an increasing demand for care, especially among the poor (Streatfield PK, personal communication May 2011). The burden of noncommunicable diseases is likely to be both significant and costly in Bangladesh. The extent to which the government should cover the costs of treatment has major budgetary implications and needs to be debated.

Another concern is that even if Bangladesh achieves the MDG target for improving nutrition (MDG1), the prevalence of malnutrition will still be more than 33%, because the baseline was so high. Other challenges that Bangladesh must overcome are described in Box 3.4. In addition, access to employment, housing and basic services (such as safe drinking water and sanitation) by the poor in urban areas is a growing concern. Socioeconomic inequalities in health and access to basic services have yet to be adequately addressed by policy-makers[65].

In order to continue making improvements in the health of the population, the Government of Bangladesh must re-commit to relatively low cost and less complex interventions. Efforts to increase skilled birth attendance should continue to be scaled up. Hard-to-reach rural and urban slums should be

> **Box 3.4 Remaining and future challenges in Bangladesh**
>
> Skilled attendance at birth remains very low (18%), and the number of home births is very high (85.3%). Concomitantly, non-medically indicated caesarean sections are rising, driving up the cost of health care and potentially endangering the health of the mother and her baby.
>
> More than 40% of children younger than 5 years of age are either underweight or stunted, or both[32], and about 17% are wasted.
>
> Injuries account for more than one third (38%) of all classifiable deaths among children between 1 and 17 years of age. The leading causes of injury-related death among children are drowning (59.3%), road traffic accidents (12.3%), animal bites (9.3%) and suicide (8.0%)[62].
>
> Approximately 20 million people in Bangladesh are exposed to excessive levels of arsenic in drinking water[13,63], which is associated with an increased risk of hypertension, diabetes and skin, lung, bladder and kidney cancers.
>
> The leading causes of death are from noncommunicable diseases, especially heart disease and diabetes. However, the health system is not prepared to prevent, treat or manage these illnesses[42,64].

targeted for primary health care with an emphasis on proven successful interventions that currently are not equitably shared across the population, such as childhood immunization. Furthermore, because of the increasing role of the private sector in providing health services and medical products to the population, the government should develop new techniques to engage with and oversee quality, distribution and the effectiveness of this important player. However, this largely unregulated sector, while saving lives, may also encourage costly and unnecessary procedures, potentially driving poor households into further poverty. Caesarean sections, an important source of revenue for providers, have risen dramatically in recent years, reaching levels beyond medical need in subgroups of the population. This may be but one example of how perverse financial incentives in an unregulated private sector can drive up unnecessary health care costs, potentially endangering the health of the population[19].

To address Bangladesh's most pressing health challenges, the government will need to apply the same principles that it has used so effectively at the community level in lowering the fertility rate, increasing life expectancy and reducing infant and child mortality. These principles are political commitment, working with the non-state sector and embracing innovative, low cost solutions.

Building on past success in areas such as family planning, child mortality and immunization, with an eye on efforts by neighbours in India and Thailand, key players within Bangladesh see universal coverage as an attainable goal for continuing to achieve 'good health at low cost'.

ACKNOWLEDGEMENTS

ICDDR,B gratefully acknowledges the contributions of the Rockefeller Foundation and of our partners from the London School of Hygiene & Tropical Medicine for making this work possible. The authors express our sincere gratitude to the many past and present health leaders in Bangladesh who served as key informants to this work as well as the grassroots workers who shared their valuable time and knowledge with us.

REFERENCES

1. Blood AK. *The cruel birth of Bangladesh.* Dhaka: University Press; 2002.

2. Islam S, ed. *History of Bangladesh 1704–1971.* Volume 1, *Political History.* Dhaka: Asiatic Society of Bangladesh; 1992.

3. Paul S. Potential Bangladesh and road to one-party rule. *Modern Ghana.* 4 April 2009 (http://www.modernghana.com/news/209806/1/potential-bangladesh-and-road-to-one-party-rule.html).

4. Kissinger declines comment on 'basket case'. *Bangladesh News.* 27 January 2008. (http://www.independent-bangladesh.com/20080127989/business/kissinger-declines-to-comment-on-basket-case.html).

5. WHO. *WHO Bangladesh Country Cooperation Strategy 2008–2013.* Dhaka: WHO Country Office, Bangladesh; 2007.

6. WHO Regional Office for South-East Asia. *11 health questions about the 11 SEAR countries.* New Delhi: WHO Regional Office for South-East Asia; 2007.

7. Anam S, Kabir R, Rai P. *Staying alive: urban poor in Bangladesh.* Dhaka: UNICEF; 1993.

8. Bangladesh Bureau of Statistics. *Report of the household income and expenditure survey 2005.* Dhaka: Government of the People's Republic of Bangladesh, Ministry of Planning; 2007.

9. NIPORT, MEASURE Evaluation, ICDDR,B and ACPR. *2006 Bangladesh urban health survey.* Dhaka: National Institute of Population Research and Training, MEASURE Evaluation, International Centre for Diarrhoeal Disease Research, and Associates for Community and Population Research; 2008.

10. Streatfield PK, Karar ZA. Population challenges for Bangladesh in the coming decades. *Journal of Health, Population, and Nutrition* 2008; 26(3):261–72.

11. Koehlmoos T et al. *Understanding the role of evidence in policy making in Bangladesh.* Report 1: *an analysis of interviews with health sector decision makers.* Geneva: Alliance for Health Policy and Systems Research; 2009.

12. World Bank. *World development indicators* [online database]. Washington, DC: World Bank; 2011 (http://data.worldbank.org/country/bangladesh, accessed 17 July 2011).

13. UNICEF. *Arsenic mitigation in Bangladesh.* New York: United Nations Children's Fund; 2008 (http://www.unicef.org/bangladesh/Arsenic.pdf, accessed 16 May 2009).

14. CIA. *The world factbook.* [online database]. Washington, DC: Central Intelligence Agency; 2010 (https://www.cia.gov/library/publications/the-worldfactbook/geos/bg.html, accessed 19 July 2011).

15. WHO. *National health accounts 2009, country health information.* Geneva: World Health Organization; 2011 (http://www.who.int/nha/country/en/, accessed 17 July 2011).

16. WHO. *World health statistics.* [online database]. Geneva: World Health Organization; 2010 (http://www.who.int/whosis/whostat/en/, accessed 17 July 2011).

17. UNICEF. *Multiple indicator cluster survey (MICS)* [online database]. New York: United Nations Children's Fund; 2011 (http://www.unicef.org/statistics/index_24302.html, accessed March 2011).

18. Expanded Programme on Immunization (Bangladesh). *Bangladesh EPI coverage evaluation survey, 2009.* Dhaka: Directorate General of Health Services, Ministry of Health and Family Welfare, Bangladesh; 2009.

19. NIPORT, MEASURE Evaluation, ICDDR,B and ACPR. *Bangladesh maternal mortality and health care survey 2010: preliminary results.* Dhaka: National Institute of Population Research and Training, MEASURE Evaluation, International Centre for Diarrhoeal Disease Research, and Associates for Community and Population Research; 2011.

20. UNICEF. [online database] New York: United Nations Children's Fund; 2011 (http://www.unicef.org/infobycountry/kyrgyzstan_statistics.html#76, accessed March 2011).

21. UNESCO Institute For Statistics [online database]. Montreal: UNESCO Institute for Statistics; 2011 (http://stats.uis.uncesco.org, accessed 17 July 2011).

22. Bangladesh Bureau of Statistics. *Statistical pocketbook of Bangladesh 2008.* Dhaka: Government of the People's Republic of Bangladesh, Ministry of Planning; 2009.

23. Management Information Systems. *Health bulletin 2008.* Dhaka: Government of the People's Republic of Bangladesh, Ministry of Health and Family Welfare; 2009.

24. Peters DH, Kayne RD. *Bangladesh health labor market study.* Baltimore, MD: Johns Hopkins Bloomberg School of Public Health; 2003.

25. World Bank. South Asia Human Development Sector Unit & HD Network Health, Nutrition and Population Team. *Bangladesh private sector assessment for health, nutrition and population (HNP) in Bangladesh.* Washington, DC: World Bank; 2003 (Report 20075-BD).

26. Larson CP et al. Childhood diarrhoea management practices in Bangladesh: private sector dominance and continued inequities in care. *International Journal of Epidemiology* 2006; 35(6):1430–9.

27. Mahmood SS et al. Are 'village doctors' in Bangladesh a curse or a blessing? *BMC International Health and Human Rights* 2010; 10:18.

28. Bhuiya A, ed. *Health for the rural masses: insights from Chakaria.* Dhaka: International Centre for Diarrhoeal Disease Research, Bangladesh; 2009 (ICDDR,B Monograph no. 8).

29. ESCAP. *Statistical yearbook for Asia and Pacific 2009.* New York: United Nations; 2010.

30. NIPORT, Mitra and Associates, and ORC Macro. *Bangladesh demographic and health survey 2004.* Dhaka: National Institute of Population Research and Training, Mitra and Associates and ORC Macro; 2005.

31. NIPORT, Mitra and Associates, and Macro International. *Bangladesh demographic and health survey 2007.* Dhaka: National Institute of Population and Training, Mitra and Associates, and Macro International; 2009.

32. Chen LC et al. Maternal mortality in rural Bangladesh. *Studies in Family Planning* 1974; 5(11):334–41.

33. Khan A, Jahan FA, Begum SF. Maternal mortality in rural Bangladesh: the Jamalpur district. *Studies in Family Planning* 1986; 17(1):95–9.

34. NIPORT, ORC Macro, Johns Hopkins University and ICDDR,B. *Bangladesh maternal health services and maternal mortality survey 2001*. Dhaka: National Institute of Population Research and Training, ORC Macro, Johns Hopkins University and International Centre for Diarrhoeal Diseases Research; 2003.

35. Chowdhury ME et al. Causes of maternal mortality decline in Matlab, Bangladesh. *Journal of Health, Population, and Nutrition* 2009; 27(2):108–23.

36. Robinson WC, Ross JA, eds. *The global family planning revolution: three decades of population policies*. Washington, DC: World Bank; 2007.

37. Sundewall J, Forsberg BC, Tomson G. Theory and practice: a case study of coordination and ownership in the Bangladesh health SWAp. *Health Research Policy and Systems* 2006; 4:5.

38. Reich M. Bangladesh pharmaceutical policy and politics. *Health Policy and Planning* 1994; 9(2):130–43.

39. Chowdhury Z. *The politics of essential drugs. The making of a successful health strategy: lessons from Bangladesh*. Dhaka: University Press; 1996.

40. DGDA MoHFW. *List of local allopathic pharmaceutical manufacturers*. Dhaka; Directorate General of Drug Administration and the Ministry of Health & Family Welfare; 2010 (http://www.ddabd.org/download/List%20of%20Pharma ceutical%20Manufacturer.pdf, accessed 9 November 2010).

41. Perry HB. *Health for all in Bangladesh: lessons in primary health care for the twenty-first century*. Dhaka: University Press; 2000.

42. Levine R. *Case studies in global health: millions saved*. Sudbury, MA: Jones & Bartlett; 2007.

43. Smillie I. *Freedom from want: The remarkable success story of BRAC, the global grassroots organization that's winning the fight against poverty*. Sterling, VA: Kumarian Press; 2009.

44. BRAC. *Who we are* [web site]. Dhaka: Bangladesh Rural Advancement Committee; 2010 (http://www.brac.net/content/who-we-are, accessed 20 December 2010).

45. Bangladesh Health Watch. *The state of health in Bangladesh 2007. Health workforce in Bangladesh; who constitutes the health care system?* Dhaka: James P Grant School of Public Health; 2008.

46. Ahmed SM et al. Socioeconomic status overrides age and gender in determining health-seeking behaviour in rural Bangladesh. *Bulletin of the World Health Organization* 2005; 83(2):109–17.

47. Bhuiya A. Village health care providers in Matlab, Bangladesh: a study of their knowledge in the management of childhood diarrhoea. *Journal of Diarrhoeal Diseases Research* 1992; 10(2):10–15.

48. Uddin MJ et al. Child immunization coverage in rural hard-to-reach areas of Bangladesh. *Vaccine* 2010; 28(5):1221–5.

49. Uddin MJ et al. *Effectiveness of combined strategies to improve low coverage of child immunization in urban Bangladesh.* Dhaka: International Centre for Diarrhoeal Diseases Research, Bangladesh; 2008 (ICDDR,B Working Paper No. 169).

50. Arefin SE et al. Effect of the integrated management of childhood illness strategy on childhood mortality and nutrition in a rural area in Bangladesh: a cluster randomised trial. *Lancet* 2009; 374(9687):393–403.

51. Alam B et al. Audit of comprehensive emergency obstetric care facilities under public health sector in Bangladesh. Paper presented at: *ASCON XII. 12th Annual Scientific Conference XII*, 9–12 February 2009. Dhaka: International Centre for Diarrhoeal Diseases Research.

52. Koehlmoos T et al. *Rapid assessment of demand side financing experience in Bangladesh.* Dhaka: International Centre for Diarrhoeal Diseases Research, Bangladesh; 2008 (ICDDR,B Working Paper No. 170).

53. Bhuiya A, Chowdhury M. Beneficial effects of a woman-focused development programme on child survival: evidence from rural Bangladesh. *Social Science & Medicine* 2002; 55(9):1553–60.

54. Chowdhury SN, Moni D. A situation analysis of the menstrual regulation programme in Bangladesh. *Reproductive Health Matters* 2004; 12(24 Suppl):95–104.

55. Rothman RL et al. Influence of patient literacy on the effectiveness of a primary care-based diabetes disease management program. *Journal of the American Medical Association* 2004; 292(14):1711–16.

56. Bangladesh Bureau of Statistics. *Adult literacy rate of population 15+ by sex. Sample Vital Registration System.* Dhaka: Government of the People's Republic of Bangladesh, Ministry of Planning; 2010 (http://www.bbs.gov.bd/PageSVRS_Rpt_4_10.aspx?page=%2fPageReportLists.aspx%3fPARENTKEY%3d102, accessed 5 February 2010).

57. United Nations. *Literacy rates of 15–24 years old, both sexes, percentage. Millennium development goals indicators* [Internet]. New York: United Nations Statistics Division; 2009 (http://unstats.un.org/unsd/mdg/SeriesDetail.aspx?srid=656, accessed 2009).

58. Laskar MS et al. Factors associated with contraceptive practices of married women in Bangladesh with respect to their employment status. *European Journal of Contraception & Reproductive Health Care* 2006; 11(3):220–7.

59. Mahmood K, ed. *Meet Bangladesh*, 3rd edn. Dhaka: Department of Films and Publications, Ministry of Information; 1987.

60. World Bank. *Dhaka: improving living conditions for the urban poor.* Dhaka: World Bank Office Dhaka; 2007 (Bangladesh Development Series Paper No. 17).

61. Swedish International Development Cooperation Agency. *Reality check Bangladesh 2008: Listening to poor people's realities about primary health care and primary education.* Stockholm: Swedish International Development Cooperation Agency; 2009.

62. Institute of Child and Mother Health, Directorate General of Health Services, The Alliance for Safe Children, UNICEF. *Bangladesh health and injury survey: key findings on child injuries.* New York: United Nations Children's Fund; 2005.

63. Kaufmann R et al. *Addressing the public health crisis caused by arsenic contamination of drinking water in Bangladesh.* Washington, DC: World Bank South Asia Health, Nutrition, and Population Unit; 2002.

64. Abegunde DO et al. The burden and costs of chronic diseases in low-income and middle-income countries. *Lancet* 2007; 370(9603):1929–38.

65. Koehlmoos TP et al. Homeless in Dhaka: violence, sexual harassment and drug-abuse. *Journal of Health, Population, and Nutrition 2009*; 27(4):52-61.

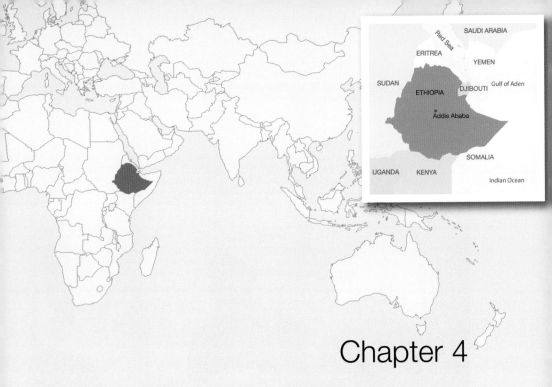

Chapter 4

ETHIOPIA: PLACING HEALTH AT THE CENTRE OF DEVELOPMENT

Hailom Banteyerga[1], Aklilu Kidanu[1], Lesong Conteh[2] and Martin McKee[3]

1 Miz-Hasab Research Center, 2 Imperial College London, 3 LSHTM

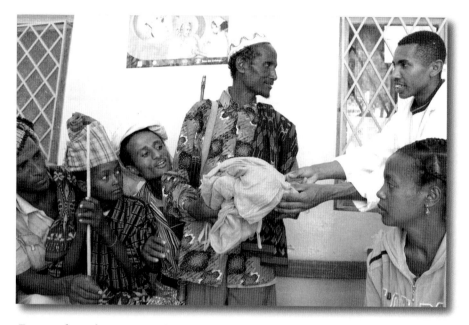

Farmers from the remote and inaccessible areas walk many hours to receive bednets during the distribution of long-lasting insecticide nets to prevent malaria.
The Gorgo Kebele health post in Ankober Woreda, Ethiopia

■ **Key messages**

- Ethiopia has demonstrated that low-income countries can achieve improvements in health and access to services if policies, programmes and strategies are underpinned by ingenuity, innovativeness, political will and sustained commitment at all levels. An example is the development and rapid implementation of the Ethiopian Health Extension Programme.

- Ethiopia demonstrates the role of good governance based on inclusiveness, participation, shared ownership and accountability. The Ethiopian Health Sector Development Programme includes civil society, the private for-profit sector, donors and the government at all levels of programme development, implementation, monitoring and evaluation.

- Ethiopia has been working within the spirit of the Paris Declaration on Aid Effectiveness and the International Health Partnership (IHP) to strengthen its health system. Ethiopia has created synergies where possible, so that global initiatives in HIV/AIDS, malaria and tuberculosis have created a favourable environment for developments in maternal and child health. This approach has made it possible to develop innovative modalities to make progress towards the Millennium Development Goals (MDGs), such as the expansion of disease prevention, the engagement of households in the Health Extension Programme, and the promotion of women as leaders in household-based health delivery.

- Ethiopia, once associated with poverty, ill health, ignorance and backwardness, has recognized that development is not achievable unless poor health is addressed in a timely manner. Health is a focal element of the poverty reduction strategy papers, the Programme for Accelerated and Sustainable Development to End Poverty and the Programme for Progress and Transformation in Ethiopia.

- Development partners have assisted Ethiopia in building the capacity to develop realistic plans, accountable and transparent procedures, and workable strategies that lend themselves to monitoring and evaluation. Donor funding has enabled Ethiopia to achieve a system of planning where districts generate data for their respective plans and the collective plans of districts create the national plan. It is no longer expert-driven or cut-and-paste planning – it is participatory and data driven. This is in the spirit of 'good health at low cost', and "less is more".

■ Introduction

It was Ethiopia, in the 1980s, that brought home to many in richer countries (quite literally, on their television screens) the scale of suffering afflicting many African countries. Advances in the technology of newsgathering enabled reporters to transmit real-time images of children dying from starvation to viewers in countries where food was plentiful. Those images provoked a remarkable and quite unexpected response in the richer countries. Famines in poor countries were not new but they had never been so visible. Ordinary people told their political leaders that something must be done, but they also did a great deal themselves, with the Live Aid concert only the most visible manifestation. Never again would politicians be able to dismiss events in "a far-away country between people of whom we know nothing"[1].

Yet there were also those who despaired that anything could really change. The post-colonial history of Africa offered few signs of encouragement[2]. Only a handful of countries were democratic and, even in those, the institutions of state were often weak. Colonial-era borders did not respect ethnic divisions, creating the ideal conditions for civil war. There were few opportunities for education and, anyway, most of those who could obtain qualifications soon left, creating severe shortages of trained workers that affected all sectors, but especially health where the rich world acted as a magnet for those with professional qualifications[3]. And in much of the continent, humans and animals alike were at risk of debilitating and often fatal diseases, such as malaria for humans.

Ethiopia exemplified these problems. One of only two countries in Africa to retain its independence in the 19th century colonial scramble for Africa, although briefly occupied by Italy in the 1930s, it had almost everything going against it. For much of its history it has been a land-locked state, with considerable but unrealized agricultural potential, and few easily exploited natural resources. It is exceptionally diverse, ethnically and linguistically. It was isolated from developments elsewhere, in part by its geography but also as a consequence of the expulsion of Jesuit missionaries in 1632. From the mid-18th century until 1855 (the *Zemene Mesafint* or Age of Princes), the country was effectively divided between warlords from the main ethnic groups. Slavery was abolished only in 1942, but Ethiopia's feudal system, which persisted until the fall of the empire in 1974, continued to concentrate power in the hands of the aristocracy and impede development, especially in rural areas.

Health care was rudimentary. In 1896, the Russian Red Cross established a treatment facility in Addis Ababa to treat those injured in the battle of Adowa, in which Ethiopian forces defeated Italian invaders. In 1910, this was replaced by a hospital which formed the basis of a limited government health system, run by

Box 4.1   Ethiopia at a glance

Population[4]   74 million. Africa's second most populous country. 84% of population live in rural areas.

Geography   Located in east Africa, varied topography and vegetation. High levels of food insecurity.

Ethnic composition   Exceptionally diverse ethnically and linguistically. Four ethnic groups make up almost 75% of population (Oromo, 34.5%; Amhara 26.9%; Somali 6.2%; Tigrayan 6.1%). 30% of the population is nomadic[5].

Government   Federal republic. 1970s and 1980s were periods of military rule with high levels of internal and external conflict. The end of military rule in 1991 brought about relative political stability and economic liberalization.

Health system   Health expenditure per capita (constant 2005 Int$)[6]: 39.87
Density of physicians, nurses and midwives per 10000[7]: 2–3
Decentralized health system, and significant geographical barriers to access. Ambitious health worker extension programme has improved access to primary health care, but high levels of out-of-pocket payments. Coverage of key interventions is low but improving: estimates of deliveries with skilled attendance vary between 6%[5] and 24.9%[8], 65.5% of infants fully immunized)[8].

Economic, demographic and social development		
GDP per capita (constant 2005 Int$)[9]		330
Economic growth per anum since 2004[9]		9–14%
Population living on less than $1.25 a day (2005)[9]		39%
Population below the national poverty line (2004)[9]		38.9%
Gini index (2007)[9]		33
Infant mortality rate (2009)[9]		67[a]
Maternal mortality ratio (2008)[10]		150[b]
Adult HIV prevalence (aged 15–49)[11]		2.3%
Life expectancy (2009)[9]		54 (men) 57 (women)
Adult literacy (2008)[9]		30%
Ratio girls to boys in education[c] (2009)[9]		88%
Access to improved water source (2007)[8]		60%
Internet usage per (2009)[9]		0.5%

Note: [a] Per 1000 live births; [b] Per 100000 live births; [c] primary and secondary education.

the Ministry of the Interior until 1948. Elsewhere, health care, where it existed at all, was provided in clinics and hospitals run by missionaries, while the American Government funded a malaria eradication programme. A large proportion of the population used traditional and spiritual healers.

This poor situation became even worse in the 1970s. Ethiopia's already vulnerable economy suffered in the 1973 oil crisis and, like its neighbour Somalia, it became caught up in the Cold War, when the United States and the USSR fought their battles by proxy in Africa and Asia. In 1974, Emperor Haile Selassie was deposed in a Soviet-backed coup led by the hard-line Marxist Mengistu Haile Mariam, who established a one-party communist state which he renamed the People's Democratic Republic of Ethiopia. At first, the ruling junta, or *Derg*, invested in the health sector, expanding primary care by using community health workers and making immunization compulsory. Infant mortality fell by about 40%. However, initial optimism soon dissipated; civil war broke out, with the opposition led by the Tigrayan People's Liberation Front, as well as war with Somalia over the disputed Ogaden area. The regime soon unleashed a wave of terror (including the deliberate use of hunger as a weapon), backed by several thousand troops from Cuba, the German Democratic Republic and North Korea. Yet there was more to come. Always vulnerable to climatic events by virtue of its location, Ethiopia suffered a series of catastrophic droughts affecting up to eight million people, of whom about a million died, some, as noted above, in front of foreign television cameras.

The situation was, however, about to change. Popular discontent, coupled with the withdrawal of assistance from the USSR and its satellites, meant that the regime's days were numbered. In 1989, the Ethiopian Peoples' Revolutionary Democratic Front (EPRDF) was formed from a number of ethnically based opposition groups and, in 1991, a transitional government was established. A new constitution was agreed upon in 1994, establishing a bicameral legislature and an independent judiciary. In May 1995, Ethiopia's first democratic elections took place, with Meles Zenawi, a Tigrayan and leader of the EPRDF, elected as Prime Minister and Negasso Gidada, an Oromo, as President.

Ethiopia's fortunes have changed remarkably in the past two decades. Although still among the poorest countries in the world, it has experienced sustained economic growth. Its inclusion in this book is justified because the country has put in place the prerequisites for improved population health. Over 85% of the population now has access to primary health care, a figure that has increased particularly rapidly in the past few years following the implementation of an ambitious Health Extension Programme. Between 2004 and 2008, the percentage of births with a skilled attendant present doubled, and the percentage of women receiving antenatal care and of infants fully immunized increased by over 50% (Table 4.1). There is still a great deal to do, but compared with the situation two decades ago and despite its continuing lack of resources, Ethiopia has made considerable progress. In the remainder of this chapter we will examine what made this progress possible.

Table 4.1   Selected indicators of health outcomes in maternal and child health, 2004 and 2008

Indicator (%)	2004	2008
Deliveries attended by skilled birth attendant	12.4	24.9
Pregnant women receiving antenatal care	40.8	66.3
Women receiving postnatal care	13.6	34.4
Infants fully immunized	44.5	65.5

Source: Adapted from reference 8.

▇ Ethiopia and its people

After Nigeria, Ethiopia is the second most populous country in Africa, with a population of 74 million, although it is only the tenth largest by area, at 1 100 000 km² (Box 4.1). It is bordered by Eritrea to the north, Sudan to the west, Djibouti and Somalia to the east, and Kenya to the south. Ethiopia sits astride the African Rift Valley. The north-western part of the country is mountainous, with many high plateaus, while the lowlands in the south-west are dominated by savannah and desert. This topography has created a great diversity of vegetation, from tropical jungles to deserts, with corresponding variations in settlement patterns and agriculture. Eighty-five per cent of the population live in rural areas.

Ethiopia is one of the poorest countries in Africa and although it has experienced a high rate of growth since 2004 (9–14% nominal GDP growth per annum), it remains behind its east African neighbours (Figure 4.1). Its economy has been dominated by agriculture, especially coffee production. Ethiopia is the ancestral home of coffee, which is now its largest export commodity, although it is also a major livestock producer. Among other things, Ethiopia's recent economic growth has been fuelled by vertical integration, so that its leather is now made into designer products in Ethiopia rather than in Europe, and by diversification, for example taking advantage of its good water supply to produce flowers for western markets. However, other initiatives have been less successful, including attempts to increase production of its gold reserves and arrangements to market coffee with a western coffee outlet, which involved registering as trademarks

Figure 4.1 GDP per capita in selected east African countries

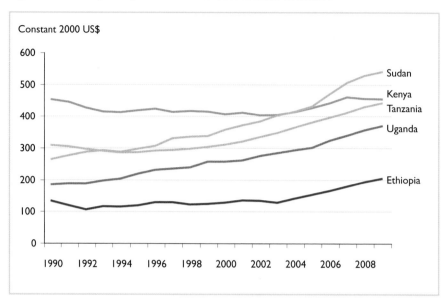

Source: Reference 9.

three of its specialist coffee brands. Its exports per capita still lag well behind those of some of its neighbours, such as Kenya.

It is impossible to understand Ethiopia without considering the diversity of its people. Although almost two thirds of its population is Christian (of whom about two thirds are Ethiopian Orthodox), all three Abrahamic religions are represented, with approximately a third Muslim and a small number of Jews (the remnants of a substantially larger population that was evacuated to Israel in the 1980s). Four ethnic groups make up almost 75% of the population (Oromo, 34.5%; Amhara 26.9%; Somali 6.2%; Tigrayan 6.1%), but there are many smaller ones, some numbering fewer than 10000 people, and 84 different indigenous languages. About 30% of the population is nomadic, but there has also been large-scale urbanization in recent years. The authors of the 1994 Constitution recognized the challenges posed by this diversity, which had often been a cause of conflict in the past, and created a federal state in which the nine *kililoch* (singular *kilil*, or regions) and two chartered cities have a high degree of political autonomy. The regions are further subdivided into zones within which are 802 *woredas* (districts) and over 1700 *kebeles* (neighbourhoods). Since 2002, a number of functions, including aspects of health planning, have been trans-ferred from the regional level to the *woredas*.

▓ Better health?

Like virtually all of Africa, data on population health in Ethiopia are extremely limited and are derived primarily from the periodic demographic and health surveys that capture the health of mothers and children, supplemented by data on the incidence of and mortality from selected communicable diseases.

These data reveal that, from a very poor starting point in 1990, Ethiopia has made considerable progress. Thus, under-5 mortality, where Ethiopia was once among the worst performers in the region, has improved rapidly, overtaking Sudan, Tanzania and Uganda (Figure 4.2). Importantly, these gains have been seen in all parts of Ethiopia (Figure 4.3).

Some of this improvement reflects the success that Ethiopia has achieved in tackling a number of communicable diseases, in particular malaria. Over two thirds of the Ethiopian population live in malaria-prone areas. The United States government-funded malaria eradication effort achieved a degree of control in the 1970s, but was discontinued in 1985 as a consequence of political differences with the Ethiopian regime. This was followed by a rapid increase in transmission. However, since the late 1990s, major strides have been made. By 2007, deaths from malaria among children had fallen by 51% compared with the

Figure 4.2   Under-5 mortality in selected east African countries

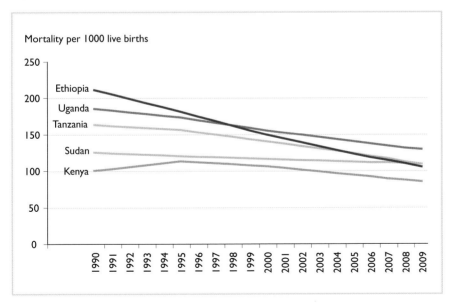

Source: Adapted from reference 9.

Figure 4.3 Change in under-5 mortality in the regions of Ethiopia, 2000 and 2005

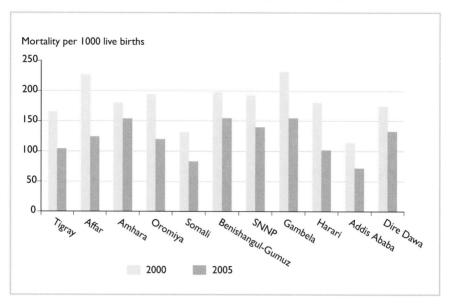

Sources: Adapted from references 5 and 12.

Figure 4.4 Percentage of children under 5 years of age sleeping under insecticide-treated bednets, most recent year available

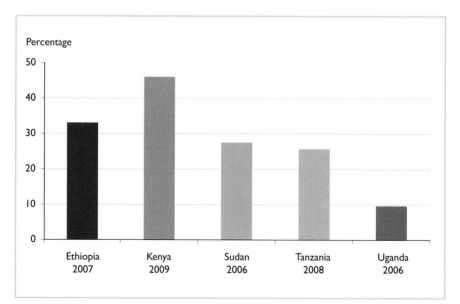

Source: Adapted from reference 9.

Box 4.2   Priorities in the prevention and treatment of malaria in Ethiopia

- Early diagnosis of fever cases and treatment of malaria cases within 24 hours of illness onset.

- Selective vector control to protect communities through provision of an average of two long-lasting insecticide-treated mosquito bednets per household in areas of malaria. Over 20 million bednets have already been distributed.

- Scaling up of artemisinin-based combination therapy.

- Training in the use of bednets by health workers.

- Increased indoor residual spraying in epidemic-prone areas; over 60% coverage has been achieved[13.]

- Provision of diagnostic equipment to health centres and hospitals, enabling rapid diagnosis and treatment by health extension workers.

- Educational interventions to raise awareness of the importance of rapid treatment when malaria symptoms arise, using electronic, print, and face-to-face methods, with a prominent role for health extension workers.

- Engagement with the private sector to ensure low cost treatment and with a nongovernmental organization (NGO) working on malaria prevention and control.

---

average during 2001–2004[13], a much greater decline than was seen with non-malaria deaths (8%). A major factor in this decline has been the increased use of insecticide-treated bednets, from only 3% in 2005[5] to a current 33%, a rate that is among the highest in the region (Figure 4.4).

This is, however, only one factor in the reduction of malaria deaths, and the Global Fund has made a major investment in a comprehensive programme of prevention and treatment (Box 4.2)

Ethiopia, like the rest of sub-Saharan Africa, has been severely afflicted by the HIV/AIDS pandemic. In 2002, the Ethiopian Government declared AIDS to be a public health emergency. By 2009, the estimated HIV/AIDS prevalence among adults had reached 2.3%, when it was estimated that about 1.1 million Ethiopians were living with HIV/AIDS[11]. In 2000, services were essentially non-existent but, by 2008, there had been a major expansion to include 483 antiretroviral therapy (ART) centres, 1469 voluntary counselling and testing sites, and 877 sites that provided a short course of antiretroviral therapy to prevent mother-to-child transmission of HIV (PMTCT).

Ethiopia has been less successful in tackling tuberculosis. It ranks seventh on the list of 22 high-burden countries, with an incidence of all forms of tuberculosis at 356 per 100 000, with smear-positive disease in 135 per 100 000. The prevalence of all forms of tuberculosis is 533 per 100 000 and the prevalence of HIV among tuberculosis patients is 21%[14]. Ethiopia's National Tuberculosis and Leprosy Control Programme began to implement DOTS (directly observed treatment, short-course) on a limited scale in 1991 and, by 2007, DOTS coverage had been integrated into routine practice, but it is estimated that only about 60–70% of the population has access to treatment because of the poor health infrastructure in many rural areas. Diagnostic services remain weak and it is estimated that only about 28% of cases are detected, compared with the WHO target of 70%. However, the treatment success rate is now estimated to have almost reached the WHO target, after a temporary decline around 2003. With assistance from the Global Fund, a major investment is currently under way.

Nevertheless, there has been considerable progress in tackling many of the underlying determinants of health and, especially, access to water and sanitation, with an increase in the use of improved drinking water sources from 23% in 1997 to 60% in 2007[8] and a rise in the use of improved sanitation facilities from 12.5% to 37% in the same period. Nutrition has also improved: the prevalence of stunting among children fell from 52% in 2000 to 27% in 2005, while the proportion underweight declined from 47% to 38%[5]. There has also been increased access to primary care, with one government-run primary health centre serving 5000 people, on average, in 2007, down from 17 000 in 1995. The number of outpatient department visits per 10 000 population per year has increased correspondingly, from 0.27% in 1999 to 0.305% in 2008, and, as noted previously, there has been a considerable increase in immunization rates[15].

■ What has Ethiopia done to improve health?

The current Ethiopian Government has placed high priority on improved population health, seeing it as a key element of its policies to alleviate poverty (its Programme of Accelerated and Sustained Development and Ending Poverty (PASDEP)). This has facilitated considerable synergy among policies in the health and other sectors. It has also ensured that there is effective participation by a wide range of stakeholders, bringing together elected representatives, the private sector and development partners. This marks a major departure from the past.

The Ethiopian health care system is multitiered. The first tier, at village level, is the health post. It provides basic sanitation services and health education. Clinical services are provided at the next tier, the health centre, which typically serves a population of about 100 000. Some health centres are able to provide interventional obstetric care, and this capacity is now being rolled out more widely. Staff at the health centre are usually responsible for five or more individual health posts. Patients requiring more than basic treatment are referred to district zonal or regional hospitals. A district hospital will typically serve a population of about 250 000 and will provide basic surgical care. More complex cases can be referred to the regional hospitals or, in a few cases, to the top tier, the federal facilities in the capital.

Innovations can be seen in all tiers. The *woredas* have assumed greater importance in planning the delivery of local services, facilitated by the Health Extension Programme, which has enabled a substantial scaling up of primary care provision while ensuring local engagement. These initiatives have, in turn, been supported by a number of regional national developments to strengthen the health infrastructure. For example, a programme has been initiated to upgrade health facilities at both primary and secondary level. In addition, a Pharmaceutical Fund and Supply Agency has been created as an autonomous agency operating a revolving drug fund, and the Ethiopian Health and Nutrition Research Institute has been strengthened and is now an autonomous agency responsible for developing laboratory services throughout the country. All of these activities have taken place within an overall framework that sees health improvement as a key element in alleviating poverty. We will now look at each of these in turn, beginning at the lowest level.

The Health Extension Programme

Like many other countries in Africa, Ethiopia has suffered a severe shortage of trained health workers[3]. The Health Extension Programme was designed to address this problem. Launched in 2003, it involves the selection of women who have completed ten years of formal education and who are willing to work in their own communities. Training is provided in four modules: health, prevention of communicable diseases, hygiene and environmental sanitation, and health education. Each is tailored to local needs. For example, in addition to family planning, reproductive health, and prevention and treatment of sexually transmitted diseases, family health addresses traditions such as early marriage, abduction of brides and hazardous delivery practices.

The creation of a cadre of health extension workers has greatly expanded access to a range of basic, but potentially life-saving interventions, including vitamin A supplementation, distribution of insecticide-treated bednets, integrated management of childhood illness, basic obstetric and neonatal care (thereby increasing the availability of skilled birth attendants), and immunization and contraception.

> *What we see from independent studies is that the Health Extension Programme is helping a lot in maternal and child health. Prevention of malaria, tuberculosis, HIV; environmental and personal hygiene: all these are there in the Programme. I remember assisted delivery was at 5%, and now we are reporting 24%. Information is important. Health extension workers are giving information to women so that they deliver in facilities. Family planning is increasing, which is good for child and maternal health, particularly spacing. Vaccination is being reported at 85%, which is critical to child survival. Malaria is being managed by health extension workers not only by distributing bednets, but also by conducting rapid tests for diagnosis of malaria. Community ownership of health is one of the major changes of attitude that is playing a role in achieving good health. People diagnosed for tuberculosis have increased as well. This is because of increased community awareness. Environmental and household hygiene is improving, which is essential for good health. Overall knowledge in health at community and individual level is increasing through the Health Extension Programme.*
>
> *Veteran in health policy and planning*

The Health Extension Programme has scaled up rapidly. Although the first workers were trained in 2004, by 2009, their numbers had increased to over 30 000. One factor in this success has been the mobilization of widespread support in Ethiopian society. Health extension workers have been well received by users[16]. While the programme is led by health officials at *woreda* and *kebele* levels, they have been supported by elders and religious leaders in the community, by agricultural extension workers and by schools. Development partners have provided considerable assistance in the form of basic equipment, such as delivery beds, first aid kits, scales, essential medicines, bednets, and rapid testing kits. The United Nations Children's Fund (UNICEF) and the United States Agency for International Development (USAID) have also supported the training of health extension workers.

A 2009 evaluation concluded that the Health Extension Programme has been successful in expanding coverage at low cost, although other research has shown that many health posts were operating at less than optimal efficiency[17]. So far, the programme has been implemented mainly among settled agricultural communities. Consequently, it is now being extended to urban and nomadic settings. Both involve some modification to the basic model. Thus, in Addis Ababa, nurses will play a greater role, with responsibility for an average of 500 households, while workers recruited from nomadic communities will require only primary education and will be supported by mobile health teams.

Let me start with what we have learned from the health extension
workers, both during the field visit … and at this meeting. They passion-
ately described the vision they share for better health for the people of
Ethiopia. We saw and they told us about the preventive and life-saving
services they provide, especially for women and children. Their enthusiasm,
dedication, capacity, desire to save and improve lives is impressive. They,
in turn, need support, rewards, and reliable referral routes into the rest of
the health service – especially for emergencies in pregnancy and childbirth.
Dr Jenny Amery, Head of Profession, Health – UK Department for
International Development (DFID) ARM 2009

The operation of the Health Extension Programme has been facilitated by a
major investment in information systems. At district level, this involves the
creation of a family folder. All households are given a folder in which their
demographic data, health status and use of services is recorded. So far, 18 million
family folders have been printed and distributed to health posts. The information collected is integrated within systems for management and evaluation. At
the same time, several hospitals are introducing modern information systems,
ranging from simple, locally produced software packages[18] to modern systems
incorporating smart card technology, although there is still some way to go to
ensure that health workers record high-quality data[19].

We have opened training of monitoring and evaluation (M&E) leaders
at MSc level in cooperation with Jimma University. We are strengthening
health management information systems (HMIS). At health posts, health
extension workers are expected to use the family folders. They should
know how to record the data in the family folders to show the health
history of each family. There is also the smart card, which is being piloted
in hospitals. We have also assisted in the identification of common indica-
tors, about 108 of them to be used in HMIS. You see, there are two essen-
tial kinds of health information: surveillance data, which should be done
daily, and routine HMIS. Health extension workers, woredas, regions
and the Federal Ministry of Health have to work with both. We are
strengthening both. If you want to have a good HMIS, you need experts
and full time staff. We are training M&E leaders at MSc level. We have
graduated so far 100 of them. Middle-level technicians in M&E who are
full time are also needed. For this purpose, we are training over 1000 in
health informatics in the regional colleges. In fact, we have enrolled 1030
students who will take the training for three years. We are also training
biostatisticians in health at MSc level at Mekele University.
Development Partner

An obvious problem with the Health Extension Programme model is that of career progression for its staff, which could threaten its long-term sustainability. This has been addressed by developing a career ladder which will allow the health extension workers to progress through three levels of increasing competencies, with the expectation that, in time, the programme will extend its activities to the management of other health problems and, in particular, chronic illnesses, while its staff will also assume greater managerial responsibilities. It also leaves open the possibility for health extension workers to retrain as health professionals and managers.

District-based planning

Ethiopia has established a mechanism of *woreda*-based planning that seeks to meet local needs within a context of national targets that focus primarily on maternal and child health and the prevention of communicable diseases. There is a strong emphasis on integration of services within the territory of the *woreda*, recognizing the dangers of fragmentation created by vertical programmes in many other parts of Africa. The *woreda* structures have played an important role in capacity building and mobilizing grassroots engagement with the health system.

This model has benefitted from a number of related initiatives, including the development of a Marginal Budgeting for Bottlenecks tool. This uses tracer conditions to identify the obstacles to achieving health goals, which may lie within the health system itself, such as shortages of human resources, institutional weaknesses, poor geographical access or inadequate supplies, or which may reflect characteristics of the population, including health-seeking behaviour. Working with all the relevant individuals and organizations (including the private sector) within the *woreda* helps to identify where action is needed. This may be anywhere from the Federal Ministry of Health to local facilities. The *woreda* plans feed into the national core plan, in which the development partners participate though a Joint Steering Committee, and which identifies national priorities and indicators of success. Progress on these indicators is monitored and evaluated monthly at the level of the *woreda* using routine administrative data. The data are brought together to inform progressively more detailed quarterly, semi-annual and annual reviews at higher levels.

> *The* woreda *planning combines top-down and bottom-up processes of planning. Direction comes from the Federal Ministry of Health. Indicators are selected from the Health Sector Development Programme and Millennium Development Goals. The Ministry discusses with the regions. The regions reflect on the selected indicators and targets to be*

achieved, regions add and/or reprioritize indicators which, in turn, are discussed with zones and woredas. Zones and woredas do the same: add reprioritized indicators and targets. Finally, a comprehensive woreda plan is developed. The plan has activities under each indicator, target and cost. The resource gap is indicated as well. The woreda plan is a tool reflecting the needs of the receiving communities. It is a tool for harmonization and alignment in that it does not give space for alternative parallel plans. Stakeholders and development partners fully participate in assisting woredas to develop their core plans.

Planning and policy expert

A geographical perspective is important, given the growing role of the private sector in the delivery of health care in Ethiopia. It includes both for-profit and not-for-profit operators, who have carved out distinctive niches at various levels. In the main cities, private hospitals provide a range of specialist services to those who can pay for accelerated treatment in better facilities; in some cases, such as for abortions, they are perceived as offering a greater degree of privacy.

The growth in international development assistance, and, in particular, that provided by the Global Fund and PEPFAR, has also played a part in encouraging the growth of private providers, especially those operating in the area of HIV/AIDS. This includes for-profit providers in the main cities and not-for-profit organizations throughout the country. Among the largest of the latter is the Christian Relief and Development Association, which runs approximately 350 facilities.

There are private for-profit health facilities that are franchised and accessing donor funds. ART is being given in all private hospitals. Many private clinics offer VCT. The private sector is getting test kits. In the last two years, scale up of ART by involving private hospitals has increased, especially hospitals in Addis Ababa. Prevention of mother-to-child transmission of HIV has started in the last two months, and it is not yet satisfactory. We are also involved in training, such as management of hospitals. We are also subcontracted in the monitoring of health facilities with regards to identifying gaps in their health delivery services. The private sector is getting training free of charge. … The private/public mix DOTS have started in 30 private facilities. Tuberculosis patients get drugs free of charge. The Minister of Health has been encouraging and is trying to strengthen the private sector through the association of private practitioners in health.

Informant from the private for-profit sector

Figure 4.5 **Physician population in selected east African countries, most recent year available**

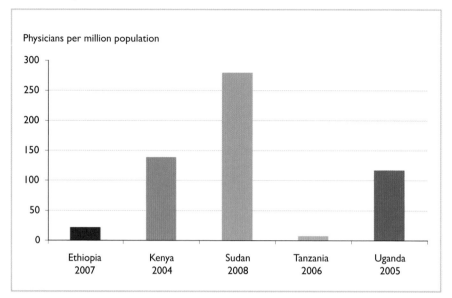

Physicians per million population

Source: Adapted from reference 9.

Building a modern health workforce

Ethiopia has a severe shortage of health workers, with far fewer physicians than in some neighbouring countries (Figure 4.5), and health workers are often poorly distributed in relation to need. The creation of a cadre of health extension workers, described above, is one way of beginning to address this shortage, but the government has taken a number of other measures, drawing on assistance from its development partners and especially the US Centers for Disease Control and USAID, and technical support from WHO.

The higher education market has been liberalized and private high schools have been allowed to train nurses, laboratory technicians and pharmacists. This has produced a considerable expansion in middle-level health professionals. More recently, a few private schools have begun to train general practitioners. Major efforts have been made to provide enhanced training to health workers treating patients with AIDS, but there have been many problems in retaining trained staff at facilities[20].

Task shifting is increasingly seen as a means of tackling the shortage of physicians. Health officers and nurses in the community are being trained to deliver services once performed by hospital doctors. This has been a major factor in the ability to scale up ART and PMTCT programmes, delivering them in health centres that lack doctors[21]. In turn, health extension workers are providing health promotion and disease prevention activities once carried out by nurses. There are other examples of new ways of working, such as specialist outreach, in which surgeons travel from central to peripheral hospitals, a policy that has been shown to be cost-effective[22].

Training of health officers, who provide intermediate care in health centres, has been accelerated. In 2009/2010, over 5000 were enrolled. They are required to staff the much-expanded number of health centres currently under construction. Each health centre is designed to be staffed by two health officers and two midwives, as well as nurses and support staff.

Physician training has been expanded, with an increase in medical schools from three to seven. The government is encouraging the remaining 16 universities to open medical schools. Training in evaluation and health informatics, from diplomas to MSc level, is also being expanded.

Expansion and upgrading of health care facilities

Ethiopia entered the 1990s with a very limited health care infrastructure, with even fewer major facilities than in 1974. Since then, there has been a major programme of investment to bring services closer to the population they serve, primarily reflecting a concern about the adverse impact of distance on uptake of services. The government has adopted a standard that, in principle, would see most people having to travel at most 10 km to the nearest facility. The results are clear. The 72 hospitals in 1991 (down from 82 in 1974) have increased to 183. There has been an accompanying programme to improve the capacity and quality of hospitals (Box 4.3). The 153 health centres in 1991 were expected to increase to 3200 by the end of 2010. This process has been accompanied by a substantial reduction in older and poorly equipped clinics, some of which have been upgraded to health centres, while others have been turned into health posts for health extension workers, which now number 14 000. The overall result is that access to a local health facility has increased from 38% in 1991 to 89.6% in 2010 (Federal Ministry of Health Office of Public and External Relations, personal communication, 2010).

Availability of essential drugs

Health workers can do little without adequate and reliable supplies of essential drugs. In the past, access to medicines in rural Ethiopia was extremely limited. This has been transformed by the creation of the Pharmaceutical Fund and

> **Box 4.3   Measures to improve hospital capacity and quality**
>
> 1. Expansion of medical, nursing and midwifery training, enabling increased staffing of health facilities since the early 2000s.
>
> 2. Improvement in the geographical distribution of the health workforce. Incentives have been introduced to attract doctors to remotely located hospitals and to retain them there. These include salary top-ups, housing, overtime payments and scholarships for specialized training. The regions now compete to hire doctors. Our informants report that this is attracting substantial numbers of doctors to the public sector, especially in remote areas.
>
> 3. Better regulation of health and health-related services and products. The Drug Administration and Control Authority, which oversees the use of medicines, has become more active in monitoring locally and internationally produced drugs to ensure their safety.
>
> 4. Implementation of standard operating procedures for pharmaceutical supplies, including provisions to buy medicines from the private sector.

Supply Agency. The delay in the procurement of drugs has been reduced from 360 days to 60 days[23] and essential medicines are much more easily available than in some neighbouring countries (Figure 4.6). This reduces wastage of expired drugs and improves the sustainability of supply. The Agency has worked closely with the Global Fund and PEPFAR to ensure adequate supplies of medicines for AIDS, tuberculosis and malaria, as well as for treating opportunistic infections. It has also constructed distribution hubs within a maximum of 160 km from health facilities and has introduced standardized distribution systems with assistance from USAID[23].

Clearly, there is very little point in making medicines available in pharmacies if the population cannot afford them. However, although availability of essential drugs has improved, about one in six patients still has to obtain drugs from the private sector, where they are about twice as expensive[25]. Consequently, the Ethiopian Government has put in place a number of measures designed to ensure that essential drugs are either free or heavily subsidized. Certain medicines should be provided free to everyone. These include vaccinations and treatment for acute watery diarrhoea, malaria, tuberculosis and HIV/AIDS. Those who are very poor are entitled to receive a range of other medications free on production of a certificate from the *kebele* administration where they live. Other essential medicines are provided at hospital and health centre pharmacies with heavy subsidies. These include antibiotics for acute infections. The cost is substantially less than that for the same preparations purchased in the private sector. However, patients still face considerable costs in obtaining diagnoses[26].

Figure 4.6 Median availability of selected generic medicines in public facilities in east African countries, various years, 2001–2009

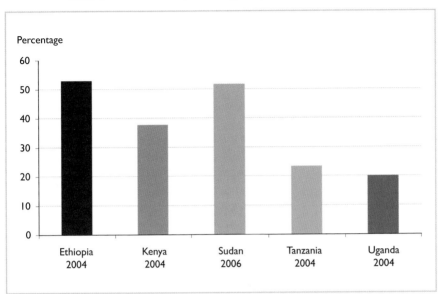

Source: Adapted from reference 24.

How has Ethiopia achieved this?

Ethiopia has come a long way in two decades. In the following section, we examine how it has done so. In particular, we look at how health fits within its broader vision for development and how it has raised money to expand its health care system.

Developing a plan

From the early 1990s, the Ethiopian Government recognized the key role that must be played by health improvement in the country's economic development. Hence, it featured prominently in the first Sustainable Development and Poverty Reduction Programme, which evolved into the current strategy, PASDEP. Intersectoral action is at the heart of this strategy, which links health to progress in other sectors such as education, water, agriculture, rural development, gender equality, tourism, trade and industry development, urban development, governance and capacity building[27]. Thus, the Health Extension Programme was designed with input from key stakeholders in the environment, water and education[28].

PASDEP is closely linked to the Health Sector Development Programme, initiated in 1997 and renewed every five years since then. The current programme places a high priority on maternal and child health, sanitation and expansion of services.

> *The development is not only in health, but also in other sectors. There is fast development in education even more than health, infrastructure, road construction, water which are contributing to health. It is a multisectoral development in all areas. All the sectors have a five-year development strategy and plan... With the Health Sector Development Programme and the overall PASDEP, there were no negative consequences visible.*
> *National health research informant*

Paying for health system development

Ethiopia still spends much less per capita on health than other countries in east Africa, and although this figure has increased in recent years, it has done so at a slower pace that in some of its neighbours, so the gap has widened (Figure 4.7).

Ethiopia still has a long way to go before it can ensure universal free access to health care for its population. Over 80% of health expenditure is still out of pocket (Figure 4.8). Consequently, the developments described above should be viewed as work in progress and as an investment for the future.

Ethiopia's additional resources have come largely from the international community, so the share of overall health expenditure from external resources has grown rapidly (Figure 4.9). Indeed, a recent study using *National Health Accounts* data reported a decrease in government funding for health between 2002 and 2006 of an amount equivalent to 1·4% of GDP, while during this same period, Ethiopia benefited from a rise in international health aid of 1.2% of GDP[29,30]. It has been estimated that, between 2003 and 2009, Ethiopia received over US$ 3.2 billion from the Global Fund, over US$ 1 billion from PEPFAR, and over US$ 70 million from the World Bank's Energy Sector Management Assistance Programme. Further substantial funding has come from United Nations organizations, the GAVI Alliance (formerly the Global Alliance for Vaccines and Immunisation) and bilateral development agencies, in particular those of Ireland, Spain, Italy, and the Netherlands. Most of these funds have been provided to the health and education sectors.

The importance of international donor agencies in funding the Ethiopian health care system has led to their much greater involvement in the governance of the Health System Development Programme.

Figure 4.7 Per capita expenditure on health in selected east African countries

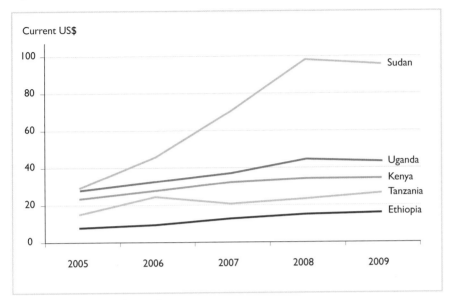

Source: Adapted from reference 9.

Figure 4.8 Share of health expenditure that is out of pocket in selected east
          African countries, 2000–2009

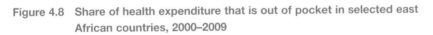

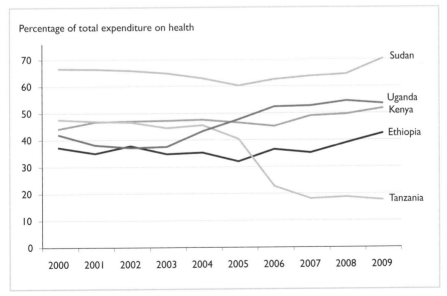

Source: Adapted from reference 9.

Figure 4.9   Share of government health expenditure from external sources, selected east African countries, 2000–2009

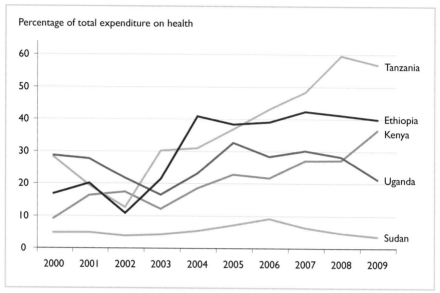

Source: Adapted from reference 9.

What development partners need is openness, accountability and results. I think this is being done to their satisfaction. This is the reason why support from development partners, whether bilateral or multilateral, is increasing. Although Ethiopia is receiving considerable amounts of external funding, no development partner has ever imposed policy or programme changes. They are all working with the policy and programme frameworks prepared by the government through broad consultations with stakeholders, especially the regions and districts. The role of development partners is to assist and speed up the implementation of sector programmes as we have for example in the implementation of the Health Sector Development Programme.

Government official

There are a several reasons why the Ethiopian Government has been able to benefit from substantial increases in development assistance, especially from the United States. One factor that cannot be ignored is its geopolitical position in the Horn of Africa, which has allowed it to support American foreign policy, most notably in 2006 when, with American backing, its armed forces moved into Somalia in support of the Somali Transitional Federal Government, which was under attack from the Islamic Courts Union and affiliated militias. However, the Ethiopian Government has also developed a reputation as a reliable partner, establishing rigorous systems to account for the use of funds. The Ministry of Finance and Economic Development has well-established procedures that comply with internationally accepted standards of financial management and accounting. It is also seen as being able to get things done, employing new management techniques where necessary, such as the Business Process Re-engineering initiative being led by the Ministry for Capacity Building and now applied in the health sector.

There is political commitment, innovative leadership and cultural change as a result of access to education and other services, and activities are grassroots-focused. The donor support to the country, especially to the health sector, is enabling the country to put its plans into practice, as we see it in health. Without the Global Fund, it would have been difficult to scale up activities in health. Although the country has not been blamed for corruption even during the past regimes, the democratization process and a participatory approach to decision-making and evaluation of outcomes and activities where development partners have a say is reducing incidences of deliberate misuse or poor use of resources. Development partners have confidence in national systems and programmes. For example, Ethiopia has the best financial system, which is very strict in accounting and fund utilization. Development partners are putting their monies in the National Treasury because they are confident in the financial systems. There are some funds off-budget which directly go to sectors or implementing agencies. We insist that the fund used in the sector should be known in order to avoid duplication of funding. This is being done. In the health sector, the partners work from one plan and they share their responsibilities for implementing activities. Therefore, there is harmonization and alignment of programme activities. This helps in the effective use of resources.
Informant, Ministry of Finance and Economic Development

Ethiopia has also benefited from improvements in systems of governance. Data from the World Bank's Worldwide Governance Indicators reveal that, between 1996 and 2008, government effectiveness increased from 14% to 40%, regulatory quality from 5% to 20%, rule of law from 19% to 34%, and control of corruption from 9% to 30%. These quantitative improvements are consistent with the comments by many of those interviewed for this study. However, there are also some concerns, again identified by our interviewees, who described over-centralized control by the government and an unwillingness to accept dissenting views[31,32]. This is apparent in the worsening of some governance indicators between 1996 and 2008, with voice and accountability declining from 24% to 10%, and stability and absence of violence from 17% to 6%.

The role of other sectors

The health system is only one of many contributors to better population health. Another is basic sanitation. In 2002/2003, only 28.4% of the population had access to safe water. By 2007/2008, this had increased to 59.5%[8]. However, in the long run, a key role will be played by education, especially of girls. This is a priority for the government. Primary school enrolment has now reached 91%, with the ratio of girls to boys reaching 92%. Improved female education is going hand in hand with investment in female empowerment. Traditionally, the status of woman in Ethiopia has been very low and their health has suffered from the persistence of a number of unsafe practices, including female genital mutilation. There has been significant progress in removing legal barriers to women's rights and in placing gender equality within policies in all sectors, although it will take longer to address deep-seated cultural beliefs.

The status … of women in Ethiopia … is low. The 1993 policy on women … outlines a strategy for dealing with the problem. The women's office was formed in the office of the prime minister headed by a minister and reaching down to the lowest government administration. The constitution … gave women equal status in terms of accessing resources, services, political and social participation and protection from harmful practices such as early marriage and genital cutting and mutilation. … the criminal code was revised to protect women … All sectors were required to mainstream gender… Parity has been achieved in primary education, and participation of women in secondary and tertiary education has improved. Women are beneficiaries of the micro-credit system. Employment of women has improved in the public sector. The Health Extension Programme is … creating job opportunities for women. Small industries are benefiting women. … The improvement in infrastructure such as roads, electricity and water is of great benefit to women. The development efforts that aim at poverty reduction very much benefit women as they suffer most from poverty.

Researcher

■ The political context

Peace and stability: a bedrock of progress

The 1970s and 1980s were not good times to live in Ethiopia. Military rule in the country was accompanied by widespread repression and conflict, both internally and with its neighbours and, as if this was not enough, Ethiopia was ravaged by drought and resulting famine. The country slipped ever further behind its neighbours, who were themselves beset by many problems. The defeat of the military government in 1991 heralded a new era in Ethiopian politics. The Transitional Government of Ethiopia was committed to healing the fractures in Ethiopian society and creating the peace and stability that were recognized by all Ethiopians as a prerequisite for development.

Almost at once it began the task of creating a government of national unity that brought all of the warring groups into the government. It also set about resolving the Eritrean issue. Eritrea had been colonized by Italy, as Italian Somaliland, in the 1890s. Italian forces were expelled in 1941 by troops from the British Commonwealth, which then ruled it under a United Nations mandate until 1951, when it was transferred to Ethiopian sovereignty. However, there had been a long standing and widely supported movement for independence. This had been opposed by the Emperor and the military government, but the new transitional government agreed to a referendum under international supervision. Eritrea became independent in 1993.

Recognizing the complexity of Ethiopian society, the drafters of the new constitution established a federation of nations, nationalities and peoples, which included the right of secession. The new country would be a democratic state, with elections every five years to a bicameral legislature, with clear separation of powers among the legislative, judiciary and executive branches of government. The constitution contains a number of checks and balances in response to the inevitable challenges that arise in a complex multi-ethnic country. Political parties are still linked to ethnicity. The EPRDF, for example, brings together four major ethnically based political groups: the Tigrayans, the Amhara, the Oromos, and the coalition of different ethnic groups of the south. The two largest opposition parties are also coalitions combining universal and ethnically defined parties, while other smaller parties are linked to single ethnic groups, such as Somalis, Oromos and Gambela. This is beginning to change with the emergence of political parties based on ideology rather than ethnicity, but it will take time.

Political changes have been accompanied by liberalization of the economy. The transitional government began a programme of economic reforms in 1992 that laid the ground for a structural adjustment programme, implemented in 1996. This led to the privatization of major industries and devaluation of the currency. Compared with the experience of other countries undertaking structural adjustment programmes, Ethiopia fared relatively well. It has been able to attract a growing volume of inward investment, especially from India, China, Saudi Arabia and Turkey.

> *The development we see in health started with the introduction of the policy of decentralization, devolution of power to regions and districts under the present government. During the military government, there was a socialist type of macroeconomic policy. I cannot say it was socialist but socialist-oriented. Under this orientation, the government at the centre believed that it could do everything on behalf of the people. It felt that it could deal with poverty and backwardness by centralizing power. It was a highly centralized system. The government controlled everything. It was government centred. As a result, there was no participation of the private sector and other civil societies. The international community did not believe in the policy, and development aid was not there, apart from humanitarian aid. The government was left alone and could not implement its development goals.*
>
> *Informant, Ministry of Finance and Economic Development*

Vision and leadership

Despite outward appearances, Ethiopia has a revolutionary government. The current generation of political leaders honed their skills in the revolutionary student movement or in the armed struggle against the military government. They achieved power by defeating a militarily powerful army supported by one of the world's superpowers, the USSR. Many of them had been elite students at Addis Ababa University, with a clear vision of what needed to be done to bring Ethiopia into the modern age. Yet they were also fully aware of the task that faced them, as many had lived for up to 17 years in rural areas, mobilizing local communities in the struggle for democracy. This gave them both the expertise and the mandate for an ambitious programme of reform. It also provided them with a clear understanding of the importance of intersectoral action and the ability to work with anyone, in the public or private sector, within Ethiopia and abroad, who could help them to bring about their country's development.

Those interviewed for this study identified the pivotal role that has been played by the Ethiopian Prime Minister, who is seen as someone who combines technical expertise in economics and development with political skills. He is credited with the ability to take ideas from many sources and bring them together effectively. This has helped to ensure a sense of ownership of policies by those charged with implementing them. He is viewed as having taken a robust stance against corruption and expects high standards of performance from government officials. He is seen as understanding the geopolitical context in which Ethiopia finds itself, using this to benefit his country. Other interviewees highlighted the positive role played by the current Minister of Health, who is seen as a close ally of the Prime Minister and someone who has been able to mobilize support for health in other ministries.

> *The programme is a government and party programme. It is an EPRDF agenda. The party has structure down to the lowest level of government. They speak the same language. The leader of the party is the Prime Minister of the country, for it is the ruling party that forms the government. It has been in power since it overthrew the military government in 1991. The current Minister of Health is an also a wonderful leader and manager. He has effectively succeeded in making the development partners fully engaged in the health sector development programme, and also the private sector. More than anything, the party is committed and evaluates its members by the performance they show if they are to stay in leadership positions. Outside the government, the Millennium Development Goals in health are also moving the government to meet them. Ethiopia enjoys the trust and support of the international community, particularly the west.*
>
> *Team Leader, Policy and Programmes, Federal Ministry of Health*

■ Conclusions and lessons learned

Just over two decades ago, the situation in Ethiopia seemed hopeless. It was beset by war, famine and corruption. Yet out of that horror sprang hope that things could be different. This hope was seen in the actions of a new generation of Ethiopians who assumed political leadership. It was also seen in the actions of millions of people outside Ethiopia who found ever more imaginative ways to raise money to help their fellow humans and, as importantly, put pressure on their political leaders to help too.

This hope is well on the way to turning into a reality. Ethiopia is still desperately poor; many of its people still live a precarious existence, ever aware of their vulnerability to events beyond their control, in particular the extreme weather that has afflicted them so often in the past. Yet many things have improved. An

Ethiopian born today is twice as likely as one born 20 years ago to survive to his or her fifth birthday. There is a new generation of health extension workers who can help at a baby's birth and who can provide basic care if he or she later becomes ill. However, that child's risk of falling ill has also reduced, due to better nutrition and improved access to clean water.

What allowed Ethiopia to move along this trajectory? One factor to emerge clearly from this analysis is the importance of peace and stability. This has not been easy. Ethiopia is an incredibly diverse society and, as our research for this project shows, high levels of ethnic diversity make it more difficult to achieve good health outcomes[33]. However, although it is more difficult, it is not impossible, as illustrated by examples in this region of countries, such as Tanzania, that have overcome this challenge to create societies in which everyone, whatever language they speak or wherever they worship, can participate. Unfortunately, others, such as Kenya, have been less successful.

The 1994 Ethiopian Constitution enshrines the principle of self-determination for Ethiopia's different communities and establishes a strong federal system that combines national leadership with regional self-determination. Crucially, this has meant that the political system is broadly representative of the major groups and is not, as it might have been, controlled by the Tigrayan people, who led the revolution against the military regime.

Stable, participative government has provided a basis for policies that foster economic growth. However, unlike the situation in many other parts of Africa, Ethiopia has striven to ensure that as many of the gains as possible are retained for the benefit of its citizens. This has not always been successful; its experience with a well-known coffee company exemplified the unequal struggle between poor industries and multinational corporations. However, it is at least trying.

Like other countries in Africa, Ethiopia's health system has faced a workforce crisis. It was clear that an expansion of physicians to levels that were adequate would take decades, especially given the lure of higher salaries and better conditions abroad. Its system of health extension workers seeks to fill some of the gap, reaching out to provide basic care for the rural poor. Of course, challenges remain, such as widening coverage to urban areas and to nomadic populations, but others, such as career development, are being addressed.

Finally, it is impossible to ignore how Ethiopia has benefited from very large sums of development assistance, in large part a result of geostrategic considerations. This is, however, a mixed blessing, as the challenge now is to find sustainable sources of funding. Fortunately, with few exceptions, it seems that donations by rich countries are relatively resistant to the economic crises they have faced in the past, and by extension, those they are facing now[34]. Yet there is no room for complacency.

What lessons can Ethiopia offer other countries with few resources? One is the importance of political commitment at all levels, to nation building, good governance, and to health and its determinants. Another is that policy and programme development strategies must be inclusive of all stakeholders and should target the people. The Ethiopian experience shows that taking the community as a potential producer of health, instead of as a potential consumer of medicines and curative services, is a way forward to achieve better outcomes in health. It is critical to ensure the participation of the private for-profit sector, non-profit NGOs and development partners as well as stakeholders from all relevant sectors in the design and implementation of reforms, ensuring effective intersectoral linkages and shared ownership. A third is the use of appropriately skilled workers and technology to achieve maximum coverage, even if this is still basic.

There are, inevitably, many remaining challenges. Many of these relate directly or indirectly to geography. One is food security. Although Ethiopia is especially vulnerable, given its location and climate, nowhere is now immune from a world where a substantial share of world food is traded globally, much controlled by a small number of multinational corporations and with prices influenced almost as much by speculators as by supply and demand.[35]

A second relates more precisely to topography. Ethiopia has a very poor transportation infrastructure, with inevitable consequences for the delivery of health care. Improved emergency obstetric care, necessary to make serious inroads into maternal mortality, will depend on an improved road network.

A third is access to clean water and sanitation. Although this has improved, it will be difficult to deliver effective sanitation to the 84% of the population living in scattered rural settlements.

A fourth relates to the wider region. Ethiopia's neighbour Somalia has effectively been divided into separate mini-states, with large parts under no effective government. Ethiopia's border with Eritrea, until recently the setting for conflict, remains disputed.

A fifth concern relates to the close relationship between the governing party and the government. While this has created considerable stability, it is incompatible with a pluralist democracy in the long term. Finally, perhaps the most important challenge, alluded to above, is how to establish a sustainable system of paying for effective health care for all.

ACKNOWLEDGEMENTS

I would like to acknowledge the immense technical support received from Professor Martin McKee. Without his support, the chapter would not have assumed its present shape. Special thanks go to Miss Katie Callaham who did her internship at Miz-Hasab Research Center and Dr Abraham Endeshaw from the Federal Ministry of Health. Miss Callaham helped in the processing of data obtained from WHO, World Bank, and Ministry of Health publications. Dr Abraham reviewed the work on behalf of the Ministry and validated the report. The Miz-Hasab Research Center is appreciative of the cooperation it received from all stakeholders in health, especially the leadership of the Federal Ministry of Health, and is grateful to the Rockefeller Foundation and the London School of Hygiene & Tropical Medicine for giving it the opportunity to work on this project. Finally, the commitment and skills in guidance demonstrated by Dr Dina Balabanova as lead researcher on the project have been admirable.

Hailom Bangteyerga Amaha (lead researcher of the Ethiopia chapter)

REFERENCES

1. Chamberlain N. Prime Minister on the issues. *The Times*, 28 September 1938; 10.

2. Meredith M. *The state of Africa: a history of fifty years of independence.* London: Free Press; 2006.

3. Chen L et al. Human resources for health: overcoming the crisis. *Lancet* 2004; 364(9449):1984–90.

4. Population Census Commission. *Summary and statistical report of the 2007 Population and Housing Census. Federal Democratic Republic of Ethiopia.* Addis Ababa: Population Census Commission; 2008.

5. Central Statistical Authority, MEASURE DHS and ORC Macro. *Ethiopia demographic and health survey 2005*. Addis Ababa: Central Statistical Authority, MEASURE DHS and ORC Macro; 2005.

6. WHO. *National health accounts, country health information*. Geneva: World Health Organization; 2011 (http://www.who.int/nha/country/en/, accessed 17 June 2011).

7. WHO. *World health statistics 2010*. Geneva: World Health Organization; 2010.

8. Planning and Programming Department. *Health and health related indicators*. Addis Ababa: Federal Ministry of Health; 2008.

9. World Bank. *World development indicators* [online database]. Washington, DC: World Bank; 2011 (http://data.worldbank.org/indicator, accessed 13 July 2011).

10. Hogan MC et al. Maternal mortality for 181 countries, 1980–2008: a systematic analysis of progress towards millennium development goal 5. *Lancet* 2010; 375(9726):1609–23.

11. Federal HIV/AIDS Prevention and Control Office. *Report on progress towards implementation of the UN Declaration of Commitment on HIV/AIDS 2010*. Addis Ababa: Federal HIV/AIDS Prevention and Control Office; 2010.

12. Central Statistical Authority and ORC Macro. *Ethiopia Demographic and Health Survey 2000*. Addis Ababa: Central Statistical Authority and ORC Macro; May 2001.

13. Federal Ministry of Health. *Annual performance report of HSDP-III*. Addis Ababa: Federal Ministry of Health; 2009.

14. Federal Ministry of Health. *Health sector strategic plan (HSDP-III)*. 2005/6–2009/10. Addis Ababa: Federal Ministry of Health; 2005.

15. Health Planning and Programming Department. *Health and health related indicators 2008/9*. Addis Ababa: Planning and Programming Department, Federal Ministry of Health; 2010.

16. Negusse H, McAuliffe E, MacLachlan M. Initial community perspectives on the Health Service Extension Programme in Welkait, Ethiopia. *Human Resources for Health* 2007; 5:21.

17. Sebastian MS, Lemma H. Efficiency of the health extension programme in Tigray, Ethiopia: a data envelopment analysis. *BMC International Health and Human Rights* 2010; 10:16.

18. Wong R, Bradley EH. Developing patient registration and medical records management system in Ethiopia. *International Journal for Quality in Health Care* 2009; 21(4):253–8.

19. Abate B, Enquselassie F. Information use in patients' referral system at Tikur Anbessa Specialized Hospital, Addis Ababa, Ethiopia. *Ethiopian Medical Journal* 2010; 48(2):123–35.

20. McNabb ME et al. Tracking working status of HIV/AIDS-trained service providers by means of a training information monitoring system in Ethiopia. *Human Resources for Health* 2009; 7:29.

21. Assefa Y et al. Rapid scale-up of antiretroviral treatment in Ethiopia: successes and system-wide effects. *PLoS Medicine* 2009; 6(4):e1000056.

22. Kifle YA, Nigatu TH. Cost-effectiveness analysis of clinical specialist outreach as compared to referral system in Ethiopia: an economic evaluation. *Cost Effectiveness and Resource Allocation* 2010; 8(1):13.

23. Banteyerga H et al. *The system-wide effects of the scale-up of HIV/AIDs, tuberculosis, and malaria services in Ethiopia.* Bethesda, MD: Abt Associates; 2010 (Health Systems 20/20 project).

24. WHO. *Statistical information system* [online database]. Geneva: World Health Organization; 2011 (http://apps.who.int/whosis/database/, accessed 2011).

25. Carasso BS et al. Availability of essential medicines in Ethiopia: an efficiency-equity trade-off? *Tropical Medicine & International Health* 2009; 14(11):1394–400.

26. Mesfin MM et al. Cost implications of delays to tuberculosis diagnosis among pulmonary tuberculosis patients in Ethiopia. *BMC Public Health* 2010; 10:173.

27. *Ethiopia: Building on progress. A plan for accelerated and sustained development to end poverty (PASDEP).* Addis Ababa: Ministry of Finance and Economic Development; 2006.

28. Dercon S et al. The impact of agricultural extension and roads on poverty and consumption growth in fifteen Ethiopian villages. *American Journal of Agricultural Economics* 2009; 91(4):1007–21.

29. Lu C et al. Public financing of health in developing countries: a cross-national systematic analysis. *Lancet* 2010; 375(9723):1375–87.

30. Ooms G et al. Crowding out: are relations between international health aid and government health funding too complex to be captured in averages only? *Lancet* 2010; 375(9723):1403–5.

31. Anon. Ethiopia's elections: five more years. *The Economist*, 20 May 2010.

32. Anon. Correspondent's diary: a country of grey and gold. *The Economist*, 28 May 2010.

33. Powell-Jackson T et al. Reducing child and maternal mortality: democracy and economic growth in divided societies. *Social Science and Medicine* 1002; 73(1):33–41.

34. Stuckler D et al. Does recession reduce global health aid? Evidence from 15 high-income countries, 1975–2007. *Bulletin of the World Health Organization* 2011; 89(4):252–57.

35. Lock K et al. Potential causes and health effects of rising global food prices. *British Medical Journal* 2009; 359:269–72.

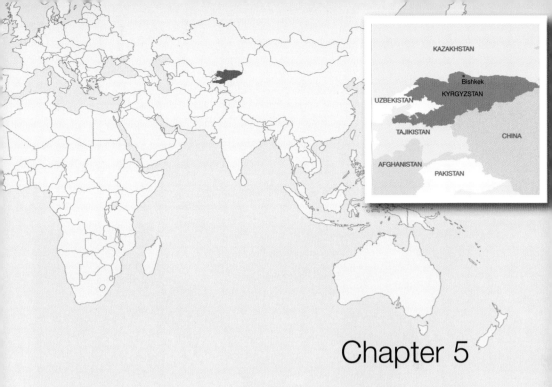

Chapter 5

KYRGYZSTAN: A REGIONAL LEADER IN HEALTH SYSTEM REFORM

Ainura Ibraimova[1], Baktygul Akkazieva[1], Gulgun Murzalieva[1] and Dina Balabanova[2]

1 Health Policy Analysis Center, 2 LSHTM

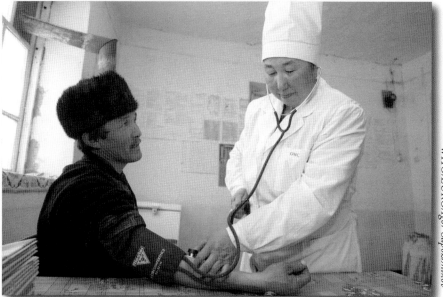

WHO/EURO/Igor Sapozhnikov

A doctor examines a patient at the Kirov Primary Health Care Centre in Uzgen. About 1500 people live in Uzgen – a remote region of Kyrgyzstan.

■ Key messages

- Kyrgyzstan is a small country facing considerable geographical, political and economic challenges that limit its ability to invest in improving health. However, it inherited some positive features of the Soviet system, which sought to achieve universal coverage and equity; independence and the transition to democracy provided an opportunity to reform the health system.

- A comprehensive reform plan to strengthen the overall health system was formulated and implemented in the early 1990s, soon after independence. The plan radically redesigned the way health care was financed and delivered, focusing on primary care and prioritizing maternal and child health and communicable and noncommunicable diseases.

- Presidential support, coupled with strong leaders in the health sector, was critical in promoting continuous, strategic and proactive political engagement throughout the reform process. However, implementation was successful because of capacity on the ground, most notably by experienced and committed administrators and technocrats.

- Good governance, a political culture of openness and efforts to promote accountability within a top-down decision-making culture were the most significant contextual factors. The policy process was inclusive and involved proactive coordination and synergies among government, donors and community representatives.

- Health system leadership was demonstrated through robust legislation and regulation that were introduced early in the change process. Policies were informed by evidence and promising innovations, the impact of the reform was regularly monitored, and the health system was redesigned as necessary.

- Major successes of the health system reform that are already improving health include revitalizing primary care, increasing coverage of essential interventions, expanding financial protection, mobilizing resources for the health sector through greater efficiency and more equitable resource allocation, and strengthening health system responsiveness.

- Achievements also point to a well-educated population, empowerment of women, solidarity and improvements in infrastructure.

■ Introduction

Kyrgyzstan is an example of a *Good health at low cost* country for many reasons, especially its ability to protect its population from catastrophic health expenditure. A small, land-locked country in the heart of central Asia, Kyrgyzstan has major geographical and economic disadvantages[1]. It is predominantly mountainous and 90% of the land is unsuitable for agriculture, but water resources are plentiful and its main export is hydroelectric energy (Box 5.1).

The *perestroika* that began at the late 1980s under Mikhail Gorbachev initiated a political change that led to the collapse of the USSR and independence for all republics in 1991. Two revolutions followed that led to changes of government (in 2005 – the Tulip Revolution – and in 2010), the latter accompanied by serious ethnic violence in the south, and a coalition government that was elected in December 2010[1]. The transition to independence was extremely painful for the country from an economic standpoint. Heavily dependent on Moscow's subsidies during the Soviet period, by 1995, the country's real GDP had dropped to about half its 1989 level[9]. This led to a dramatic decline in living standards, rising unemployment and increased levels of poverty that were not mitigated by social sector spending. However, these trends were later reversed, and since 2000, the country has experienced stable economic growth.

A strong economic recovery since 2007 underpinned the government's ability to implement wide-ranging reform and promote socioeconomic development. Politically, Kyrgyzstan has been known as an island of democracy in the central Asian region since independence in 1991. However, since the mid-2000s, the country has experienced considerable political turmoil and uncertainty.

Despite political and economic challenges, Kyrgyzstan has made rapid progress in reorienting its health system towards primary health care, improving access, strengthening financial protection and reducing the ubiquitous out-of-pocket spending. Under government leadership, two subsequent national health plans that spanned the years from 1996 to 2010 provided a coherent framework for radical reform and donor investment in the health sector. The reforms led to a shift from specialist-oriented care to family practice; implementation of a basic benefits package; health financing reform, including introduction of contracting and a consolidated single-payer system; and liberalization of the pharmaceutical market. Rationalization of hospital provision is also under way. In other words, there has been a transition from a hierarchical and highly centralized Soviet-style health system to one that is decentralized and more responsive to the health needs of communities[9].

Throughout years of economic turmoil, reforms have benefited from sustained

---

Box 5.1   Kyrgyzstan at a glance

Population   5.3 million, rural population 64% (2009), with almost one quarter living in remote mountainous rural areas[2].

Geography   Located in central Asia, 90% mountainous, limited natural resources.

Ethnic composition   The main ethnic groups are Kyrgyz (65%), Uzbek (14%) and Russian (13%) (1999 census)[3]. Two official languages: Kyrgyz and Russian.

Government   A republic. Regarded as an island of democracy in the period from independence from the USSR in 1991 until 2005, but considerable political turmoil since then.

Health system   Health expenditure per capita (constant 2005 Int$)[4]: 151.7
Density of physicians, nurses and midwives per 10 000[4]: 80
Radical health reform targeted at strengthening of primary care and financial protection, but still high levels of out-of-pocket payments. High coverage of most key interventions (98% of women deliver with skilled birth attendant, and child vaccination rates over 90%)[5].

Economic, demographic and social development

GDP per capita (constant 2005 Int$) (2009)[2]	2073
Real GDP growth rate (2007)[6]	8.7%
Population living on less than $1.25 a day (2007)[2]	1.9%
Population below the national poverty line (2005)[2]	43.1%
Gini index (2007)[2]	33
Infant mortality rate (2006)[5]	38[a]
Maternal mortality ratio (2006)[5]	104[b]
Adult HIV prevalence, aged 15–49 (2009)[7]	0.3%
Life expectancy (years) (2009)[8]	64.8 (men) 73 (women)
Total fertility rate (2008)[8]	2.8
Adult literacy (2009)[2]	99%
Ratio girls to boys in education[c] (2008)[2]	101%
Internet usage (2009)[2]	41.2%

Note: [a] Per 1000 live births; [b] Per 100 000 live births; [c] Primary and secondary education.

---

general government expenditure on health, although to a lesser extent than some of its wealthier neighbours. Other significant contributions were effective political leadership, coordinated working arrangements with donors, continuity of reform efforts and piloting of projects prior to their scaling up[6].

Since independence, Kyrgyzstan has demonstrated good or better health outcomes and performance of the overall health system compared to the region. Because universal coverage has been achieved, at least in theory, Kyrgyzstan can be identified as a performer in central Asia and the Caucasus. This chapter demonstrates how and why this has been possible.

■ Health gains

Over the past decade, Kyrgyzstan has shown steady improvement in the health of its population. The infant mortality rate has shown continued progress according to survey data, with an almost 50% reduction from 66 to 38 per 1000 live births between 1997 and 2006[5,10] (Table 5.1). Similarly, surveys indicate that the under-5 mortality rate has decreased from 72 to 44 per 1000 live births during these same years. Trends in official data are more difficult to interpret because of known under-registration in the past and the adoption of WHO live birth criteria in 2004. However, there is a process of convergence between official statistics and surveys, reflecting improved registration of infant deaths, facilitated by a change in attitudes to monitoring and evaluation. Of the children

Table 5.1   Maternal, infant and child mortality by source

	1997	2000	2003	2005	2006	2007	2008	2009
Infant mortality rate per 1000 live births								
WHO/surveys	66.0[a]	61.3[b]			38.0[c]			
RMIC	28.2	22.6	20.9	29.7	29.2	29.8	27.1	25.0
Perinatal	n/a	n/a	n/a	32.4[d]	33.7[c]	33.0[d]	30.9[d]	
Neonatal	n/a	n/a	n/a	21.0[d]	22.5[c]	21.7[d]	19.2[d]	
Under-5 mortality rate per 1000 live births								
WHO/surveys		72.3[b]			44.0[c]			
RMIC	n/a	30.0	27.6	35.2	34.6	35.3	31.5	29.3
Maternal mortality ratio per 100 000 live births								
WHO/surveys	72.0[a]	110.0[b]		150.0[c]	104.0[c]			
RMIC				46.4	61.0	53.0	62.5	58.9	75.3
NSC			45.5	49.3	60.1	56.0	51.9	53.0	

Sources: Adapted from references 5, 8,10 and 12 ([a]Reference 10; [b]Reference 8; [c]Reference 5; [d]Refernce 12).

Notes: NSC: National Statistical Committee; RMIC: Republican Medical Information Center, Ministry of Health; n/a: Not available.

Figure 5.1   Life expectancy at birth

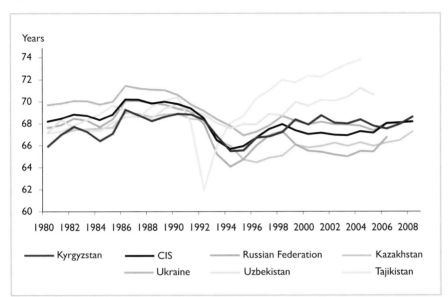

Source: Reference 8.

under one who die, 30% do so on the first day of hospital admission. More than 50% of under 5-deaths are children aged between 1 and 2 years and occur at home. These figures suggest that hospitalization for serious medical conditions is often delayed due either to poor parental awareness of symptoms requiring immediate and urgent medical attention, or to barriers to accessing care[11].

Table 5.1 also shows that the maternal mortality ratio is less encouraging. It varies from year to year, but its overall stagnation reflects the influence of economic, social and cultural factors and possibly health system deficiencies[12]. The main medical causes of maternal mortality are bleeding and hypertension (47% and 25%, respectively, in 2006)[12]. The sharp increase in maternal mortality ratio in 2009 mainly reflects the improved registration system in Kyrgyzstan. On a positive note, the total fertility rate has declined steadily from 4.1 in the 1980s to 2.8 in 2008[8], which is likely to be beneficial for sustaining improvements in maternal and child health.

Other health system indicators show positive trends over time[13]. Life expectancy is recovering since the mid-1990s when socioeconomic problems were at their worst (Figure 5.1). It remains at an average level for the Commonwealth of Independent States (CIS). Surprisingly, it is higher than countries with much

Figure 5.2   Standardized death rate, tuberculosis, all ages

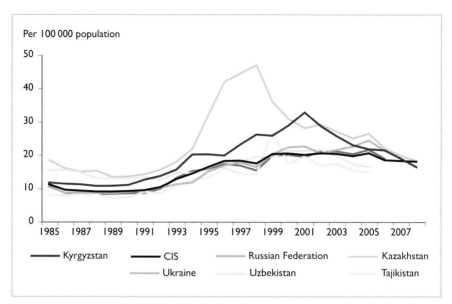

Source: Reference 8.

greater resources, such as Russia and Kazakhstan. Recent analysis has shown that adult mortality (between the ages of 20–59) has been lower than in Russia despite the fact that Kyrgyzstan is much poorer (gross national income (GNI) per capita in Kyrgyzstan was about 13 times less than in Russia in 2008) and has suffered a more severe crisis of transition[14]. This is attributed to Russia's higher burden of external and cardiovascular causes of death, particularly those strongly related to culturally determined patterns of alcohol consumption.

Mortality from tuberculosis declined from 11 per 100 000 in 2005 to 8.7 in 2009 (Figure 5.2). There have been similar declines in the central Asian region since 2000, but Kyrgyzstan has improved despite its relatively high incidence.

The burden of diseases of the circulatory system remains high in Kyrgyzstan, although the mortality rate has declined significantly since 1995 and it remains substantially below the CIS average (Figure 5.3). Although it has slightly decreased in the past 10 years, mortality from stroke in Kyrgyzstan has been consistently the highest in the region in those under 65; 30% of the population over 17 years had elevated blood pressure in 2007. Poor quality of care at the hospital level has hindered improvements in this area[15,16].

Figure 5.3   Standardized death rate, diseases of circulatory system, aged 0–64

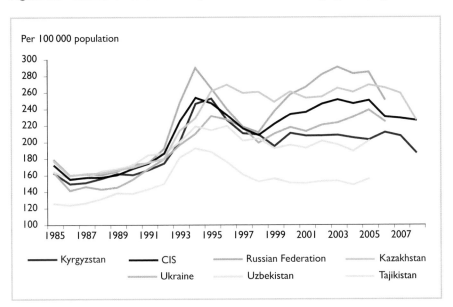

Per 100 000 population

| | Kyrgyzstan | CIS | Russian Federation | Kazakhstan |
| | Ukraine | Uzbekistan | Tajikistan | |

Source: Reference 8.

▪ Improvements in access to care

Kyrgyzstan has made significant progress on a range of intermediate health system goals, such as expanding coverage of essential care (especially in the areas of maternal and child health) and increasing financial protection and equity. These are expected to improve population health over time. Coverage by antenatal services remains high at 97% and often exceeds the WHO-recommended four visits per pregnancy. Antenatal care coverage is only slightly less in rural than in urban areas, at 95.4% and 99%, respectively[5]. A contraceptive prevalence rate of 47.8% (2005), associated with fewer unplanned pregnancies, abortions and deliveries along with longer intervals between births, has reduced the number of pregnancy-related deaths[17].

The percentage of institutional deliveries in the region remains high since this was universal practice during the Soviet period. Kyrgyzstan has maintained a stable rate of approximately 98% of births at specialized maternity hospitals over the past decade, although there are issues related to the quality of care in many regional and rural facilities. Even in villages, most women deliver in facilities and have access to qualified staff, despite high out-of-pocket payments associated with inpatient deliveries[18], and the fact that many rural areas are geographically isolated.

Health gains since 1991 are also explained by skin-to-skin contact immediately after birth and exclusive breastfeeding, which were not considered key to child health care under the Soviet system but were prioritized after transition. It is reported that 89% of women initiate breastfeeding on the first day, and 70% within an hour after birth[10]. Rates of exclusive breastfeeding in early infancy also show improvements, although rates of exclusive breastfeeding at six months remain low[12].

During the Soviet era, vaccination of children in Kyrgyzstan was well organized and free of charge. Kyrgyzstan has managed to maintain childhood immunization coverage of 98–99% despite shortages of funds and population migration that is amongst the highest in central Asia. Support from the Global Alliance for Vaccines and Immunisation has been vital in ensuring free access to vaccinations, and in 2005, the government began co-funding the procurement of vaccines, covering 60% of all costs in 2008, which is high by regional standards. New initiatives, such as information campaigns by the Republican Immunization Centre and door-to-door visits by primary health care staff and village health committee volunteers, have helped to increase population awareness and target vulnerable groups.

As a mountainous country with limited access to fruits and vegetables, there is a high risk of iron deficiency anaemia, iodine deficiency and stunting. Kyrgyzstan has mitigated these risks by piloting innovative initiatives to reduce under nutrition. The government and donors have targeted micronutrient insufficiency through the successful promotion of breastfeeding, vitamin D supplementation for children 6–24 months and new mothers, and food fortification for children 6–24 months. These practices were included in physician training programmes and implemented by maternity ward doctors and trained village health committee volunteers. They are also promoted by the mass media.

> *… This is recognized by neighbouring countries as one of the best practices in this area. The Kyrgyz team has now been invited to share their experience …*
>
> *Donor representative*

■ What has Kyrgyzstan done to improve health and access to services? The role of the health system

This section briefly examines features of the former Soviet model of health care and changes in Kyrgyzstan following the collapse of the USSR. It then focuses on the two reform programmes implemented after independence and discusses their implications on health gains and on access to affordable health care.

The inheritance

From the Second World War until the mid-1980s, the Soviet Semashko model of health care focused on increasing the health system's capacity to deliver universally accessible health services funded and managed by the state and free at the point of delivery.

In order to achieve these objectives, the USSR developed a rigorously planned and supervised system with nearly universal coverage and distribution of facilities to reduce geographical barriers to primary care. Maternal and child health and control of communicable diseases were strategic priorities and had high staffing levels, even if many staff had limited training. However, serious challenges began to emerge from the 1960s, leading to a deterioration in population health and access to care[1]. These included severe underfunding of the health sector and persistence of a system that linked financing to cumbersome infrastructure, bed and staff quotas, rather than activities. This was compounded by political interference in the health system and top-down management with no incentives for quality improvement[19]. The system was overly medicalized and primary health care and prevention were of low priority in both financial allocations and medical education.

In the mid-1980s, the Soviet leadership sought to liberalize the economy and introduce market mechanisms in the public sector, such as full or partial self-financing of some health facilities and user fees for some services. However, the principle of state-guaranteed free health care was maintained as a constitutional entitlement.

It is a widely shared view among study respondents that, despite its shortcomings, this model provided affordable and accessible essential care that brought about considerable health gains during the Soviet period. Indeed, many practices from the Semashko model underpin subsequent health reforms in Kyrgyzstan, such as free access to key services, resulting in nearly universal institutional deliveries and child vaccinations. In fact, a shared institutional memory and values (fairness and equity) may have helped to retain positive health system characteristics, such as universal coverage, after the initial system collapse following independence.

Post independence: rapid change and comprehensive reform programmes

Following independence in 1991, Kyrgyzstan was quicker than its neighbours to embrace change and develop its own health policy. The process of democratization and institution building took place as the country's economy collapsed, severely depleting resources in the health care system. The *Manas* reform programme (1996–2006) radically restructured the health system. Momentum was sustained with the *Manas Taalimi* programme (2006–2010).

These comprehensive programmes sought to address multiple determinants of health to attain health targets. Figure 5.4 shows the phases of reform and political events which impacted on health and accessibility of basic health services. Within these strategic plans there were also specific vertical programmes that were prioritized and benefited from the broader health system strengthening. For example, maternal and child health was an early reform priority and, despite radical changes in financing and delivery systems, continuity was maintained with each intervention or policy building on its predecessor. Consequently, improvements in health and access to services have already been seen (Box 5.2).

This section explores two components of the reform programmes that are considered key to implementing a wide range of successful interventions, and have positively influenced health and health indicators in the Kyrgyz Republic: (1) restructuring of delivery: strengthening primary care and hospital downsizing and (2) new financing mechanisms to improve accessibility and efficiency.

Transformation of service delivery

Post-independence, it became clear to policy-makers that, given the changing political and economic realities, urgent measures were needed to prevent a complete collapse of the health system. This led to a decisive move to implement a package of radical changes in service delivery early in the reform process, demonstrating an effort to increase access to care, including: (1) a shift from a specialist-dominated model to a comprehensive family medicine model of primary care; (2) the training of more mid-level cadres and community health workers; and (3) the rationalization of hospital infrastructure.

Development of family practice

The core principle of reform was the move from specialist-based primary health

Figure 5.4   Timeline of reforms and major political events, 1997–2009

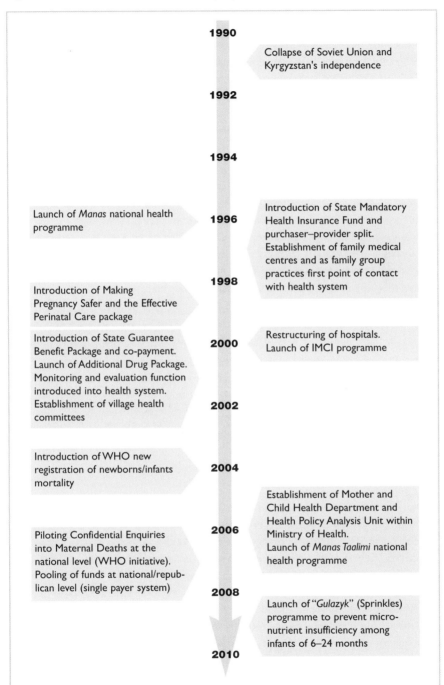

See Box 5.2 for explanations of structural and regulatory changes for maternal and child health

Box 5.2   Structural and regulatory changes for maternal and child health

Improvements in mother and child health can be traced to practices starting during Soviet times. After independence, Kyrgyzstan started introducing internationally recognized approaches that often challenged established practice. The government mobilized support nationally and among donors and, in 2000, the Ministry of Health endorsed the IMCI to reduce infant and child mortality and improve quality of primary health care, particularly diagnosis and referrals. In 2001, WHO conducted national training on IMCI algorithms and supported trained staff. IMCI has been included in family practitioner training since 2003.

In 2006, the Ministry of Health established a dedicated National Mother and Child Health Unit and the tertiary Republican Centre for the Protection of Mother and Child Health. In 2006, the National Strategy on Reproductive Health 2006–2015 was enacted but hampered by financial constraints. The Effective Perinatal Care Package – evidence-based clinical protocols, quality monitoring and supervision – was piloted in a few oblasts in 2005 and subsequently scaled up to half of all maternity facilities. As a result, newborn mortality fell significantly in facilities and pilot sites using the package, while effective management of the third stage of labour increased from 12% to 91%[12].

Monitoring and evaluation has been increasingly emphasized. In 2004, Kyrgyzstan introduced an international definition of live births and a facility-based register of newborn, child and maternal mortality. Efforts were made to improve maternal mortality data. However, some discrepancies between official data and independent sources still exist. Since 2007, a national committee has conducted an annual review of all pregnancy- and delivery-related deaths to identify system deficiencies. This process has been well publicized in the media, in contrast to the culture of secrecy in the past.

These developments led to the endorsement of the Ministry of Health Perinatal Care Improvement Programme in Kyrgyzstan for 2008–2017 embedded within *Manas Taalimi,* with the aim of raising quality of care, improving referrals and reducing regional inequalities of access and outcomes.

The reforms have been characterized by an early prioritization of mother and child health, continual refinements and a clear set of goals that remained consistent despite political changes, and these concerted efforts have seen reductions in infant and child mortality. Valuable achievements have been safeguarded (e.g. free vaccinations, near institutional deliveries) and the health system has been flexible enough to embrace Making Pregnancy Safer and IMCI, acquire new skills and foster radical change of institutions. Change involved a rapid cycle of piloting, evaluating and scaling up new models of care and partnerships among the Ministry of Health, donors, primary care providers and communities. Current challenges include obsolete equipment and staff shortages, leading to poor quality emergency obstetric care, especially in rural areas. Poor living conditions, access to water and sanitation are common in rural areas: a major cause of pneumonia in children.

care delivered through polyclinics[a] to a family medicine model, and there was consensus that this represented the foundation for subsequent health system reforms.

The family medicine model was introduced in 1997 and extended to the whole country by 2000, providing universal coverage of essential primary care. This transformation involved training a new cadre of family practitioners on a massive scale. Family medicine curricula for postgraduate and undergraduate levels were produced with the support of development partners (such as WHO, USAID and the World Bank) and a comprehensive retraining programme for doctors and nurses is ongoing, based on international evidence-based standards. The training programme and improved access to medical information increased staff motivation.

> …*Nearly all doctors and about 95–96% nurses and* feldshers *[paramedics] were retrained in the Family Medicine Programme. All this… made a positive impact on performance.*
>
> *Ministry of Health experts*

In order to facilitate the transition to a family medicine model, all health facility managers (and many general practitioners) underwent training in the main reform strategies and regulations. This strengthened the reform process at district and local levels.

Reorienting the system towards primary health care also involved changing processes, such as referral procedures, communication channels and peer support. Previously, primary health care practitioners were subordinate to secondary care facilities and had little autonomy regarding treatment and referrals. Some of these practices have persisted. For example, family doctors often avoid treating patients needing chronic care because of lack of support from specialists, resulting in disrupted follow up and poor outcomes[20,21].

Financial incentives to improve the quality of primary health care have been introduced. The Mandatory Health Insurance Fund monitors "socially significant diseases"[b] normally treated at primary care level, such as hypertension, asthma, pneumonia and so on. Underperforming family practices are investigated

---

[a] Polyclinics are urban multipurpose facilities providing primary and first-line specialist care at city and district levels, covering designated catchment areas. Under the former USSR, polyclinics were staffed by district physicians and several specialists with basic training, but often served as a referral point for hospital care and were often bypassed.

[b] Diseases accounting for the highest rates of mortality, morbidity and disability.

and remedial measures, either through additional support or fines, are taken. Responsiveness (measured through patient surveys) has improved, with patients consistently providing high scores for various quality indicators in most family practices[6,18].

While recognizing the positive effects of large-scale change, health worker retention is perceived as a major threat to efforts to improve health. Before independence, the Ministry of Health assigned medical graduates to compulsory service in rural areas for five years, but, according to many respondents, after the transition, financial and non-financial incentives to attract and retain personnel in remote areas have failed. Remuneration of health workers has remained low by national standards; a general practitioner's salary is the equivalent of US$ 80 a month, below the minimum monthly consumption basket per person, forcing many health professionals to leave the health system or look for additional sources of income[22]. While planned reductions in health care workers through early retirement and reallocation created savings in some areas, currently, shortages and uneven distribution of staff are visible.

The health workforce is getting older and only 20% to 30% of all graduates are employed in rural areas, with many migrating to urban areas or abroad. The shortage of personnel in rural primary health care facilities has increased the workload for remaining staff, undermining their retention. In addition, wealthier neighbouring countries, such as Russia and Kazakhstan, seek to attract highly trained doctors and nurses through better salaries and more attractive benefit packages and working conditions. Migration is facilitated by the widespread use of the Russian language. The relocation of staff from rural to urban areas in search of better work conditions has exacerbated the shortages in rural areas.

> ...We have spent a lot of World Bank money – about US$ 3.5 million – to retrain former internists and paediatricians to become family doctors at family group practices (FGPs). But more than one thousand of them went abroad. We have now 56 FGPs without any doctors and in 158 FGPs we have just one doctor instead of three or four, serving up to 12 000 people instead of 1500 as planned. This affects accessibility and quality. The fact that these people are hired in Russia, and given a residence permit and housing, demonstrates that they are quite well-trained and experienced.
>
> *Ministry of Health representative*

The respondents demonstrated a widely shared belief that developing a well-integrated family practice is complex and will take time. Training the new cadre is important but has to be accompanied by better infrastructure and laboratory diagnostic capacity at primary health care facilities, especially in rural areas, to reduce the bypassing of first-line facilities. Reorienting the system towards comprehensive primary health care has unintentionally increased the workload of family doctors, with limited capacity to support them, while reducing the workload of district specialists. Reporting on vertical programmes has also increased dramatically, decreasing doctors time to treat patients.

Vital role for mid-level cadre and community workers

The role of front-line health workers has been critical in rapidly scaling up family practice. Approximately one quarter of Kyrgyzstan's population is located in remote rural areas, and settlements with populations of 500 to 2000 people are still served by *feldsher*–midwifery posts, which were widespread in the Soviet system. They are staffed by at least one paramedic (*feldsher*), and in larger villages, by a midwife and a nurse. They provide basic curative, antenatal and postnatal care, vaccinations and health promotion. Deliveries take place in the nearest general health care centre or district hospital. Most of the posts have been renovated and re-equipped, and staff has been retrained, contributing to improved accessibility and quality of health services in remote areas.

Kyrgyzstan is unique in the former USSR in its use of non-medically trained community workers organized in village health committees. These committees have played a vital role in the health reform programme, supporting service delivery in underserved areas. The initiative, funded by the Swiss Agency for Development and Cooperation, the Swedish International Development Cooperation Agency and USAID, started in 2001, and by 2009, there were more than 1400 such committees, covering about 86% of all villages and about 2.5 million people (almost half the population). Village health committees are independent community-based organizations whose members work as volunteers. They are trained by primary care staff to implement health and prevention activities prioritized by their communities, including promotion of iodized salt and good nutrition, control of brucellosis, hygiene education, the reduction of alcohol abuse, hypertension control and sexual and reproductive health.

The work carried out by village health committees is believed to have had a positive effect on the health of the population, contributing to an increase in exclusive breastfeeding during the first six months, for instance, and a decrease in goitre prevalence among school students[13]. Committee members are valued locally by both the residents and the authorities and they have given rural communities some decision-making power over local health services. Village health committees are seen as innovative low-cost mechanisms to implement priority public health initiatives and create sustainable partnerships between rural communities and the government health system.

Rationalization of infrastructure

Throughout the *Manas* programme (1996–2006), primary care infrastructure was strengthened mainly through government and donor funding. At the same time, there was a major restructuring of obsolete and excessive infrastructure in the hospital sector. Hospital rationalization was among the first priorities, along with the linking of budget allocation to actual performance rather than to inputs such as beds. Hospitals were given an opportunity to decide which part of their infrastructure they should downsize to reduce utility costs, and were given incentives to improve efficiency, measured by bed turnover. From 2000 to 2003, 42% of buildings and 35% of floor space were reduced[23], the largest initiative of its kind in the former USSR. This, combined with planned facility closures, significantly reduced recurrent expenditure and led to an increased share of resources for patient treatment and care rather than for hospital maintenance (this allowed the budget for care under the basic benefits package to increase from 20.4% of hospital expenditure in 2004 to 32.7% in 2007).

New financing mechanisms

Together with restructuring health service delivery, changes in health system financing have been the cornerstones of post-Soviet reform. There has been widespread agreement that improving the population's financial protection and access to care have been consistent policy goals from the start and among Kyrgyzstan's most important achievements. Financial protection was seen as necessary to promote equitable use of essential services as well as to reduce the financial burden caused by paying for health care. The results have been impressive. By 2005, almost universal coverage was provided for all citizens of Kyrgyzstan (through insurance or budgetary funds) with specified vulnerable groups entitled to essential services at no charge. As a result, access to care is expanding. Out-of-pocket and informal payments[c] are declining and becoming more equitable. However, these changes cannot be attributed to increased resources invested in the health sector. Kyrgyzstan's total health expenditure per capita has been consistently the second lowest, after Tajikistan, among the CIS countries (Figure 5.5). Public health expenditure as a percentage of total government expenditure in Kyrgyzstan has remained relatively stable over time, and is also among the lowest in the region, even below countries that have suffered conflict and extreme economic shocks, such as Georgia and Armenia. This suggests that health improvements cannot be explained simply by more government resources spent on health (as a share of GDP or of the public budget).

---

[c] Informal payments are defined as unofficial monetary or in-kind transactions, mainly in the public sector, between a patient and a staff member for services that are officially free of charge.

Figure 5.5   Total health expenditure, WHO estimates

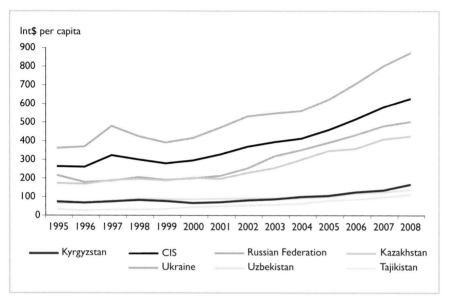

Source: Reference 8.

The next section explains some of the factors that promoted positive results, implemented within the framework of the *Manas* and *Manas Taalimi* programmes. These include:

- providing mandatory health insurance and a basic benefits package;

- addressing out-of-pocket payments for services;

- and improving risk-pooling arrangements through improved resource allocation.

Mandatory health insurance

The most fundamental change to financial protection was the shift from a Soviet-style system financed through general government revenues to a system that combines general taxation and mandatory health insurance. The Kyrgyz experience is in contrast with other CIS countries, which had limited success in implementing health insurance.

The Kyrgyz Mandatory Health Insurance Fund (MHIF) was established in 1997 with the aim of safeguarding resources for health care. Premiums are deducted via a payroll tax (2% paid by the employer), or allocated by the government for those who are unable to contribute. Farmers working on their own land are required to contribute the equivalent of 5% of their land tax for health insurance. Health insurance coverage is over 80% despite the large rural population working in agriculture.

As reported by senior designers of the reform programme, the strategy's core goal was to ensure equity and accessibility of health services for the poorest in the country, including those in rural and remote regions. This was supported by a shift from reliance on arbitrary top-down state funding to a solidarity-based model based on cross-subsidies among population groups:

> *A principle of solidarity, where the rich pay for the poor, the young pay for the old, the employed pay for the unemployed, and the healthy pay for the sick – we were talking about health insurance. And all these things seemed to be impossible, but we achieved them.*
> *Former senior policy-maker in the Ministry of Health*

In conjunction with mandatory insurance, a State Guaranteed Benefits Package (SGBP)[d] was introduced in 2000, ensuring free health services for certain population groups who previously had to pay (formally or informally) to access them. The SGBP is revised annually, with a number of subsidized categories or levels of compensation gradually expanding. Initially, free services were provided for infants and pregnant women, and for childbirth. In 2007, the package was extended to children under 5 and those over 75.

The SGBP seeks to promote essential primary care services for all, and hospital services for certain groups of people; it also defines citizen's rights to receive free care. The SGBP represents an increasing share of public health expenditure, rising from 26.4% in 2004 to 37.9% in 2007. The regional distribution of expenditures under the SGBP has also become more equal. Along with the SGBP, an Additional Drug Package[18], which subsidizes essential drugs in outpatient facilities, has much popular support and been crucial in increasing demand for primary care and access to essential drugs in remote areas.

The introduction of the basic benefits package was a result of effective intersectoral collaboration between parliamentarians and civil society. It was a political decision agreed upon by multiple actors rather than one made by the Ministry of Health. Moreover, the SGBP was financed from multiple sources. The Ministry of Finance provided funds for the population groups covered and the MHIF introduced it.

---

[d] The SGBP is a regulatory document issued by the state that defines the scope of health services provided to citizens free of charge or on an exempted basis.

Shifting from a tax-based system to a mixed system funded by tax revenue and mandatory insurance, institutionalizing universal coverage, and providing a guaranteed essential care package have been key to improving access to essential services and increasing equity.

Implementation of the SGBP and the Additional Drugs Package has been hampered by migration, which leads to women not being registered at their place of residence, and consequently, not registered in a health facility at all. According to the Law on State Guaranteed Benefit Package, within the framework of *Manas Taalimi*, a pregnant woman should be registered automatically even without registration of her home address; nevertheless, awareness of this policy is low.

Tackling direct payments for care

During the communist regime, there were few direct payments for health care. However, after independence, out-of-pocket (including informal) payments became endemic[24]. Such payments have often served to fill resource gaps in public budgets and have been critical for sustaining basic health care provision. Kyrgyzstan has an intermediary position in the region in terms of out-of-pocket and informal payments, lower than Tajikistan, whose system collapsed in the 1990s, and Georgia, where health care is predominantly privately financed (Figure 5.6). Payments are most widespread for inpatient care[25]. Despite some recent declines, there are concerns that these payments may limit access to care despite universal coverage. A household survey conducted in 2007 showed that those households reporting it "difficult" or "very difficult" to find the money to pay for health care employed coping strategies such as reducing consumption, using savings, borrowing money from relatives, and depleting household resources[25].

Informally paying for health care is particularly damaging as it can reverse achievements in financial protection. Kyrgyzstan has undertaken the only documented measures in central and eastern Europe and the former USSR seeking to reduce the burden of informal payments. This involved changing provider payment mechanisms, tighter accountability, complaints channels and the introduction of formal co-payments nationwide[26].

As a result of these initiatives, informal payments in Kyrgyzstan significantly declined in real terms between 2001 and 2006, especially for medicines and supplies. Seventy per cent of all hospitalized patients paid medical personnel in 2001 and 52% paid in 2006; 81% of hospitalized patients paid for drugs in 2001, and 51% in 2006[18]. The main reason for the decrease is efficiency savings created by budget pooling (single payer). Reductions in informal payment were

Figure 5.6   Total private households' out-of-pocket payments on health as a percentage of total health expenditure

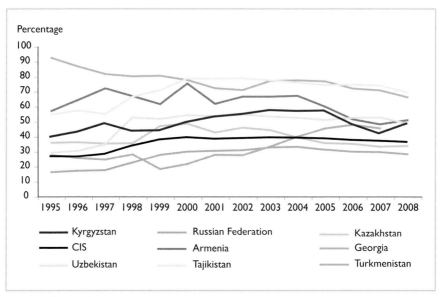

Source: Reference 8.

not fully offset by the introduction of co-payments, with 40% of patients paying both co-payments and informal payments[18]. However, declines of this magnitude are not seen in other parts of the region and are shown to have a significant impact on affordability. Despite the still high level of out-of-pocket payments, visits to family practices increased by 36% and hospitalization rates rose by 18% in 2005–2007. However, informal payments still made up 26–34% of total health expenditures for hospital care in 2006[18]. The persistence of these payments indicates that there is a funding gap that is still not covered by public funding and co-payments. It may also point to lack of trust in the official system and cultural preferences[18]. Nevertheless, despite temporary setbacks, there is a longer-term decline in informal payments that is not apparent in other countries in the region. Health expenditure is also becoming more equitable and financial and geographic barriers to care have decreased; the share of those who needed but did not seek care in the past month because care was "too expensive" or "too far" fell from 11.2% to 3.1% between 2001 and 2006[13]. In fact, the largest reductions in financial burden on the patient were among the poorest quintile (out-of-pocket health expenditure for this group was 7.1% of the annual household budget in 2004 compared with 4.9% in 2006)[6].

Improved resource allocation

There have also been steps to ensure that available funds are used optimally. A major component of reform was strengthening risk pooling at regional level. Since 2001, the MHIF has been responsible for pooling the health budget funds at *oblast* level (single payer system), merging funding streams from insurance, state and regional budgets into a single pool in order to address socioeconomic and health differences[27]. In addition, amendments to existing laws were rapidly enacted to support defragmentation of funding, which permitted a surprisingly quick implementation process.

Major advances were undertaken in purchasing, and both the MHIF and Ministry of Health became purchasers in their areas of responsibility. These changes aim to ensure that all services in the SGBP are covered by the government budget. There have been efforts to move to strategic purchasing based on projections of the need for medical services.

Changes in resource allocation and the introduction of contracting have also taken place. Under the Soviet system, hospitals were financed according to the number of beds, and staff and managers had limited autonomy to allocate resources according to need[28]. The shift to mandatory social insurance involved the testing and introduction of progressive payment methods for health services. First, case-based payments in hospitals and capitation in primary care were introduced. However, the increased coverage of the population and the existence of multiple financing sources (budget, insurance, local) prompted introduction of a single payer system in 2001–2004, creating single pools of funds at *oblast* level that included local budget funds and transfers from the national budget and reducing fragmentation. Uniform provider payments methods were introduced, which provided incentives for strengthening primary care, for example through an integrated capitation payment for services in family practices. This may have encouraged extensive hospital downsizing. Initially, the new financing mechanisms were piloted in two *oblasts*, and after 2004, were scaled up nationally. This set of sophisticated initiatives places Kyrgyzstan ahead of many countries with similar income levels that spend more on health care. It also shows coherence among different reform components seeking to uphold access and equity. However, despite the far-reaching transformation of health system financing, progress is still limited by relatively low public health spending (despite some increases since 2006), mainly used to cover utility and some operational costs (medical supplies, drugs and salaries), with almost no resources for preventive interventions and equipment. Despite intentions to allocate resources according to need, the financing of peripheral primary health care services is limited.

■ Political context

This section describes a set of wider policy factors – political and economic – that enabled Kyrgyzstan to design and implement the ambitious reforms of the health system described in the previous section. These factors help to explain the improvements in health and access to essential services relative to the income level of the country.

The pressure to reform

As one of the 15 countries of the former USSR, Kyrgyzstan's policies in the health and social sectors historically reflect Soviet principles stipulating free comprehensive health care for all, subsidized from Moscow. In the early 1990s, trade agreements and guaranteed subsidies ended, triggering a severe economic crisis, and by 1995, the country's real GDP was approximately half its 1989 level. Government spending decreased by 67% between 1990 and 1996[29]. Since 2001, the country has been classified as a low-income country with a GDP per capita of US$ 433[29]. Interestingly, while this decline was accompanied by a reduction in absolute income levels and a rise in poverty[30], Kyrgyzstan had the most rapid decrease in inequality in the former Soviet countries, as measured by the Gini index[2].

The fall in public spending threatened its many achievements in health, education and social protection. Hospitals did not have enough resources to function, and allocated less and less from their budgets to primary care (at the time, regional hospitals allocated resources to all facilities in their regions). The primary care situation became critical: in addition to high staff turnover, there were no supplies or drugs, malfunctioning equipment and restricted emergency transportation. Only limited diagnosis and treatment were possible.

Resources available to the health sector fell from 4% of GDP in 1991 to 1.9% of GDP in 2002[23]. A huge infrastructure and a large number of doctors meant that most state funding had to be spent on utilities and staff salaries (75–91% of the total health budget). Water supply and sanitation were often inadequate; bed linens and food in hospitals were not available. Lack of funds for medication (90% of drugs are imported), maintenance and the procurement and operation of new laboratory and diagnostic equipment resulted in severe deterioration in the quality of health services, particularly in rural areas. The health system was meeting people's needs less and less. Prompted by the serious situation in the health sector and the concurrent economic crisis, the Ministry of Health implemented the *Manas* (1996–2006) and *Manas Taalimi* (2006–2010) programmes, which involved radical restructuring of the health system. These structural reforms were widely regarded as the only way to keep the system afloat.

> *It was a coercive measure; the country faced a difficult economic situation right after its independence, health-financing reforms were needed due to fragmentation and duplication of health care delivery, inefficient methods of financing and the need to maintain bulky infrastructure....*
>
> Government expert

Donors played an important role supporting reforms, particularly in health financing; however, neither the design nor the implementation was donor driven. To develop *Manas Taalimi*, the Ministry of Health, together with WHO, hired a qualified team of six independent experts who worked closely with the Ministry. The strategy was developed during six months of extensive consultations at all policy-making levels.

Kyrgyzstan's health sector reacted more rapidly than other sectors to the political, social and economic changes taking place and was among the first of the former Soviet countries to introduce a long-term reform programme.

Political independence as a window of opportunity

After independence, the rebuilding of the state institutions and social reforms were seen as a "historical necessity" (a phrase used by a key informant in an interview) and were supported at the highest political level. Political momentum enabled the country to make ambitious changes more rapidly than neighbouring countries. In the health sector, powerful individuals and the elite lobbied for health sector reforms, with the understanding that if the status quo was maintained, the health system would deteriorate even more than during the initial post-independence collapse of 1994/1995. As a result, in mid-1996, there was political impetus for radical steps to be undertaken, as the first President, Askar Akayev, declared health system reform a priority.

Early in its independence, Kyrgyzstan was perceived as one of the most politically open countries in central Asia, with a quickly emerging civil society. The country has become a regional centre for donors and international organizations. In 1998, Kyrgyzstan was the first CIS country to be accepted into the World Trade Organization and it was also the first country of the former USSR to introduce its own currency. The first President's policy of engagement with the global health community and interest in evidence-based strategies helped to attract international assistance. The public administration's openness and pragmatism played an important role in the rapid implementation of comprehensive and evidence-based reform programmes and ensured that those programmes were consistent with international targets. For example, efforts and close communication by the government and key donors ensured that *Manas Taalimi* was aligned with the achievement of the Millennium Development Goals (MDGs).

However, since independence, there have also been occasions when political events threatened to disrupt public sector reforms. During President Askar Akayev's final years, the openness policy and democratic changes were challenged. In March 2005, a popular revolt against perceived corruption and authoritarian policies, coupled with controversial parliamentary elections, forced Akayev to resign (the Tulip Revolution). In April 2010, Kyrgyzstan's second president and government were overthrown amid widespread allegations of corruption, dictatorship, nepotism and a worsening economy. In May and June 2010, ethnic conflict led to killings and destruction; international involvement was sought. Despite political and ethnic turmoil, in October 2010, parliamentary elections were held, leading to a coalition government in December 2010.

It is remarkable that, despite these political challenges, health sector reforms were not disrupted and continuity and institutional stability have been maintained. Kyrgyzstan's major strategic documents, including the Comprehensive Development Framework until 2010, the National Poverty Reduction Strategy for 2003–2005 and the Country Development Strategy, indicate that development of the health system was a priority among other public sectors. In addition to a clear political commitment to improving health, existing managerial capacity was crucial. For set periods, there were restrictions on firing civil servants and technical experts, allowing many health system administrators to remain in place and continue the long-term reforms.

Legal and regulatory change as key facilitating factors

A legal framework built on three main laws has helped to guarantee sustainability of health reforms, even during times of political upheaval and economic difficulties[31–33]. One law regulates the provision of health services to the population[31]; a second regulates how health organizations (facilities) operate[32]; and a third regulates new arrangements for the flow of funds and new provider payment mechanisms[33]. Additionally, all changes to the health system were introduced through the development and formal approval of regulatory documents and norms and standards.

This supportive legal and regulatory framework enabled the comprehensive *Manas* reform. With strong support from the first president and knowledgeable and committed individuals and interest groups in the health sector, Kyrgyzstan was able to enact legislation rapidly, paving the way for mandatory insurance. In other former Soviet countries, a slow and inefficient legislative process obstructed reform implementation. It should be noted that, along with donors' support, the International Monetary Fund (IMF) also bolstered the implementation of health financing reforms. When the MHIF could not obtain its payroll money from the Social Fund, which gathered payroll tax on behalf of the MHIF, the IMF intervened with the condition that unless the Social Fund transferred funds to the MHIF, the country would not receive further support from the IMF.

Some laws addressed the wider determinants of health. For example, laws were adopted that obligated flour manufacturers to fortify flour with iron and salt with iodine. Similarly, a law on the protection of breastfeeding and regulation of marketing of substitutes of breast milk was approved in 2006[34], the result of lobbying by health system representatives, lawyers, the nongovernmental sector, researchers, paediatricians, parliamentarians and community representatives.

The timely introduction of other laws facilitated health reforms. Thus, some of the modifications in health financing were made possible due to the adoption of the law on *Financial and Economic Foundations of Local Self-Government* (2003)[35], simplifying the budgeting process. This allowed the introduction of the single payer system, which is core to the health system reform.

Effective research-to-policy channels

Another important factor was the introduction of an effective research-to-policy process, which helped to shorten the lag between innovation and implementation (Figure 5.7). The policy process in the health sector over two decades has passed almost two full cycles, going from defining the problem and identifying the options available, to making political decisions, to piloting innovative designs and learning from evidence, to evaluating and redesigning, to scaling up and, finally, to embedding the reforms in the legal, regulatory framework. In 2000, the monitoring and evaluation function was undertaken with technical assistance from the WHO and financial assistance from the United Kingdom Department for International Development (DFID); in 2006, the Health Policy Analysis and Monitoring Unit was integrated into the Ministry of Health's structure. Knowledgeable and committed individuals in the health sector facilitated the incorporation of monitoring and evaluation into routine operations, meeting policy-makers' demand for evidence to use in policy formulation and monitoring.

The Health Policy Analysis Center, a public–private institute established in 2009, conducts health policy and systems research in close collaboration with

Figure 5.7   Features of the policy cycle in Kyrgyzstan

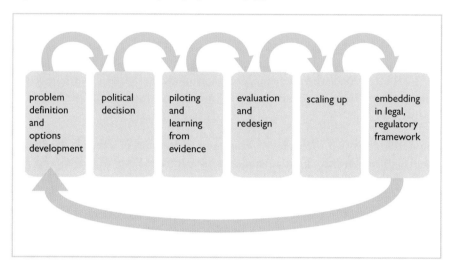

government and donors to inform policy development. Monthly and annual monitoring of performance of health facilities aims to identify problem areas, understand the reasons and improve the situation. These analyses were possible due to investment in multilevel information systems, standardized protocols for reporting and networks for data sharing.

Until recently, the existence of a dedicated unit to connect the policy process with monitoring and evaluation was unique in Kyrgyzstan among the CIS countries. The same function now has been replicated in Tajikistan (2007), Azerbaijan (2008) and the Republic of Moldova (2010), with assistance from WHO-EURO and input from the Health Policy Analysis Center.

Nature of the policy process

Sustained progress in health reform in Kyrgyzstan is the result of a number of characteristics of the political process, including comprehensiveness, continuity, accountability and transparency, intersectoral cooperation, multi-stakeholder engagement and donor coordination.

The comprehensive *Manas* reform programme demonstrated vision and, despite its broad system-wide objectives, had achievable goals and clearly operationalized objectives not found elsewhere in the region. According to the majority of respondents, creating essential structures and mechanisms (especially in health financing) enabled faster and more effective reform implementation, helping to gain support among key stakeholders and increasing motivation among front-line providers. The changes in health financing demonstrated vision and ambition, as well as the ability to sequence multiple steps along the path towards the main goal.

Continuity was also widely seen to have been important in promoting sustainability. Despite political volatility threatening to derail the reform process (new policy-makers/parliamentarians came into power in 2002 and 2006 and there was political unrest), the reform process has continued with support from powerful individuals such as the first president, along with committed technical experts who remained involved during the entire period. For example, it was emphasized that *Manas Taalimi* (2006–2010) was:

> *... based on continuity and targets cultivating the achieved results under the Manas programme and further development of the sector*
>
> Ministry of Health experts

Accountability and transparency were explicitly built into the policy process across all public sectors soon after independence. As a result, indicators of equity, transparency, accessibility and responsiveness of the health system were monitored throughout the *Manas* programme and were shown to have improved[6]. In 2000, transparency was identified as an important issue in the health and finance sectors. In 2002, the government responded with a five-year governance and financial management project funded by DFID. This aimed to increase accountability and transparency of public expenditures through improving budget formulation, enhancing revenue collection and strengthening internal audits. This led to a considerably simplified public health budget in 2006.

The successful implementation of *Manas* was supported by social development programmes and other initiatives beyond the health system. All respondents interviewed described comprehensive intersectoral cooperation, facilitated centrally by a Coordination Council set up by the government and chaired by the vice prime minister, and at *oblast* level, through Coordination Commissions for Health Administration.

There are many documented cases of multi-stakeholder engagement and effective donor coordination explicitly promoted by the government. The health reform programmes were initiated by the Ministry of Health, supported by development partners, and priorities were identified through a consultative process. The *Manas Taalimi* programme was implemented in the framework of a sector-wide approach (SWAp), the first of its kind in former Soviet countries[36].

Implementation was evaluated twice a year during joint annual reviews, and recommendations were discussed at health summits.

These processes enabled strong partnerships among government and non-government sectors and international organizations, and encouraged participation by local communities and the mass media. This has facilitated understanding, acceptance and support by the population. It is a widely shared view that bringing all the donors active in the health sector to a common platform under government leadership has helped to improve efficiency in investments in health systems, achieve synergies across the sector and emphasize the joint responsibility for the gradual expansion of pilot projects.

Effective coordination and collaboration was unique in this region to Kyrgyzstan, partly explained by knowledgeable and committed individuals in the health sector who were able to exert political influence. A culture of pragmatism and a supportive institutional environment, combined with mutual trust among actors and interest in partnerships and joint action, were also commonly reported by key stakeholders.

◼ Beyond the health system: what can explain Kyrgyzstan's achievements?

This section reviews a number of contextual features that may have influenced health gains and effective health care reforms. Many of these factors relate to the characteristics of the country and its people.

The human factor: inspirational leaders and ideas

Kyrgyzstan's improved health outcomes and stronger health system are frequently attributed to human resource capacity at three levels. The first is the presence of strong national leaders (particularly the president) and institutions in the health sector and beyond. The first Kyrgyz President Askar Akaev was highly educated and interested in innovations and policy change.

> ...the role of personality in the history of the country is a cornerstone for promoting the changes in the country.... It is important how the leader in this or that sector is educated and committed to reforms. If he/she is then the changes could be developed and introduced quickly in the country.... An example is Askar Akaev, first President of Kyrgyzstan
>
> Respondent from the former governor's office

Second, a number of powerful individuals and elites lobbied for reforms in the health sector, reflecting concerns about severe deterioration and even collapse of the health system. Third, there was strong capacity in the Ministry of Health and other executive agencies, aided by relatively low turnover and intensive efforts in capacity building by donor agencies. As mentioned above, charismatic actors with a long-term commitment in the health system played an important role in sustaining the reform process.

> *...during 1997–2005, a few times the reforms were under threat because new parliamentarians, policy-makers came to power who were not aware about health reforms. The strong technical team in the health sector that was in place at that time did not let them destroy what had been done already via educating them about the rationale behind the health reforms...*
>
> *Donor representative*

It is the predominant view that well-educated, motivated and committed individuals, trained during the former Soviet period, were instrumental to reforms soon after independence and to sustaining momentum often in difficult circumstances. In many rural areas of the country, older health care professionals effectively sustained a basic service.

> *We probably have to pay them credit that 70% of all health professionals are people with an old Soviet mentality, and they are very dedicated to their work. Notwithstanding the fact that they have been wearing the same shoes for 15 years, that they have holes in their purses, and that they cannot afford to spend money for fun, they cannot turn their backs on their patients. Therefore, probably by virtue of their education ... they cannot leave their jobs and their quite modest salaries, and they bear the burden, although at the same time this is their calling, and they do that throughout their whole life ...*
>
> *Ministry of Health official*

Economic growth

After the crisis of the 1990s, Kyrgyzstan benefited from significant economic growth, resulting in increases in income and a decline in poverty rates between 2000 and 2007 (Figure 5.8). Sound economic policies have ensured macroeconomic stability. In 2007, economic growth was particularly strong: real GDP growth rate of 8.7% was the highest recorded in the previous ten years. Growth did not benefit all population groups equally, as it was accompanied by a 20% rise in consumer prices, particularly for food, which usually hits the poorest

Figure 5.8 Trends in GDP per capita and poverty rate, 2000–2009

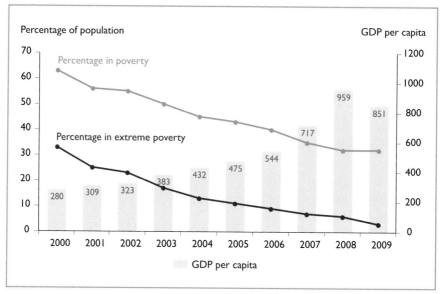

Source: Adapted from reference 6.

groups. However, recent household surveys indicate that poorer households increased their consumption more than other income groups[6].

The more promising economic situation and the resulting improvement in water and sanitation, nutrition and living conditions may explain, on the one hand, decreases in child mortality. On the other hand, maternal mortality, which is more dependent on the health system and has been associated with high informal payments, has stagnated.

Empowerment of women

The role of women in Kyrgyz society has increased during the past decade. In 2007, a special amendment was made to the "Election Code of the Kyrgyz Republic", mandating the inclusion of women in government structures. There is now a minimum quota of 30% representation of women in parliament and the auditing chamber[37,38]. In 2008, Kyrgyzstan had more women in parliament (26.6%) and government (21%) than any other central Asian country[39]. In many cases, female parliamentarians have helped to prioritize health issues.

This represents considerable progress considering that in 2005 there were no women in parliament and just one woman in a senior government position[39]. In

2010, Roza Otunbayeva was elected President of Kyrgyzstan, the first time a woman has held such a position in central Asia; and the Constitutional and the Supreme Courts of Kyrgyzstan are headed by women. In public institutions and in the judicial system, representation is almost equal, although women occupy more junior positions than men.

Freedom of movement for women and physical access to health facilities is relatively good, which may be the reason for the high utilization of maternal and child services, and for nearly universal births in health facilities.

Historically, due to the influence of the Muslim religion, some central Asian countries shared the belief that education was necessary for men but not women. However, in Kyrgyzstan, these beliefs have not been prevalent, and families have invested equally in the education of girls and boys. The literacy rate is almost 100%, with only small regional and ethnic variations. For the 2006/2007 school year, net enrolment in primary education was about 88% and enrolment in secondary education was approximately 85% (similar for both sexes)[39]. In 2002/2003, just over a half of the students enrolled in higher education were women[40].

Alongside these achievements, however, are concerns about the actual quality of the schooling provided[41,42]. Stereotypes still prevail and women who pursue higher education typically choose gender-specific training, opting for education, health care and social sciences. There are also equity concerns because enrolment, attendance and educational performance of children are lower in rural areas compared with urban areas. Other problems include low teachers' salaries, a shortage of free textbooks, deteriorating infrastructure of schools and poor quality in rural areas.

In addition, women lost many benefits following the break-up of the USSR. The government's system of support for working women is insufficient. Since independence, the closure of affordable state-run child care services means that women are faced with a double burden of caring for their children and working to contribute to the family income often with limited support from employers. Social benefits have been eroded in value (in 2008 the child benefit was US$ 15 per child per month)[40]. Maternal mortality and reproductive health are impacted by the severe workload of pregnant women, who are traditionally responsible for household duties and care for family members, combined with income-generating activities in the informal sector.

Early and consanguineous marriages also have a negative influence on maternal and child health and education opportunities. These are growing, with severe consequences for pregnancy and morbidity. There are 11 to 12 marriages registered officially each year in which the bride is under 16 years and about 300 cases when a bride is under 17; however, there are indications that many marriages in this age group are not registered with the authorities[40]. Raising the minimum age of marriage from 16 to 17 years is currently being considered.

On the positive side, the total fertility rate has shown a dramatic decline: from 4.9 in 1970, to 3.6 in 1991, and to 2.8 in 2008[8]. This is unprecedented in central Asia. In addition, there are signs of progress regarding lowered fertility rates in women aged 15 to 17, with a reduction of 60% in recent years. Also, in 2004, the age group between 20 and 29 years accounted for more than 60% of the births in the country[43].

The use of contraceptives has increased. Traditionally, as a result of the limited supply and affordability of contraceptives before independence, women in central Asia relied on legal abortion for birth control[41], which only requires consent of the pregnant woman to be performed[44]. Modern contraceptive use increased from 30% in 1990 to 47.8% in 2005[5], attributed to the wide dissemination of information about family planning from NGOs and other aid agencies.

However, growth in traditional and religious beliefs and values, and a weak system of improving awareness about sexual health issues, means that investment in family planning and use of contraceptives needs strengthening. In recent years, materials promoting home deliveries and refusal of contraception have started to appear in the mass media and there are reports that in 2009 these were generated by religious organizations operating in the south of Kyrgyzstan, which shares borders with more religious countries such as Uzbekistan and Tajikistan.

Trust and solidarity

Despite multiple political changes, health sector reform benefited from high levels of public trust in the country's institutions. In 2002, representative surveys showed that citizens in Kyrgyzstan trusted institutions such as the government, the parliament and the president much more than citizens in any of a group of eight former Soviet countries, which may have led to more support for reform (*Living Conditions, Lifestyle and Health Surveys*, unpublished data, 2001; authors' calculations from private area of website http://www.llh.at/, accessed 14 March 2011). However, this may have changed following the political instability in more recent years. In addition, Kyrgyzstan has been rated the most receptive country for setting up new businesses due to its regulatory framework, considered trustworthy and supportive compared with regional standards[45]. Kyrgyzstan is the only central Asian country to have both Soviet and US military bases, which may be interpreted as an indicator of political openness[46].

Social factors that contribute to good health in Kyrgyzstan include solidarity and the ability to draw on family relationships in order to access care. However, reliance on information provided through informal channels may be problematic; recent studies reveal that parents do not recognize dangerous disease symptoms in their children and seek health care late, a major concern in some areas.

Kyrgyzstan is the second most ethnically diverse country in the region[3]. All citizens of Kyrgyzstan – irrespective of their ethnicity – have access to health care services. However, the influx of refugees (for example, in the 1990s and early 2000s from Tajikistan) created barriers to accessing health care, as the migrants were not citizens of Kyrgyzstan and had to pay out of pocket. This has been addressed, for example by a joint Ministry of Health and United Nations High Commissioner for Refugees programme for the integration of Tajik refugees into the national health system in 2002–2009, with 8000 refugees included in the mandatory health insurance system[47].

■ Lessons learned and future challenges

Kyrgyzstan has maintained or slightly improved the health of its population despite periods of political and economic turmoil, including severe cuts in public spending on health. As this study has demonstrated, this was possible because soon after independence in 1991, the government and donors moved quickly to build the foundations of a strong health system. This vision was manifested in the comprehensive *Manas* and *Manas Taalimi* reform programmes, which radically restructured the health system and linked reforms to measurable outcomes. Despite two major revolutions and economic crises, as well as a change in leadership, the reform programmes provided a solid base for long-term health system strengthening, and spurred action by government agencies and donors. This contrasts with the experience in other countries of the former USSR.

The first reform plan, *Manas* (1996–2006), provided a stable and coherent framework to channel donor investment into the health sector (thereby avoiding programme verticalization), and to coordinate efforts by different national and international agencies under government leadership. *Manas* led to a shift from specialist-oriented care to family practice, implementing a basic benefits package, promoting health financing reform through contracting and a consolidated single payer system, and liberalizing the pharmaceutical market. Rationalizing hospital care has also been part of the reform. The process of policy change built on the positive features of the former Soviet model, preserving the value of universal coverage and access to affordable care for all, made reforms popular. There was an understanding that addressing health needs

---

Box 5.3 Future challenges

- High levels of noncommunicable and chronic disease

- Low public health spending

- Persistence of out-of-pocket and informal payments (despite the formal guarantee of free access to a basic package of health care)

- Growing migration (both internally and externally), which hinders access to and use of health services

- Political instability

- Health worker retention

- Need for better financial protection and equity in the system, particularly for disadvantaged population groups.

---

requires broader developmental strategies that encompass health and other sectors.

While the reforms in both *Manas* and *Manas Taalimi* focused on interventions in priority health areas, strategic elements strengthened the overall health system, enabling effective implementation, including planning and monitoring. This was made possible through consistent government leadership and support for health system reforms, the coordination of multiple actors, national ownership, a comprehensive approach – including financing as well as other health system building blocks – and community involvement. Reform design and implementation have benefited from continuity and strong human resource capacity in the health sector (both clinical and managerial) and in the government. Key figures remained in leading administrative roles and were a driving force of radical policy change. Many of these elements were unique for Kyrgyzstan among its neighbours. The health system is considered a model of good practice in central Asia and certain features are being replicated throughout the region. Nevertheless, efforts need to be continued with a heightened focus on current challenges (Box 5.3).

The Kyrgyz experience illustrates the advantages of investing in health sector development, improving the legal and regulatory framework, promoting accountability and recognizing the crucial role of strong leadership and coordination among sectors and actors. Tangible improvements have been achieved in health and affordability of essential care and in addressing the needs of disadvantaged population groups. Good outcomes can be traced to practices and political processes reflecting good governance and a political culture of openness.

By continuing this positive trend and concentrating on current challenges, achievements can be not only sustained but consolidated.

ACKNOWLEDGEMENTS

The authors are grateful to all those interviewed for providing their truthful views, experience and comments on the historical development of the health system in Kyrgyzstan. These included local and international specialists/experts working in the social and health sectors in Kyrgyzstan, NGO specialists as well as current and former policy-makers involved in health policy formulation in the government and the Ministry of Health.

Special thanks are extended Joe Kutzin and Melitta Jakab (WHO Regional Office for Europe) for providing input during preparation of this chapter and reviewing its final version.

Jenny Maisonneuve made a significant contribution to this chapter, specifically on the section on non-health factors and the role of gender.

In addition, this chapter was written by the team drawing on local and international reports, peer-reviewed and other published papers, and on the extensive experience of the principle investigator, Ainura Ibraimova, who was Deputy Minister of Health and Director of the MHIF.

Our deep gratitude is extended to the team at the London School of Hygiene & Tropical Medicine who provided technical assistance and supported this work. In addition, thanks to colleagues from the other study countries (Bangladesh, Ethiopia, Tamil Nadu (India) and Thailand) who provided their comments and inspiration while developing this chapter.

REFERENCES

1. Ibraimova A, Akkazieva B et al. Kyrgyzstan: Health system review. *Health Systems in Transition*, 2011; 13(3):1–152 (http://www.euro.who.int/__data/assets/pdf_file/0017/142613/e95045.pdf).

2. World Bank. *World development indicators* [online database]. Washington, DC: World Bank, 2011 (http://data.worldbank.org/indicator, accessed 12 July 2011).

3. CIA. *The world factbook* [online database]. Washington, DC: Central Intelligence Agency; 2010 (https://www.cia.gov/library/publications/the-world-factbook/geos/kg.html, accessed August 2010).

4. WHO. *World health statistics* [online database]. Geneva: World Health Organization; 2010 (http://www.who.int/whosis/whostat/en/).

5. National Statistical Committee of the Kyrgyz Republic/UNICEF. *Multiple indicator cluster survey (MICS) Kyrgyz Republic, 2006: monitoring the situation of children and women*. Bishkek: National Statistical Committee/United Nations Children's Fund; 2007.

6. Ministry of Health. *Evaluation of national health programme "Manas Taalimi"*. Bishkek: Ministry of Health; 2011.

7. UNICEF. [online database] New York: United Nations Children's Fund; 2011 (http://www.unicef.org/infobycountry/kyrgyzstan_statistics.html#76, accessed March 2011).

8. WHO Regional Office for Europe. *European health for all database* (HFA-DB). Copenhagen: WHO Regional Office for Europe; updated January 2011 (http://data.euro.who.int/hfadb/, accessed March 2011).

9. Kutzin J. A descriptive framework for country-level analysis of health care financing arrangements. *Health Policy* 2001; 56 (3):171–204.

10. Macro International for the Institute of Obstetrics and Pediatrics, Ministry of Health. *Kyrgyz Republic demographic and health survey*. Calverton, MD: Macro International; 1997.

11. Ibraimov A et al. *Social-medical causes of mortality of children under 2 years old, who died at home and during the first 24 hours after hospitalization*. Bishkek: Health Policy Analysis Centre; 2009.

12. Bhutta ZA, Khan YP. *Maternal and newborn health in Kyrgyzstan and Chui oblast: assessment and implications for interventions*. Karachi: Division of Women & Child Health, The Aga Khan University; 2009.

13. Ministry of Health. *Mid-term review (MTR) report: Manas Taalimi health sector strategy*. Bishkek: Ministry of Health; 2009.

14. Guillot M, Gavrilova N, Torgashova L. Divergent paths for adult mortality in Russia and central Asia: evidence from Kyrgyzstan. *2010 European Population Conference,* Vienna, Austria, 1–4 September 2011 (http://epc2010.princeton.edu/download.aspx?submissionId=100123, accessed July 2011).

15. Jakab M, Lundeen E, Akkazieva B. *Health system effectiveness in hypertension control*. Bishkek: Health Policy Analysis Unit, Centre for Health System Development; 2007 (CHSD Policy Research Paper 44).

16. Akunov N al. *Quality of prevention and treatment of cardiovascular disease.* Bishkek: Health Policy Analysis Unit, Centre for Health System Development; 2007 (CHSD Policy Research Paper 45).

17. Newport S. *A review of progress in maternal health in eastern Europe and central Asia.* New York: United Nations Population Fund; 2009.

18. Jakab M, Kutzin J. *Improving financial protection in Kyrgyzstan through reducing informal payments. Evidence from 2001–06.* Bishkek: Health Policy Analysis Unit (DFID/WHO); 2009 (Policy Research Paper 57).

19. Balabanova D, Coker R. Russia and former USSR, health systems of. In: Heggenhougen K, Quah S, eds. *International encyclopedia of public health*, Vol 5. San Diego, CA: Academic Press; 2008:627–37.

20. Hopkinson B et al. The human perspective on health care reform: coping with diabetes in Kyrgyzstan. *International Journal of Health Planning and Management* 2004; 19:43–61.

21. Abdraimova A, Beran D. *Report on the rapid assessment protocol for insulin access in Kyrgyzstan.* London: International Insulin Foundation; 2009.

22. Kojekeev K, Murzalieva G, Manjieva E. *Why are our doctors leaving? Exploring the reasons behind migration of medical personnel in Kyrgyzstan.* Bishkek: Health Policy Analysis Centre; 2008 (http://hpac.kg/images/pdf/PRP51_E.pdf, accessed July 2011) (Policy Research Paper 51).

23. Kutzin J. *Health expenditures, reforms and policy priorities for the Kyrgyz Republic.* Bishkek: Health Policy Analysis Unit (DFID/WHO); 2003 (Policy Research Paper 24).

24. Lewis M. Informal health payments in central and eastern Europe and the former Soviet Union: issues, trends and policy implications. In: Mossialos E et al, eds. *Funding health care: options for Europe.* Buckingham: Open University Press; 2002:184–205 (European Observatory on Health Care Systems Series).

25. Falkingham J, Akkazieva B, Baschieri A. Trends in out-of-pocket payments for health care in Kyrgyzstan, 2001–2007. *Health Policy and Planning* 2010; 25(5):427–36.

26. Kutzin J, Jakab M, Cashin C. Lessons from health financing reform in central and eastern Europe and the former Soviet Union. *Health Economics, Policy and Law* 2010; 5(2): 135–47.

27. Kutzin J et al. Reforms in the pooling of funds. In: Kutzin J, Cashin C, Jakab M, eds. *Implementing health financing reform: lessons from countries in transition.* Copenhagen: World Health Organization, on behalf of the European Observatory on Health Systems and Policies; 2010:119–53.

28. Fuenzalida-Puelma HL et al. Purchasing of health care services. In: Kutzin J, Cashin C, Jakab M, eds. *Implementing health financing reform: lessons from countries in transition.* Copenhagen: World Health Organization, on behalf of the European Observatory on Health Systems and Policies; 2010:155–86.

29. Kutzin J. *Patient payment policies within the context of the Kyrgyz single payer reform: a preliminary assessment.* Bishkek: Health Policy Analysis Unit (WHO-DFID); 2001 (WHO Policy Research Paper 12).

30. Falkingham J. Poverty, affordability and access to health care. In: McKee M, Healy J, Falkingham J, eds. *Health care in Central Asia.* Buckingham: Open University Press; 2002:42–56.

31. The Kyrgyz Republic. *Law of the Kyrgyz Republic "On health protection of the citizens of the KR".* No. 6, 9 January 2005. Bishkek: Toktom; 2005.

32. The Kyrgyz Republic. *Law of the Kyrgyz Republic "On health care organizations in the KR".* No. 116, 13 August 2004. Bishkek: Toktom; 2004.

33. The Kyrgyz Republic. *Law of the Kyrgyz Republic "On Single payer system in health care financing".* No. 159, 30 July 2003. Bishkek: Toktom; 2003.

34. The Kyrgyz Republic. *Law of the Kyrgyz Republic "On protection of breastfeeding and regulation of marketing of products for artificial feeding".* No. 263, 17 December 2008. Bishkek: Toktom; 2008.

35. The Kyrgyz Republic. *Law of the Kyrgyz Republic "On financial and economical foundations of local self-government".* No. 215, 25 September 2003. Bishkek: Toktom; 2003.

36. Mirzoev T, Green A, Newell J. Health SWAps and external aid: a case study from Tajikistan. *International Journal of Health Planning and Management* 2010; 25(3):270–86.

37. CEDAW. *Concluding observations of the Committee on the Elimination of Discrimination against Women.* Portugal: UN Committee on the Elimination of Discrimination Against Women; 1 April 2009 (CEDAW/C/PRT/CO/7).

38. UNDP. Kyrgyzstan: leading women's representation in parliament in Central Asia. Paris: United Nations Development Programme, Europe & CIS. 21 June 2010 (http://europeandcis.undp.org/home/show/59B1F79B-F203-1EE9-B50C3B3B A6AE287B, accessed 20 August 2010).

39. Asylbekova N et al. *United Nations in the Kyrgyz Republic: translating commitments on gender equality into actions.* Bishkek: United Nations; 2009.

40. UNDP. *The Kyrgyz Republic: The second progress report on the Millennium Development Goals*, 2nd edition. Bishkek: United Nations Development Programme; 2010.

41. Paci P (ed). *Gender in transition*. Washington, DC: World Bank; 2002.

42. East and Central Asia Regional Department and Regional and Sustainable Development Department. *The Kyrgyz Republic. A gendered transition: Soviet legacies and new risks. Country gender assessment*. Manila: Asian Development Bank; 2005.

43. Torgasheva LM, Chinybaeva RK. Population. In: Vlasova NN, ed. *Women and men in the Kyrgyz Republic: 2000–2004 gender-disaggregated statistics*. Bishkek: National Statistical Committee of the Kyrgyz Republic; 2005;37–52.

44. Wejnert B, Parrot A, Djumabaeva A. *Maternal health policies in countries in transition: Poland and Kyrgyzstan, 1990–2006*. Abingdon, NY: Routledge; 2009.

45. World Bank. *Doing business 2011. Making a difference for entrepreneurs*. Washington, DC: World Bank and International Finance Corporation; 2010.

46. Anon. Stalin's harvest. The latest outbreak of violence in the ethnic boiling-pot of central Asia will take generations to heal. *The Economist*, 17 June 2010.

47. MHIF. *Annual report of MHIF performance in 2009*. Bishkek: Mandatory Health Insurance Fund; 2010.

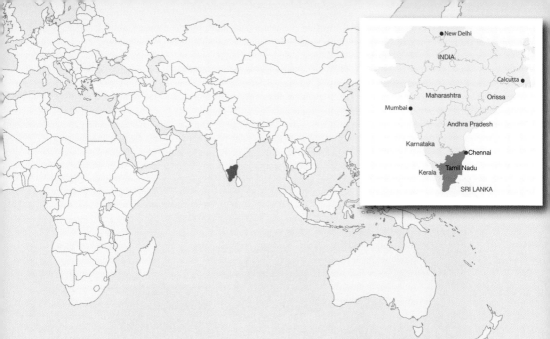

Chapter 6

TAMIL NADU 1980s–2005:

A SUCCESS STORY IN INDIA

VR Muraleedharan[1], Umakant Dash[1] and Lucy Gilson[2]

1 Indian Institute of Technology, Madras, 2 LSHTM and University of Cape Town

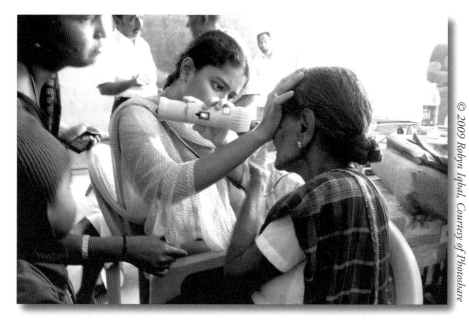

A volunteer optometrist examines a rural women for signs of glaucoma using basic instruments at a mobile medical camp in Tamil Nadu. Such mobile camps are often the only medical care and treatment that rural Indians receive each year. The vision camps are held annually in many small towns and villages as a programme which offers free eye examinations and treatment of basic vision problems.

© 2009 Robyn Iqbal, Courtesy of Photoshare

■ Key messages

- Tamil Nadu has made great progress in improving maternal, newborn and child health, performing consistently above the Indian national average.

- The Government of Tamil Nadu has had a long-term commitment to improving primary care in rural areas. Primary health care centres have expanded access to health care, providing high-quality primary care and emergency obstetric and newborn care, among other services. The inclusion of indigenous medicine has increased use of public facilities.

- A stable bureaucracy and effective managers have ensured continuity and have formulated, implemented, evaluated and adapted government policies to improve health outcomes and equity. The state is unique in India in developing a strong public health management cadre at the district level.

- At the end of the 1970s, Tamil Nadu trained and deployed village health nurses to serve rural communities more rapidly than in most other parts of India. Since then, the range of primary care services they deliver has gradually increased. The impact of this initiative on key health indicators has been clearly documented, for example through increased numbers of antenatal care visits and institutional deliveries in rural areas.

- Another innovation was the launch of a new drug distribution system in 1995 that rationalized the purchase and distribution of medicines to all public hospitals and primary health care centres. Performance reviews attest to its impact in improving the overall effectiveness of the health delivery system in Tamil Nadu.

- Since the 1990s, Tamil Nadu has had one of the most rapidly expanding private health sectors in India. Some joint public–private engagement has occurred, including health awareness raising campaigns, the contracting out of services such as laboratory diagnostics, and some corporate support for primary health care facilities. By focusing on the public sector, the Government of Tamil Nadu has been able to ensure that people have access to lower-cost alternatives to private sector health services.

- Other factors that have contributed to better health outcomes include a lower fertility rate, improved gender equality, a higher literacy rate, economic growth, rapid industrialization and improved infrastructure.

■ Introduction

With a population of 72 million, Tamil Nadu is larger than many countries[1]. It is the eleventh largest state in India by area and the seventh most populous. Most of the population, 88%, is Hindu, with Christians and Muslims constituting 11%, and other religions 1% (2008) (Box 6.1). Children under 15 years of age make up 27% of the population and 64% are aged 15–60 years. Administratively, the state has been divided into 32 districts, with approximately 45% of its population living in urban areas. Chennai (formerly known as Madras) is the state capital. The services sector makes up 45% of the economic activity in the state, followed by manufacturing (34%) and agriculture (21%).

Economically, Tamil Nadu is relatively prosperous. It ranks third among all states in India, with an average per capita income in 2007 of Rs 32733 (Int$ 3522), which is substantially above the national average. Both its literacy rate and its Human Development Index (HDI) are also significantly above the national average, as are several other socioeconomic indicators (Table 6.1). Total fertility rate reached a replacement level of 2.1 in the early 1990s, far ahead of most other states in India. Life expectancy at birth for men and women is high compared with the rest of India, and maternal, newborn and child mortality rates are among the lowest in the country.

Typically, the public health care system in India delivers modern medical services. This is true of Tamil Nadu as well, but there has been a conscious effort by the state also to provide indigenous medical services through primary health care centres. The Government of India has promoted various indigenous approaches to medicine, mostly through supporting research on them, and less through delivery of services in public facilities.

Most health spending (about 4% of state GDP) is from private sources, largely from people paying for consultations and treatment out of their own pockets. The private sector has expanded rapidly in cities, towns and rural villages since the 1980s, and now accounts for 80% of outpatient and 60% of inpatient care. Although there are few empirical data, the available literature suggests that a number of factors have encouraged the growth of the private sector in India. These include, for example, the inability of public institutions to cater to growing health care needs; huge private investment in the medical industry; a lack of appropriate regulation and regulatory bodies; and the interests of a vast network of indigenous medical practitioners, particularly in rural parts of the country[14].

Nevertheless, the state plays a significant role as a provider of health care services. The Government of Tamil Nadu spends about 1% of state GDP on health,

Box 6.1 Tamil Nadu at a glance

Population	72 million[1]. India's 11th largest state by area and 7th by population. 48% of the population is urban[2].
Geography	Located at the southernmost tip of India. Long coastline. Highly dependent on monsoon rains, with drought when they fail.
Ethnic composition	88% Hindu, 11% Christian or Muslim, 1% other[2].
Government	One of 28 states in the Federal Republic of India. India gained independence in 1947, and the current state boundaries and name date from 1969. State elections every five years, but despite changes in political leaders and parties, commitment to strengthening public health and equity has been constant.
Health system	Health expenditure per capita (public)[3]: Rs 223 (Int$5.06)[a] Health expenditure per capita (private)[3]: Rs 1033 (Int$23.48)[a]. Density of physicians, nurses and midwives per 10 000: 12.3[4]. Emphasis on improving primary health care, extensive use of multipurpose workers, as well as services for women and children. Focus on equity. Rapidly expanding private sector. Coverage of key interventions is high (90% deliveries with skilled attendance[5], 92% of infants fully immunized)[5].

Economic, demographic and social development indicators		
	GDP per capita (constant 2005 Int$)[6]	3522
	Economic growth: higher and poverty reduction faster than the India average in the 1990s[7].	
	Population living on less than $1.25/day	–
	Gini index[8]	28.3
	Infant mortality rate (2007)[9]	35[b]
	Maternal mortality rate (2004–6)[10]	111[c]
	Adult HIV prevalence rate (aged 15–49)[11]	0.25%
	Life expectancy (2001–6)[9]	67 (men) 69.8 (women)
	Total fertility rate (2006)[9]	1.7
	Literacy rate (2011)[1]	80%
	Ratio girls to boys in education[d] (2005–6)[5]	0.94
	Access to improved water source (2005–6)[5]	93.5% households
	Internet usage per 100	–

Note: [a] At 2005 exchange rate; [b] Per 1000 live births; [c] Per 100 000 live births; [d] Primary and secondary education.

which is similar to most other states in India, although very low by international standards. Although we recognize that people's access to private health services is likely to have had a significant impact on health outcomes in Tamil Nadu, this chapter focuses on government health policies and actions, and how public funds have been used to attain greater health gains than have been achieved by almost all other states in India.

Table 6.1   Comparative health indicators across major states of India, most recent year available

States/India	GDP PPP per capita in US$ (2009)[6]	Total fertility rate (2006)	Infant mortality per 1000 live births (2007)	Life expectancy at birth (years) (2001–6)		Under-5 mortality per 1000 live births[13] (2006)	Maternal mortality per 100 000 live births (2004–7)	Full immuniza-tion (2002–4)
				Male	Female			
Andhra Pradesh	3197	2.0	54	62.8	65.0	87.7	154	62.9
Assam	1875	2.7	66	59.0	60.9	85.0	480	19.3
Bihar	1068	4.2	58	65.7	64.8	84.8	312	24.4
Gujarat	3849	2.7	52	63.1	64.1	60.9	160	57.7
Haryana	5386	2.7	55	64.6	69.3	52.3	186	62.9
Karnataka	3244	2.1	47	62.4	66.4	54.7	213	74.1
Kerala	3854	1.7	13	71.7	75.0	16.3	95	81.2
Madhya Pradesh	1692	3.5	72	59.2	58.0	94.2	130	32.5
Maharashtra	4288	2.1	34	66.8	69.8	46.7	335	74.3
Orissa	2303	2.5	71	60.1	59.7	90.6	303	55.1
Punjab	4133	2.1	43	69.8	72.0	52.0	192	75.3
Rajasthan	2110	3.5	65	62.2	62.8	85.4	388	25.4
Tamil Nadu	3522	1.7	35	67.0	69.8	35.5	111	92.1
Uttar Pradesh	1462	4.2	69	63.5	64.1	96.4	440	28.1
West Bengal	2839	2.0	37	66.1	69.3	59.6	141	54.4
India	2930	2.8	55	64.1	65.4	74.3	254	47.6

Sources: References 6, 12 and 13.

This chapter presents a historical perspective on Tamil Nadu's pursuit of better health, focusing on the period from 1980 to 2005[a]. The late 1970s and early 1980s is a clear landmark for beginning the analysis, as this was when the rural health care delivery system was restructured as part of the commitment to the 1978 Alma-Ata Declaration about universal access to primary health care. Health gains and their assessment are included only up until 2005 because this is when the National Rural Health Mission was launched. This flagship programme of the Government of India, in collaboration with state governments, has already resulted in a number of architectural changes in the functioning and management of public health care facilities in rural regions of the country. There has been a substantial increase in funding to state governments to implement the programme, which is expected to lead to further improvements in health. Although it is too early to draw meaningful conclusions, its impact is beginning to be seen in a variety of ways.

The chapter highlights progress in improving health outcomes in Tamil Nadu, followed by a description of the supportive structures, policies and individuals that have been critical in strengthening the public delivery system. It then explains the most significant health policies and interventions to be implemented in the 1980s and 1990s, analysing the impact that these policies had on usage and the extent to which the poorest population groups have benefited. Next, it flags the possible contributions of certain larger socioeconomic and cultural factors. The chapter concludes with a set of lessons derived from Tamil Nadu's experience, which may be useful to other governments seeking to improve the health of their people.

Better health?

Table 6.1 and Figures 6.1–6.4 show that the relative position of Tamil Nadu on a range of health indicators has been much better than the average for India.

Between 1980 and 2005, the infant mortality rate in Tamil Nadu decreased by 60%, compared with 45% for the country as a whole. The decline was even more significant in rural areas of the state, and by 2005, infant mortality was only slightly lower in urban areas (Figure 6.2). Even though the infant mortality rate fell throughout the entire country of India between 1971 and 2005, the female–male differential in the infant mortality rate actually increased with the notable exception of Tamil Nadu, which showed the lowest gender disparity during this period[16].

---

[a] See Chapter 2 and Annex for an explanation of the methodology and data sources.

Figure 6.1 **Life expectancy (male and female) in Tamil Nadu and India, 1992–2006**

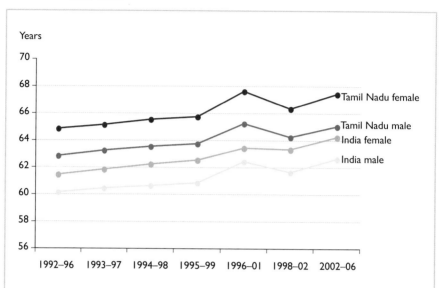

Source: Adapted from reference 9.

Figure 6.2 **Infant mortality rate in Tamil Nadu and India (rural and urban), 1982–2005**

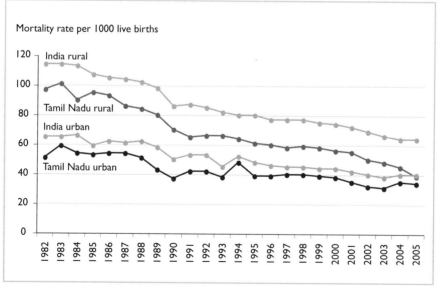

Source: Adapted from reference 9.

Figure 6.3   Under-5 mortality rate in Tamil Nadu and India, 1992–1993, 1998–1999 and 2005–2006

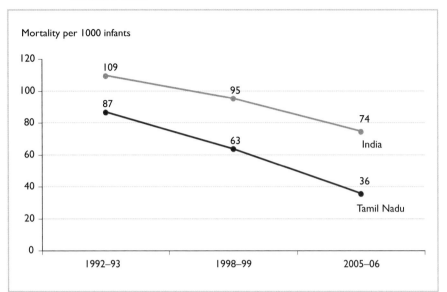

Sources: Adapted from references 5, 13 and 15.

By the mid-1990s, nearly 23% of infant deaths were due to premature births and low birth weight. Asphyxia and birth injuries accounted for another 23%, while diarrhoea and acute respiratory infections accounted for 6% and 17%, respectively[17]. In the absence of periodic and regular reporting on these causes, it is not possible to comment on trends over the years.

The under-5 mortality rate in Tamil Nadu fell by 53% between 1992–1993 and 2005–2006, compared with 32% for the country overall (Figure 6.3). In 2006, Tamil Nadu had the third lowest rate of under-5 mortality in India, with 35.5 deaths per 1000 live births in contrast to an average of 74.3 for India.

However, the most dramatic difference between Tamil Nadu and the rest of India has been in the number of women who die as a result of pregnancy or giving birth. Between 1982 and 1986, the maternal mortality rate in Tamil Nadu was estimated at 319 deaths per 100 000 live births, compared with a national average of 555 (ranging from a high of 1028 in Assam to a low of 235 in Kerala)[18]. By 2004, the maternal mortality rate in Tamil Nadu had dropped to 111 deaths per 100 000 live births, less than half of India's average of 254 and the second lowest in the country (Figure 6.4)[10].

Figure 6.4   Maternal mortality rate in Tamil Nadu and India, 1997–2006

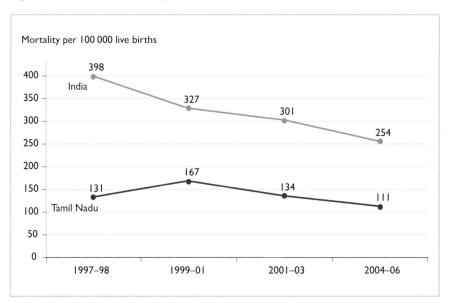

Source: Adapted from reference 10.

Since 1980, the Health and Family Welfare Department of the Government of Tamil Nadu has reported reductions in poliomyelitis, tuberculosis, malaria, leprosy, whooping cough, measles and typhoid. Guinea worm disease was practically eliminated by the mid-1980s[19] and no polio cases have been reported in the state since 2000, in contrast to some other parts of the country.

The state has achieved better than average results in implementing the Blindness Control Programme, which is funded by the Government of India. For example, in 2003, Tamil Nadu led the country in the number of cataract operations performed (592 per 100 000 population) and the prevalence of blindness due to cataracts was reduced from 1.13% in 1994 to 0.40% in 2002, while the national average only fell from 1.19% to 0.70% during the same period.

The next two sections discuss how political leadership, committed civil servants and good management practices, as well as specific policies and interventions from within the public health system, have contributed to significant improvements in health outcomes.

How has Tamil Nadu achieved this? The importance of leadership, commitment and good management in improving health

The commitment by and insight of government leaders in Tamil Nadu have made a significant contribution to the health gains in the state. Even though political leaders and parties in power have changed over the years (elections are held every five years), two aspects of the government's approach to strengthening the public health system have remained consistent since the early 1980s. First, health policies and government spending on health have emphasized improving primary care services, especially in rural, poor and disadvantaged communities. Second, political leaders have been committed to implementing innovative interventions, some of which are common across all states and funded by the central government, efficiently and effectively.

The Government of Tamil Nadu has prioritized and invested resources in primary health care, particularly for services benefiting women and children. The state's total health budget increased dramatically, from Rs 4108 million (US$ 167.9 million) in 1991/1992 to Rs 14 870 million (US$ 335.9 million in 2005/2006)[20]. In nominal terms, spending increased by 3.6 times between 1993/1994 and 2005/2006. Medical, public health and family welfare is the second-largest expenditure category in the state, next to education. Since 1990, central government has contributed approximately 20% of the state's annual health budget and the Health and Family Welfare Department of Tamil Nadu has consistently spent about 45% of its annual budget on primary health care. In Tamil Nadu, the tertiary sector's share of the budget fell from 33% in 1990 to 24% in 2002, and the secondary sector's share increased correspondingly during the same period. There are no hard data for other states, but most health officials and former health secretaries in the national government who were interviewed by the research team reported that the overall share of resources devoted to primary care within the health sector budget was not as high in other states as it was in Tamil Nadu (interviews conducted by the authors with various state officials who had managed many national programmes, and two former health secretaries in Delhi, 2010).

It is widely accepted among people interviewed as part of this study, especially those working at the central government level who were implementing common programmes in different states, that Tamil Nadu's health sector has benefited from a number of committed health secretaries who have been the drivers of the innovative initiatives discussed in the next section. The vigorous support for maternal and child care in the late 1990s and early 2000s was particularly due to the vision, commitment and leadership of senior civil servants. One example was a determined campaign by one health secretary and the Government of Tamil Nadu against female feticide in the late 1990s, making effective use of the media to generate public support for reform. The importance of the state's political and bureaucratic commitment to bridging gender differentials in mortality has received some scholarly attention[16,21].

The presence of civil servants with management skills and sufficient power and discretion to implement reforms has been an important factor in promoting continuity of policy. Bureaucratic leaders made use of modern public management methods, giving greater autonomy to agencies within the public sector[24]. The creation of quasi-governmental organizations has proved to be an effective mechanism for overcoming tardy bureaucratic producers[23]. This is well-documented in the case of the Tamil Nadu Medical Services Corporation (see below), an autonomous body managing drug procurement that has been able to implement a series of measures to improve the quality of drugs and promote rational drug use.

Other features of the process of implementing health policies that were considered important at national level are flexibility and the ability to learn lessons. There seemed to be a recognized need for central leadership and strong institutions, as well as for bottom-up innovation to ensure that policy changes translated into improved access to health services. For example, many district health authorities were immune to shifting political and state priorities and had the autonomy and flexibility to plan immunization campaigns and other primary health care initiatives, attracting support from charitable bodies where necessary.

Another example relates to efforts to reduce maternal deaths. Tamil Nadu district officers were given the authority to develop local solutions to problems that emerged from maternal death reviews, and successful local strategies were replicated in other districts. In parallel, there were collaborative processes at state level, such as the development of evidence-based guidelines to standardize treatment for potentially life-threatening complications during childbirth across the state.

Tamil Nadu is the only Indian state with a distinct public health management cadre at the district level. Everyone interviewed identified this as a vital component of effective management of the health delivery system. Most states eliminated their public health management cadre after independence in 1947, but Tamil Nadu retained it and put the staff in charge of managing primary health institutions. The staff undergo a series of training programmes in public health and allied subjects, including in managerial skills. They are also expected to qualify for a diploma in public health, which enables them to move up the career ladder. A major advantage of the public health cadre is that it provides managerial continuity at district and higher levels of primary health care, and a forceful argument to this effect has been made recently[24]. Most interviewees said that this continuity was critical for following up issues at various levels.

> *The Tamil Nadu state had a much better combination of managerial skills at various levels, from state secretariat to district health system and even below. In my six years of association with this sector, I would say no other state could boast of having such a blend of professionals. I would even say that, overall, the administrative efficiency of the state health system is far higher than that of other states of India.*
>
> *Former Secretary of the*
> *Ministry of Health and Family Welfare of the Government of India*

The presence of this cadre meant that managers were able to act quickly because they were familiar with the issues, and over time had developed a good understanding of the best ways to deal with them. Managers in other states where no public health management cadre exists are frequently transferred from one department to another within the health sector. Consequently, they are often slower to act, as it takes them longer to grasp the situation on the ground.

The combination of experienced managers at all levels of the state health system, and the greater autonomy they had, resulted in speedier allocation and more effective use of resources at facility level, thus enhancing access to health care (as will be described below). Greater access implied better protection from conditions that lead to adverse health outcomes.

The examples in the next section illustrate why Tamil Nadu has a reputation for having made more effective use of the resources it receives from the central government and for having spent resources more efficiently in comparison with most other states, a point that was made by several officials during interviews conducted by the research team.

■ What did Tamil Nadu do to improve health (1980–2005)?

Together, four complementary actions by the Government of Tamil Nadu during the 1980s and 1990s made a significant contribution to improving health, especially the health of women and children in rural areas:

1. training and deploying a new type of village health worker;

2. building a network of primary health care centres;

3. scaling up immunization; and

4. developing an innovative drug distribution system.

This section is largely based on many interviews with former officials who served during the 1980s and the 1990s. Whenever possible, officially reported data are used to validate their views and observations.

Training and deploying thousands of village health workers

As part of a new strategy to deliver primary health care in rural areas, the Multipurpose Workers Scheme was launched by the central government in early 1980 with the goal that every rural community with a population of 5000 would be served by an adequately trained health worker. In Tamil Nadu, the multipurpose workers are all women and are designated as village health nurses. This new health worker role was created to work in the community and provide antenatal and postnatal care, vaccinations, contraception and other basic maternal and child health services during regular home visits. The village health nurses are required to keep complete records, for example of all pregnant women, and encourage women to give birth in a health facility rather than at home. To help synergize the work of various cadres and improve child health status, village health nurses are expected to work closely with community nutrition workers on the nutritional meal scheme, aimed at schoolchildren.

Tamil Nadu implemented the Multipurpose Workers Scheme faster than most other states by absorbing existing maternity assistants as village health nurses and opening nearly 60 schools to train thousands more. This had an immediate and significant impact on the manner in which primary care was deployed and delivered in rural areas. Invariably, interviewed officials highlighted this as a critical factor in improving health status.

Having completed 10 years of school, village health nurses are given approximately 18 months of training in basic primary health care. A great deal of emphasis was on imparting practical skills for better management of common conditions, such as acute respiratory infections and diarrhoea. By the early 1980s, approximately 2000 village health nurses were serving rural communities and by the late 1980s, nearly 8000 of them were in place across rural areas of the state. They have improved access to essential services at community and household level, and the range of available primary care services delivered by them has gradually increased. The impact of this initiative on key maternal and child health process indicators has been clearly documented. This can be seen, for example, through the increased number of antenatal care visits and institutional deliveries in rural areas.

Building a network of primary health care facilities

When the Multipurpose Workers Scheme was getting off the ground, the central government also launched an initiative to expand the number of primary health centres and health subcentres in rural areas. The plan was for primary health centres to provide primary care, including normal deliveries, outpatient care, care for minor accidents and vaccinations, as well as to manage school health programmes and various national public health programmes, such as those for tuberculosis and leprosy. A typical primary health centre would have four to six beds, and be staffed by one or two physicians, two nurses (with the title of auxiliary nurse and midwife) with wide-ranging roles, a pharmacist, a driver and one or two assistants, depending on local conditions. Administratively, each primary health centre would have four to eight health subcentres under its jurisdiction. Each health subcentre would have one village health nurse serving a population of 5000.

Tamil Nadu embraced the concept wholeheartedly and built the facilities much faster than almost all other states. The rate of expansion was remarkable. In the early 1980s, there were only about 400 primary health centres and 4000 health subcentres across rural areas of the state. By 1990, nearly 1400 primary health centres and about 8000 health subcentres had been opened and Tamil Nadu was very close to achieving the national target of one primary health centre per 30 000 people and one health subcentres per 5000 people. Since then, these achievements have more or less been sustained. In 2005, Tamil Nadu had approximately 1500 primary health centres (one for every 33 000 people) and 8680 health subcentres (each covering a population of 5100). Only two districts had fewer primary health centres and health subcentres than the national population norms. Very few states have reached this high level of coverage through the primary health care system.

With sustained financial support from the central and state governments and from development partners, primary health services continued to improve. Several development partners contributed to the expansion of health infrastructure in Tamil Nadu. Among them, the Danish International Development Agency (DANIDA) has been the most significant in strengthening primary care[25]. DANIDA has had a presence in Tamil Nadu's health sector since the early 1980s. Although its annual budget has remained at around 1% of the total state health budget, a substantial amount has been channelled into constructing primary health centres and capacity-building exercises. DANIDA's commitment to primary health care demonstrates that development partners can make a positive, lasting impact on the system.

The rapid expansion of primary health centres was possible because of the speed and overall efficiency with which Tamil Nadu officials, compared with most other states, made use of the resources allocated from the central government. And unlike other states, innovative approaches were encouraged. In the 1990s, for example, nearly 400 primary health centres in rural regions of Tamil Nadu were constructed with in-kind contributions (in the form of labour) from local community members. An added benefit of such community participation was that it is judged to have improved utilization of the facilities.

The state government also made efforts to tap resources from industrialists by appealing to their philanthropic instincts to adopt health care institutions in their areas and make contributions towards maintenance and improvements. Since 1998, 20 different industrialists in Tamil Nadu have adopted more than 65 primary health centres and government hospitals[26,27]. The Government of Tamil Nadu also encouraged members of the legislative assembly and members of parliament to make use of the Development Fund for the adoption and maintenance of primary health centres and hospitals in their constituencies. Contributions from industrialists were used for staff, medicine, equipment, civil works, the construction of staff quarters and the maintenance of buildings. Several medical officers noted that, in the long run, such forms of assistance could not be relied upon for operating the public health facilities, but that such assistance had helped them with overall maintenance and, even if temporarily, had visibly improved the upkeep of the primary health centres. A DANIDA representative stated that adoption of primary health centres by private corporate bodies in the 1990s has had a significant impact on the overall appeal of public facilities.

Another development was the concept of the 24-hour primary health centre, which was pioneered in 1996/1997 to offer outpatient care during evening hours and to increase women's access to routine essential and emergency obstetric care. Within two years, nearly 250 primary health centres were open around the clock, and by 2008, nearly all of the state's 1500 primary health centres had joined them. The range of services provided by the centres has also grown considerably over the years and now, for example, several centres offer advanced diagnostic services and dental care. Finally, the state also provides indigenous medicine and treatments in many public health care facilities. By the mid-1990s, indigenous physicians were present in 281 primary health centres, and in several hospitals too. This is believed to have increased access to services.

In order to ensure that the performance of primary health centres could be routinely monitored and, when necessary, followed up with remedial measures, the Department of Public Health with the help of DANIDA established a monthly Institutional Services Monitoring Report System. Data on staff positions, vacancies, use of resources (such as beds and vehicles), services delivered (including inpatient and outpatient coverage, antenatal care, abortions, vaccines administered, and diagnostic laboratory tests conducted), types of delivery conducted, and so forth, are reported on a monthly basis for all primary health centres in the state.

Scaling up the immunization programme

A third successful intervention was the Universal Immunization Programme, which was rapidly scaled up across the country from 1986 with the support of UNICEF. The measles immunization campaigns that started in 1978 (with tremendous support from the Christian Medical College of Vellore, and vaccine supplied by the Rotary Club) had already had a major impact on child health. As part of the new programme, Tamil Nadu adopted a five-dose policy for polio vaccine (unlike other states, which had a three-dose policy), and significant improvements in child health followed (Jacob John, internationally recognized scholar and pioneer in the conception and design of the immunization programme in India, personal communication, August 2010).

By the early 1990s, Tamil Nadu ranked first among all states in India in the number of children vaccinated: 60% of children in rural areas and 75% of children in cities had been fully immunized, while only 6% of rural and 1.7% of urban children had received no immunization at all[28]. By that time, the state had also achieved the lowest variation in full immunization rates between the richest and poorest quintiles and between rural and urban areas (although the former had a slightly higher level of inequality than the latter). The reduction in inequity due to income and geographical location was much greater in Tamil Nadu than in other states. In addition, differences in immunization coverage by gender, both in rural and urban areas, were the lowest in India. Mass campaigns were common and, in addition to the roles played by primary health centres and health subcentres, several community organizations, including local schools and Rotary Clubs, contributed to their success. Throughout the state, village health nurses and nurses at primary health centres administered vaccinations during regular household visits, as well as on set dates over the course of the year.

By the late 1990s, 99% of rural and 100% of urban children in the state had received some immunization, while 85% of rural and 91% of urban children had received full immunization[29]. Evidence of overall health gains among children in the state was overwhelming.

The high level of immunization achieved in Tamil Nadu did not result from a discrete vertical programme, but was the product of a long-term political process that gave high priority to maternal and child health, leading to the integrated expansion of primary health centres and broader behavioural and cultural change among policy makers and the general population.

Ensuring a reliable supply of essential drugs

The most innovative development conceived by the Government of Tamil Nadu was the creation of the Tamil Nadu Medical Services Corporation (TNMSC), established in 1995 as an autonomous body to purchase and distribute medicines to all public hospitals and primary health centres.

> *This was a far-sighted vision of the then health secretary (in 1996) who had to face difficult moments as it involved huge amounts of money and the interests of many stakeholders. The state had earlier suffered from serious defects in the public eye, due to abuses of power and corruption in the drug purchase system, which had to be weeded out. The reputation of the present drug system actually helped build the overall reputation of the health delivery system*
>
> *Former district official, Tamil Nadu[b]*

Drugs overall have accounted for about 15% of the state health budget since the 1990s. Prior to the formation of TNMSC, health facilities under the jurisdiction of various departments purchased drugs on their own, with funds that came directly from one of three directorates: Medical Education, Medical and Rural Services, or Public Health and Preventive Medicine. There were persistent complaints about the misuse of funds, with frequent misappropriation of non-essential drugs and high distribution costs. Stock-outs of essential medicines were common across government health institutions at all levels. Once TNMSC was established, the three budgets were combined for drug procurement and the state's drug list was reduced to approximately 250 drugs, all generic.

Under the new system, medicines procured by TNMSC through an open-tender process are delivered directly by suppliers to district warehouses. District officers are given fixed transportation allowances to transfer these drugs to hospitals and clinics. Although the government is able to predict overall consumption within the state very well, district and subdistrict level consumption is highly variable

---

[b] This is a widely shared and accepted view of those in civil service, particularly among those in federal (central) government services who are able to compare the effectiveness of various states that implement common programmes.

and so all health care institutions (including primary health centres) are given considerable leeway in deciding which drugs they need and in what quantities. In return, all facilities are required to keep up-to-date records of their stocks and utilization. TNMSC regularly inspects district warehouses and storage facilities. It does not have its own laboratory facilities but hires the services of reputable private laboratories for quality testing.

Although its performance has yet to be evaluated systematically, TNMSC's effectiveness is widely admired and it has helped many other states begin similar drug management systems. A detailed analysis of TNMSC was published in 2000[23] and a review published in 2008 assessed TNMSC's performance and its impact on improving the overall effectiveness of the health delivery system in Tamil Nadu[30].

TNMSC has a reputation for strict quality adherence, and for being very transparent and accountable. Its well-designed computer system allows for good control of the medicines stocked in district warehouses and for the movement of medicines to be accurately tracked. Such information is uploaded on to its website on a daily basis.

A reliable supply of high-quality medicines in primary health centres has led to increased patient satisfaction and has contributed to the overall increase in demand for services across the state at all levels of the public health system. There is also anecdotal evidence that TNMSC has driven down the cost of competing drugs in the private sector, for example by a fall in price of brand name drugs for the treatment of tuberculosis (former state tuberculosis official, interview, September 2010)[31].

Once its success in managing the supply of medicines was firmly established, the scope of TNMSC was expanded to include other services. For example, its savings were used to purchase diagnostic equipment. All hospitals up to sub-district level were provided with technology for ultrasonography and other diagnostics. In later years, the government made a decision to equip all district hospitals with computer tomography scanners and a magnetic resonance imaging machine. The availability of this equipment in the public sector increased access and decreased the cost to patients, who might otherwise have sought services in the private sector or, in the case of the poor, gone without a proper diagnosis.

■ What else has Tamil Nadu done to improve health?

Services for women and children

The government's concerted efforts to train village health workers, build primary health centres and ensure they were adequately staffed, equipped and stocked with essential medicines and other supplies led to a marked increase in the use of primary health care services in Tamil Nadu, particularly by women and children and poor families from rural areas.

Several indicators of use of primary health care services in the public sector show significant improvements between 1990 and 2005. For example, almost all pregnant women received antenatal care in this sector: the proportion of women who received at least three antenatal visits increased dramatically from about 20% in the early 1990s to 95% by 2005[32].

In the early 1970s, 80% of women gave birth in their homes. By the early 1990s, this number had fallen to 42% and by 2005, it was 10% (Figure 6.5). Recently (2005–2009), the share of total deliveries in primary health centres has increased to nearly 25% and in the same period there has been a reduction from 43% to

Figure 6.5   Proportion of institutional deliveries, Tamil Nadu, 1992, 1998 and 2005

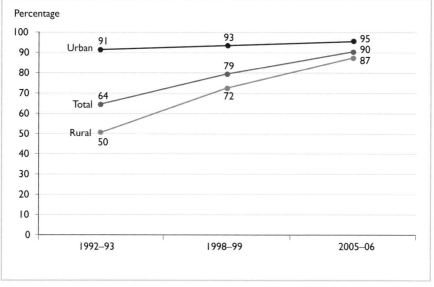

Source: Adapted from reference 33.

Figure 6.6   Share of private and public institutions in total deliveries, Tamil Nadu, 2005–2008

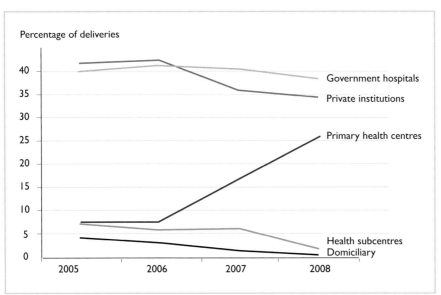

Source: Adapted from reference 33.

35% in the share of deliveries in private facilities (Figure 6.6). The beneficial effects of institutional delivery to bolster primary health care, along with other policy efforts, have led to a gradual but substantial fall in the maternal mortality rate.

As the following figures show, the average number of daily outpatient visits in primary health centres in Dharmapuri District (one of the least developed regions in the state) increased from 113 in 2004 to 153 in 2009 (Figure 6.7). Likewise, the average number of deliveries conducted per month in primary health centres increased more than three times over the same period (Figure 6.8).

Reaching the poorest

In addition to measuring the increased use of primary health services in the public sector, it is also essential to know the extent to which the benefits of public spending have reached the poorest in society. To put it differently, are the poor getting their fair share of the benefits of public spending on health care, in terms of higher use of health services and/or improved health status?

Figure 6.7   Daily outpatient attendance per primary health centre, Dharmapuri
District, 2004–2009

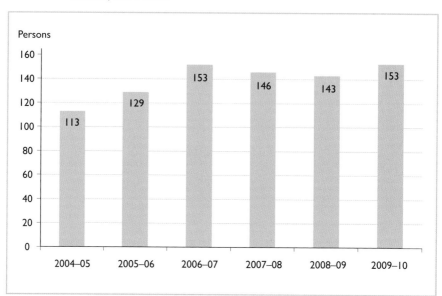

Source: Deputy Director, Health Services, Dharmapuri District, Tamil Nadu.

Figure 6.8   Average deliveries per month per primary health centre, Dharmapuri
District, 2004–2009

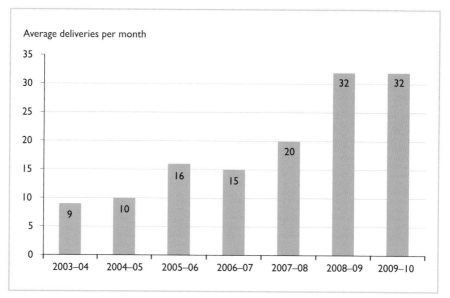

Source: Deputy Director, Health Services, Dharmapuri District, Tamil Nadu.

Figure 6.9 Distribution of maternal deliveries in public facilities, Tamil Nadu, by socioeconomic quintile, 1995–1996 and 2004

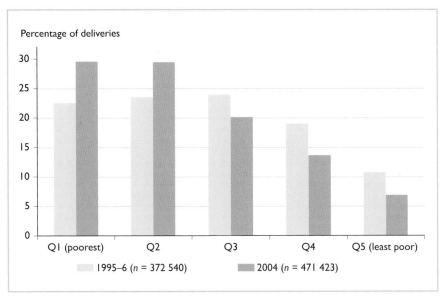

Source: Vaidyanathan G et al. (see text).

Evidence from a recent analysis on the use of public institutions for maternity and child health services shows that they are being used to a greater extent by those in poorer sections of the society (Vaidyanathan G et al. *Do the poor benefit from public spending on healthcare in India? Results from benefit (utilization) incidence analysis in Tamil Nadu and Orissa.* Unpublished draft report submitted to LSHTM, May 2010). This holds true for immunization (as discussed above) and other preventive health services that have a direct impact on maternal and child health[34]. Figure 6.9 shows that, in terms of consumption, people in the poorest quintile have used the public delivery system for maternity services more than those in the top quintile. Such results are not obvious. For example, the public health care system for outpatient care and inpatient services was more pro-rich (that is, used by better-off groups) in 1995 than in later years. And in many poor states, such as Orissa (Figure 6.10), the public system continues to be pro-rich, meaning that those who are least poor are using services to a greater extent than the poorest, although programmatic interventions may be changing this situation (Vaidyanathan G et al., as above).

In summary, by 2005, public spending on health care in Tamil Nadu had become more pro-poor than it was a decade earlier. Although, as was noted in the Introduction, the private health sector also grew substantially over the same

Figure 6.10 Distribution of maternal deliveries in public facilities, Orissa, by socioeconomic quintile,1995–1996 and 2004

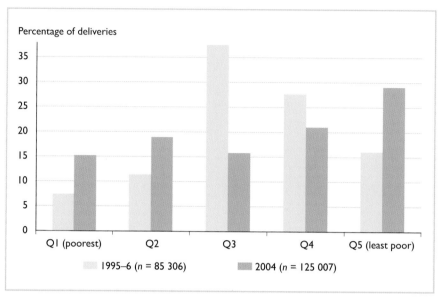

Source: Vaidyanathan G et al. (see text).

period in rural as well as urban areas, the people interviewed by the research team reported that it was the deployment of village health nurses to rural villages and the state-wide network of primary health centres that led to the vast improvement in the overall access to care.

> *Much of these changes can be attributed to the efforts of village health nurses and the overall presence and functioning of the primary health delivery system in the state.*
>
> A former Joint Director, Salem District, Tamil Nadu

■ What have other sectors contributed?

What were the most significant factors outside the health system that contributed to improved health outcomes in Tamil Nadu between 1980 and 2005? A steady decline in the total birth rate (Figure 6.11) provided the initial conditions critical for effective health care interventions in later years. In addition, an increase in female literacy and progress on women's empowerment were also essential in reducing maternal and child morbidity and mortality. More broadly, extensive improvements in roads and in other infrastructure as well as industrial economic

Figure 6.11 Birth rate, India and Tamil Nadu (rural and urban) 1971–2008

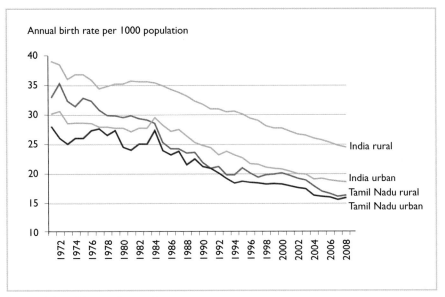

Source: Adapted from reference 9.

growth also played important roles in Tamil Nadu's health gains over this period. Chapter 10 provides a more detailed analysis of how these and other cultural and socioeconomic factors affect the health status of populations.

Scholars have examined the fertility transition in south India during the 1970s and 1980s and have put forward several competing and complementary explanations on the reasons for the changes. These are still being debated today[21,35].

Literacy, age of first marriage and contraception use are three of the most widely accepted reasons for a declining fertility rate. Compared with India's average literacy rate in 2001 (75% for males and 54% for females), Tamil Nadu's rates of 82% for males and 65% for females indicate a fairly high level of literacy. The average age for females at marriage in Tamil Nadu is close to 20 years, older than in the rest of India; there is also a relatively high rate of contraception use, at about 50%.

The social reform movement in Tamil Nadu (particularly from the 1940s to the 1960s) also played an important role in raising the low status and limited autonomy of women in general. For example, as mentioned above, the state has the distinction of having the lowest gender differential in infant mortality and in overall mortality figures. One of the most complex issues addressed in the academic literature relates to women's empowerment. Discussions are ensuing as to whether or not women in Tamil Nadu experience greater autonomy than those in other parts of the country, and whether or not such autonomy has had any effect on the fertility rate.

In one study, researchers examined dimensions of women's autonomy in Punjab in Pakistan, in Uttar Pradesh in north India and in Tamil Nadu in south India[36]. They explored the contextual factors underlying observed differences and assessed the extent to which these differences could be attributed to religion, nationality or north–south cultural distinctions. Their findings suggest that while women's autonomy, in terms of decision-making, mobility, freedom from threatening relations with husband, and access to and control over economic resources, is constrained in all three settings, women in Tamil Nadu fare considerably better than women elsewhere in India, irrespective of religion. They argue that in the patriarchal and gender-stratified structures governing the northern portion of the subcontinent, women's control over their lives is more limited than in the southern region. There are, however, contrary views and some have suggested that observations of greater female autonomy in Tamil Nadu should be interpreted with circumspection[37,38].

The government's Family Welfare Programme has had a greater impact in this state than elsewhere in India. Mass media and the cinema have played a role promoting the benefits of a small family, which has contributed to changing cultural preferences and values.

In Tamil Nadu, a larger cross-section of people has access to maternal and child welfare services than in most other states in India. The Noon Meal Scheme, introduced to schoolchildren in the early 1980s, has been particularly successful.

Two other developments help to explain Tamil Nadu's low total fertility rate and better health outcomes compared with most other states in India: infrastructure development and industrialization.

Improvements in infrastructure and industrial economic growth not only directly affect production and consumption but also generate positive externalities, such as better health[39–44]. Since the early 1970s, compared with other developed states in India, Tamil Nadu has consistently performed better with respect to infrastructure development. A recent study shows that Tamil Nadu's Infrastructure Overhead Capital Index, which includes transportation facilities (roads and railways), irrigation, electricity and telephone mainline, ranked second in 1971/1972 and 1981/1982 among all major Indian states. It fell to fifth place in 1991/1992, but rose to third by the late 1990s[45].

A study based on demographic and health survey data for more than 60 low-income countries found that access to electricity significantly reduces child mortality, independent of any income effect[46]. This is because electricity is not only essential for hospitals to function and for the delivery of health services but also for cooking at home with clean energy, which, in turn, improves health outcomes by reducing indoor air pollution and the incidence of respiratory illnesses.

Improved transportation networks contribute to easier access to health care, particularly in rural areas. A study using cross-section regressions found that road infrastructure (as measured by the length of the paved-road network) had a significant effect on a number of health indicators, including infant and maternal mortality rates[44].

Water and sanitation should be added to these factors because much of the morbidity and mortality among children results from waterborne infections (dysentery and diarrhoea are the major causes)[19].

Four major features of industrialization in Tamil Nadu are noteworthy. First, Tamil Nadu is one of the leading states in India in industrial development. The state's share of the manufacturing sector in the national GDP has remained high at 14% in 1980/1981 and at about 17% in 2007/2008. Second, Tamil Nadu had the highest number of registered manufacturing factories (15–16%) for seven successive years, starting in 1997/1998. Third, Tamil Nadu ranks second behind Maharashtra in the percentage of people engaged in various activities of production. The state's share of the national total has consistently increased, from about 10% in early 1980s to about 14% during the period 2001–2005. Finally, Tamil Nadu is behind only Maharashtra and Gujarat in fixed capital, productive capital, gross value of output and net value added.

Economic development resulting from industrialization provides increased work opportunities and income growth and creates capital for public- and private-sector investment. These, in turn, improve material circumstances in the population and the ability to purchase goods and services that are health enhancing, particularly for child health[47].

It is important to highlight the contributions of nongovernmental organisations (NGOs) in the implementation of key national disease control programmes in Tamil Nadu. The state officials working on these programmes have consciously sought to engage NGOs in controlling the prevalence of HIV/AIDS and tuberculosis. The state, as many other states, has benefited from the creation of autonomous bodies such as Tamil Nadu State AIDS Control Society, with considerable financial support from external development partners since mid-1990s. The Society's early disease control strategy was largely implemented through NGOs. More than 400 NGOs have received funds to implement health interventions over the last eight years (Ramasundaram S et al. *HIV/AIDS control in India: lessons from Tamil Nadu.* Unpublished research report draft submitted to ICRIER, New Delhi, 2001). It is important to emphasize the willingness of the public authorities in the state to collaborate with NGOs in addressing HIV/AIDS and tuberculosis. In the early 1990s, the state had the second highest prevalence of HIV in India. The rapid absorption of funds from the Government of India and other funding agencies through a network of NGOs has helped to control and reduce the prevalence of HIV, and this can be largely attributed to the public–private partnership model.

Several discussions with both district officials and NGOs point to the overall increase in income, along with higher literacy, a greater role of media and extensive improvement in public transportation facilities as factors that have made the public health system respond positively to the health care needs of the population.

■ Lessons learned and future challenges

Several lessons can be drawn from Tamil Nadu's experience over 25 years that may be helpful to other countries.

The focus in Tamil Nadu on primary health care ensured that a substantial share of the health budget was allocated to this level of care. The Ministry of Health established the physical infrastructure for effective primary care and set norms for public health facilities required to provide primary care to the local population. Field staff were recruited, with an emphasis on engagement of female health workers. Efforts were made to integrate complementary programmes at field level (including water, sanitation, nutrition and so forth).

The Government of Tamil Nadu developed and implemented an autonomous drug distribution system to ensure there was no delay in the purchase and movement of essential medicines for primary care. Other innovative delivery and financial management systems were adopted, such as 24-hour health facilities and the creation of autonomous bodies (quasi-governmental institutions) to bypass bureaucratic hurdles that would limit the effective delivery of essential care.

A number of other enabling conditions have contributed to Tamil Nadu's public health successes. These include political commitment at the highest level and support from the Government of India. At the same time, the state and district administrations have been involved in the design and implementation of strategic policies and programmes. They have been active participants in large part because the Government of Tamil Nadu has worked to ensure that it has in place an adequate number of health personnel, from the field level up to district and state levels, who are trained and experienced in managing public health challenges. Recognition needs to be given to the work culture and commitment of field staff and all levels of management.

Outside of the health system, several cultural and socioeconomic factors have contributed to Tamil Nadu's achievements, such as a low fertility rate, better literacy, progress on women's empowerment and higher incomes.

Nevertheless, it should be noted that Tamil Nadu cannot claim to be in good health in all respects, and several pressing health challenges need to be tackled more effectively. Perhaps the greatest remaining challenge is addressing the alarmingly low nutritional status of adults and children, as in other states of India. High levels of malnutrition and undernutrition indicate that the state has had less success with policies aimed at tackling some of the broader determinants of health that fall outside the health sector. In fact, Tamil Nadu fares worse than many other states and the overall average in India with regard to average calorie and protein intake, and the number of babies who are underweight at birth.

In addition, more could be done to lower the maternal mortality rate. Nearly 60% of maternal deaths are from sepsis after delivery, postpartum haemorrhage, pulmonary embolism, anaemia and jaundice. A large number of maternal deaths continue to occur during transit (due to a lack of transportation, as in other parts of the country); at home, where 10% of women give birth; or even in maternity centres, due to the lack of skilled health personnel. All of these problems can be prevented through judicious policy interventions.

Likewise, Tamil Nadu's infant mortality rate, although low compared with other states, could be even lower. About 60% of infant deaths occur at the early neonatal and post-neonatal stages (as in other states of India) and most could be prevented. Official estimates for 2008 show birth asphyxia and low birth weight accounted for many infant deaths in the state. While the aggregate infant mortality rate has fallen over the years, the relative contributions of asphyxia and low birth weight continue to be high (28% and 40%, respectively, in 2008) and pose serious challenges to policy makers.

Apart from the conditions covered by the Millennium Development Goals, Tamil Nadu, like all other states in India, needs to face the increasing burden of noncommunicable diseases. The Government of Tamil Nadu should pay special attention to providing basic care to people in underserved areas, namely in hilly and tribal regions, and to developing policies to bring about behavioural changes. The most worrisome issue is the increasing financial burden on the poor from illnesses that require long-term care. Another emerging trend is that, as a result of increased public awareness of health issues, people have become much more conscious of their health status than in the past. This has led to rising expectations and demands for public health services, such as care for diabetes, hypertension, cancer and mental health.

Under the National Rural Health Mission introduced in 2005, with substantial increases in the overall budgetary allocation from the Government of India and with considerable managerial autonomy delegated to executive staff and field functionaries, the state has decreased maternal mortality and infant mortality rates even further, and has also begun to meet the demand for services for noncommunicable diseases.

Efforts are being made to upgrade primary health centres with modern diagnostic facilities and, in particular, to provide them with the equipment and skilled health personnel needed to prevent neonatal, infant and maternal deaths. Like many other Indian states, Tamil Nadu has recently introduced a vast network of emergency services, which also provide emergency obstetric care. Consequently, the financial burden on the general population should decrease considerably, through reductions in out-of-pocket expenditure.

Meanwhile, DANIDA has been instrumental in establishing a health management information system, which will reduce the workload on village health nurses, on the staff at primary health centres and on first referral units for regular reporting of vital events and other information. The health management information system has already been extended to all districts. In time, it is expected to evolve into a better management decision support system.

Although Tamil Nadu still has a long way to go to address the above challenges effectively, the signs are positive that it is moving in the right direction. Its successes to date can provide useful lessons and a backdrop for the hurdles it has to face, both now and in the future.

ACKNOWLEDGEMENTS

We are extremely grateful to a large number of individuals who have contributed to this chapter. Several of them had served the Government of Tamil Nadu and Government of India during the 1980s and 1990s. Several others are still in service. Their frank and perceptive insight has helped us construct a credible account of the health sector of Tamil Nadu over the past three decades. In particular, we are grateful to the Government of Tamil Nadu for sharing with us a large number of documents and statistics.

Our special thanks to Dr Dina Balabanova of the London School of Hygiene & Tropical Medicine and her entire research team for their constant intellectual support and patient response to every single difficulty we faced at various stages of this study. Our special thanks to Wendy Wisbaum for her excellent editorial help.

We are immensely grateful to the Rockefeller Foundation for providing us with the opportunity to share the experience of Tamil Nadu with the international community and for allowing us to be part of this comparative study.

REFERENCES

1. Ministry of Home Affairs. Directorate of Census Operations – Tamil Nadu. *Census-2011. Provisional Population Total.* Chennai: National Informatics Centre; 2011 (http://www.census.tn.nic.in/state_ppt.php, accessed 31 July 2011).

2. Government of India. *Census 2001* [database online] New Delhi: Office of the Registrar General & Census Commissioner, India: 2001 (http://www.census india.gov.in/Census_Data_2001/Census_data_finder/C_Series/Population_by_ religious_communities.htm, accessed March 2011).

3. Government of India. *National Health Accounts 2004–05.* New Delhi: Ministry of Health and Family Welfare; 2009 (http://www.whoindia.org/LinkFiles/Health _Finance_National_Health_Accounts_2004-05.pdf, accessed June 2011).

4. Roa KD et al. *India's health workforce size, composition and distribution.* New Delhi: Public Health Foundation of India & World Bank; 2008 (HRH Technical Report 1).

5. International Institute of Population Sciences. *National Family Health Survey-III, 2005–06.* Mumbai: International Institute of Population Sciences; 2007.

6. Government of India. *Economic Survey of India 2010–11.* New Delhi: Government of India; 2010.

7. World Bank. Poverty Reduction & Economic Management Unit. South Asia Region. *Economic growth and poverty alleviation in Tamil Nadu. Notes on selected policy issues.* Washington, DC: World Bank; 2005.

8. Government of Tamil Nadu. *Tamil Nadu human development report 2003.* New Delhi: Social Science Press; 2003.

9. Registrar General of India. *Sample registration system.* New Delhi: Registrar General of India; 1970–2006.

10. Registrar General of India. *Sample registration system. Special bulletin on maternal mortality in India 2004–06.* New Delhi: Registrar General of India; 2009.

11. Government of India. *HIV sentinel surveillance and HIV estimation in India 2007. A Technical brief.* New Delhi: National AIDS Control Organisation, Ministry of Health & Family Welfare, Government of India; 2008.

12. Registrar General of India. *Sample Registration System.* New Delhi: Registrar General of India; 2007.

13. International Institute of Population Sciences. *National family health survey-II, 1998–99.* Mumbai: International Institute of Population Sciences; 2000.

14. Nandraj S et al., eds. *Private health sector in India: review and annotated bibliography.* Mumbai: Centre for Enquiry into Health and Allied Themes; 2001.

15. International Institute of Population Sciences. *National family health survey-I, 1992–93.* Mumbai: International Institute of Population Sciences; 1994.

16. Narayana D. Intensifying infant mortality inequality in India and a reversal by policy intervention. *Journal of Human Development and Capability* 2008; 9(2):265–81.

17. Athreya V, Chunkath SR. Gender and infant survival in rural Tamil Nadu: situation and strategy. *Economic and Political Weekly* 1998; 33(40):3–9.

18. Jejeebhoy SJ. Addressing women's reproductive health needs: priorities for the family welfare programme. *Economic and Political Weekly* 1997; 32(9/10):475–84.

19. Government of Tamil Nadu. *Annual policy notes.* Chennai: Department of Health and Family Welfare; 1985–2006.

20. Government of Tamil Nadu. *Annual State's Budget Estimates. Performance Budget.* Chennai: Health and Family Welfare Department, Chennai; 1996–2006.

21. Guilmoto CZ, Rajan SI, eds. *Fertility transition in South India.* London: Sage; 2005.

22. Kaul M. The new public administration: management innovations in government. *Public Administration and Development* 1997; 17(1):13–26.

23. Bennett S, Muraleedharan VR. 'New public management' and health care in the third world. *Economic and Political Weekly* 2000; 35(1–2):59–68.

24. Das Gupta M et al. *How to improve public health systems: lessons from Tamil Nadu.* Washington, DC: World Bank, Development Research Group; 2009.

25. DANIDA. *Country Report India: evaluation of DANISH bilateral assistance to health 1988–97*. Copenhagen: Danish International Development Agency; 1999.

26. Government of Tamil Nadu. *Adoption of primary health centres/government hospitals*. Chennai: Health and Family Welfare Department; 1998 (Order no. 349, 22 June 1998).

27. Government of Tamil Nadu. *Government Order No. 449*. Chennai: Health and Family Welfare Department; 1998 (August 1998).

28. Pande RP, Yasbeck AS. What's in a country average? Wealth, gender and regional inequalities in immunization in India. *Social Science & Medicine* 2003; 57(11):2075-88.

29. Gaudin S, Yasbeck AS. Immunization in India 1993–1999: wealth, gender, and regional inequalities revisited. *Social Sciences & Medicine* 2006; 62(3):694–706.

30. Lalitha N. Tamil Nadu Government intervention and prices of medicine. *Economic and Political Weekly* 2008; 43(1):66–71.

31. Muraleedharan VR. Private–public sector partnership in health care sector in India: a review of policy options and challenges. In: Nandraj S at al., eds. *Private health sector in India: review and annotated bibliography*. Mumbai: Centre for Enquiry into Health and Allied Themes; 2001:29–49.

32. Padmanaban P, Raman PS, Mavalankar DV. Innovations and challenges in reducing maternal mortality in Tamil Nadu, India. *Journal of Health, Population, and Nutrition* 2009; 27(2):202–19.

33. WHO Regional Office for South East Region. *Safer pregnancy in Tamil Nadu: from vision to reality*. New Delhi: WHO Regional Office for South East Region; 2009.

34. Peters DH et al. *Better health systems for India's poor: findings, analysis and options*. Washington DC: World Bank; 2002.

35. Bhattacharya P. Economic development, gender inequality and demographic outcomes: evidence from India. *Population and Development Review* 2006; 32(20):263–91.

36. Jejeebhoy SJ, Sathar ZA. Women's autonomy in India and Pakistan: the influence of religion and region, *Population and Development Review* 2001; 27(4):687–712.

37. Sundari Ravindran TK. Female autonomy in Tamil Nadu: unravelling the complexities. *Economic and Political Weekly* 1999; 34(16/17):WS34–WS44.

38. Rahman L, Rao V. The determinants of gender equity in India: examining Dyson and Moore's thesis with new data. *Population and Development Review* 2004; 30(2):239–68.

39. Brenneman A, Kerf M. *Infrastructure and poverty linkages: a literature review.* Washington, DC: World Bank; 2002.

40. Behrman JR, Wolfe BL. How does mother's schooling affect family health, nutrition, medical care usage, and household sanitation? *Journal of Econometrics* 1987; 36(1–2):185–204.

41. Lavy V et al. Quality of health care, survival and health outcomes in Ghana. *Journal of Health Economics* 1996; 15(3):333–57.

42. Lee L, Rosenzweig MR, Pitt MM. The effects of improved nutrition, sanitation, and water quality on child health in high-mortality populations. *Journal of Econometrics* 1997; 77(1):209–35.

43. Leipziger D et al. *Achieving the Millennium Development Goals: The role of infrastructure.* Washington, DC: World Bank; 2003 (Working Paper No. 3163).

44. Wagstaff A, Claeson M. *The millennium development goals for health: rising to the challenges.* Washington, DC:World Bank; 2004.

45. Ghosh B, De P. Investigating the linkage between infrastructure and regional development in India: era of planning to globalisation. *Journal of Asian Economics* 2005; 15(6):1023–50.

46. Wang L. Determinants of child mortality in LDCs: empirical findings from demographic and health surveys. *Health Policy* 2003; 65(3):277–99.

47. Gwatkin DR. Poverty and inequality in health within developing countries: Filling the information gap. In: Leon DA, Walt G, eds. *Poverty, inequality and health: an international perspective.* Oxford: Oxford University Press; 2001:217–46.

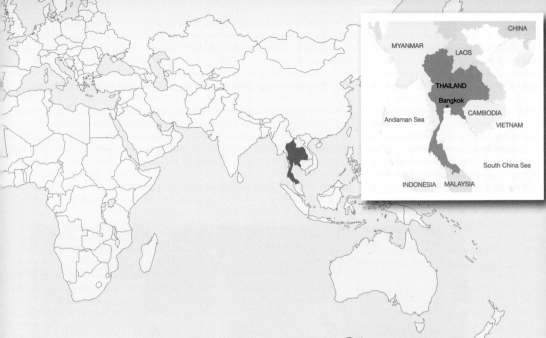

Chapter 7

WHY AND HOW DID THAILAND ACHIEVE GOOD HEALTH AT LOW COST?

Walaiporn Patcharanarumol[1], Viroj Tangcharoensathien[1],
Supon Limwattananon[1], Warisa Panichkriangkrai[1],
Kumaree Pachanee[1], Waraporn Poungkantha[1],
Lucy Gilson[2,3] and Anne Mills[3]

1 IHPP, 2 University of Cape Town, 3 LSHTM

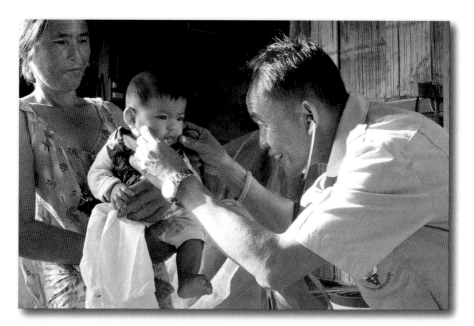

Health professional staff from the "Salah Chiang Tong Health Center" deliver outreach health services, including maternal and child care, to people in remote Karen villages in the Mae Sariang District, Mae Hong Son Province on the border between Thailand and Myanmar.

■ Key messages

- Thailand has outperformed many other countries in improving health outcomes at relatively low per capita health spending. Interventions essential to child survival and maternal health, notably free antenatal care, skilled birth attendance, family planning, and immunization, reached universal coverage by the 1990s, and all health Millennium Development Goals (MDGs) were achieved by the early 2000s.

- These services are provided mainly by the public sector – in primary health care centres and district hospitals geographically accessible to the rural poor. Longstanding policies of government bonding and rural deployment of all graduates of the health-related professions have been critical to the successful expansion of district health systems.

- Financial risk protection, introduced initially to protect the poor and vulnerable, was subsequently extended to achieve universal coverage of the entire population by 2002.

- Nine successive five-year national health plans ensured continuity over four decades of health system development. Generations of charismatic leaders and highly influential technocrats and medical leaders inside and outside of the Ministry of Public Health (MOPH), sharing a common vision of improving the health of the poorest, ensured that pro-poor, pro-rural health policies remained the priority of health system development.

- Royal Health projects, promoted by the Royal Family, contributed to comprehensive rural development, not only improving health but also empowering rural communities.

- Other contributing factors to Thailand's good health outcomes have been economic growth and poverty reduction, a high level of female literacy and a fall in the gender literacy gap.

- Thailand has developed the institutional capacity to generate evidence to inform policy, which puts it in a good position to deal with current and future health challenges.

Introduction

Thailand, a lower-middle-income country in South-east Asia with a population of 67 million, is the only nation in the region that has never been colonized. Thailand is a democratic country, with the King as head of state. Thailand is divided into 75 provinces, and there are also two special governed districts: the capital Bangkok and Pattaya. Each province is divided into districts and the districts are further divided into subdistricts (*tambons*). In 2010, there were 878 districts as well as the 50 districts of Bangkok.

One unique feature of the Thai health system is its extensive and long-term investment in a health care delivery infrastructure that reaches even the most rural and remote areas. Primary health centres, typically 1 per 5000 people, function well because the MOPH produces its own nurses and para-professionals and because rural service is mandatory for all health professionals. Thailand achieved all health MDGs in the early 2000s and introduced the concept of MDG Plus, a set of country-specific targets going well beyond the international targets. By adopting goals and targets that are customized to local needs and priorities, MDG Plus has become a central theme in Thailand's multisectoral human development movement[1,2].

Thai health spending was 4.3% of gross domestic product (GDP) in 2009. This is in line with the 4.3% of GDP spent on average by lower-middle-income countries as a group. However, when adjusted for purchasing power, Thailand's per capita health expenditure is higher, at Int$ 345 compared with an average of Int$ 145 for lower-middle-income countries. In addition, compared with other countries at a similar level of national resources, general government expenditure on health is higher (75.8% of total health expenditure), and private health expenditure lower (24.2%)[3,4]. Donor resources contribute a very small share. As shown in Figure 7.1, which correlates under-5 mortality and total health expenditure per capita in all low- and middle-income countries, Thailand performs exceptionally well.

Since the 1980s, Thailand has benefited from a growing gross national income (GNI) per capita (Figure 7.2), with US$ 3760 in 2009, which is higher than the average of the lower-middle-income group, US$ 2316. Rapid economic growth has resulted in significant poverty reduction, from 49.7% of the population in 1988 to 10.7% in 2007, although income distribution as measured by the Gini index has not improved much.

However, Thailand also made significant health investment decisions at a time when it was not propitious from an economic point of view. Universal health coverage was introduced in 2002 during an economic decline following the

Box 7.1 Thailand at a glance

Population	67 million (2009)[5], 66% of the population is rural (2009)[5], concentrated in the rice-growing areas of the central and northern regions. 94.6% of the population is Buddhist[6].
Geography	Located in South-east Asia. Densely populated central plain, highland areas in the north-east and mountain range in the north, west and south-east.
Ethnic composition	75% Thai, 14% Chinese and 11% other.
Government	A democratic country, with the King as head of state, a constitutional monarchy since 1932. Thailand was never colonized. Recent period of political unrest but successful elections completed in 2011.
Health system	Health expenditure per capita (constant 2005 Int$) (2009)[7]: 344.69 Density of physicians, nurses and midwives per 10000[3]: 17 Extensive and long-term investment in primary health care, particularly in infrastructure and health workers in rural and remote areas. Achieved universal health coverage and low out-of-pocket payments. Coverage of key interventions is high (99% of deliveries with skilled attendance, over 90% of children vaccinated[8]). Successful prevention and treatment programmes have turned a generalized HIV epidemic into a concentrated epidemic among specific groups.

Economic, demographic and social development indicators		
GDP per capita (constant 2005 Int$) (2009)[5]	7260
Economic growth: GNI 2000 to 2008[5]	5.2% per annum
Population living on less than $1.25/day (2009)[5]	10.8%
Gini index[5]	42.5 (2004)
Infant mortality rate[9]	8.3 (2010)[a]
Maternal mortality ratio[10]	47[b]
HIV prevalence (adults aged 15–49) (2009)[5]	1%
Life expectancy (2009)[5]	69
Total fertility rate (2009)[5]	1.8
Adult literacy (2005)[11]	93.5%
Ratio girls to boys in education[c]	103%
Access to improved water source (2008)[5]	98%
Internet usage (2009)[5]	25.8%

Note: [a] Per 1000 live births; [b] Per 100000 live births; [c] Primary and secondary education.

Asian financial crisis (as shown in Figure 7.2), and when Thailand was still at the lower end of the GNI per capita range of lower-middle-income countries.

Empirical evidence shows that health financing is progressive (the richer groups pay relatively more than the poorer groups) because of the dominant role of general tax financing, and the reduction in the share of out-of-pocket payments

**Figure 7.1   Correlation between under-5 mortality rate and per capita health
expenditure in all low- and middle-income countries, 2005**

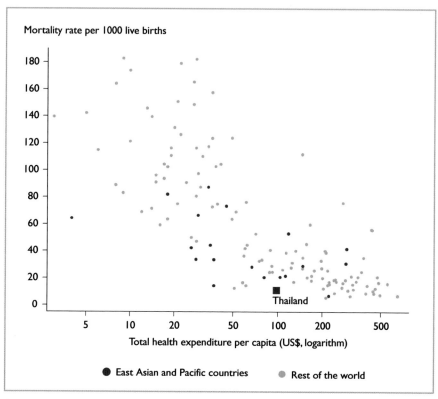

Source: Data from reference 3.

for health (to 18% of total health expenditure with a very low level of catastrophic health expenditure)[12]. Equity in utilization has resulted in public
subsidies which favour the poor[13].

This chapter examines data for the period from 1970 to 2010 as well as interviews with key policy-makers, administrators and researchers. The research team
was able to draw on the extensive knowledge of one of its members (Viroj
Tangcharoensathien) who has been involved in the process of health development
since the 1980s; however, information was validated through wider interviews.

Findings are presented in five sections. First, the improvements in health
outcomes are described, in particular relating to maternal and child health. Next,
information is provided on the coverage of specific health interventions that
contributed to such achievements. Third, evidence is provided on how health

Figure 7.2 Thailand's GNI per capita, 1970–2009, current year prices

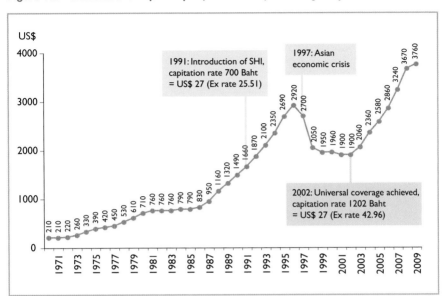

Note: SHI: Social Health Insurance.

Source: Data from reference 5.

systems supported the effective delivery of these interventions. The fourth section examines how and why over time the health system's development and other wider policy interventions were possible. Finally, the contributions of other sectors and the sociopolitical and cultural factors influencing health gains are assessed.

■ Better health?

Between 1975 and 2005, life expectancy in Thailand increased markedly, with female life expectancy outpacing male (Figure 7.3) due to the impact of AIDS in the 1990s. The 1999 and 2004 studies on the burden of disease showed that HIV is the leading cause of disability-adjusted life years (DALYs) lost for both men and women[14].

Infant mortality has fallen sharply in Thailand, from a rate of 68.0 per 1000 live births in 1970, to below 20 in 1991, reaching under 10 in 2006 (Figure 7.4). The urban–rural gap has decreased, although rural infant mortality was still 20% higher than urban infant mortality in the early 2000s. Likewise, a consistent reduction in under-5 mortality was observed, although it slowed in the mid-

Figure 7.3 Life expectancy at birth by sex, 1975–2005

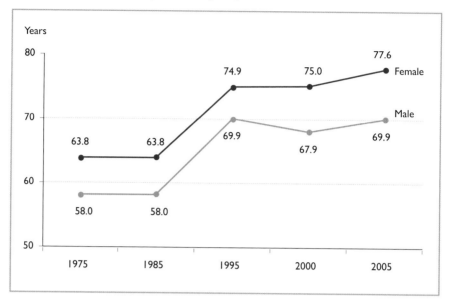

Source: Data from references 15 and 16.

Figure 7.4 Infant mortality rate, 1970–2010

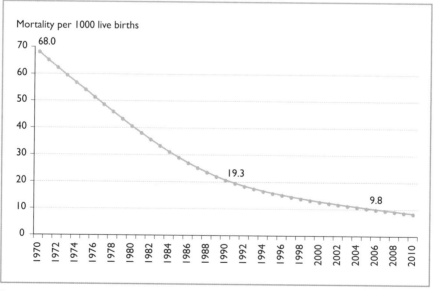

Source: Data from reference 9.

Figure 7.5   Maternal mortality ratio, 1960–2008

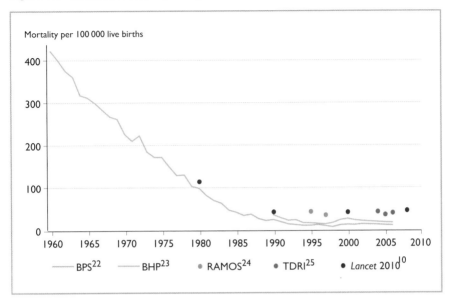

Sources: Data from references 10 and 22–25.

2000s. Provincial disparities in mortality have decreased but still persist, with higher child and infant mortality in some provinces in the north-eastern, northern and southern regions of Thailand. Nonetheless, a substantially larger reduction in child mortality has been observed among the poorer quintiles, and the excess child mortality risk between the poorest and richest quintiles decreased by 55% (95% confidence interval, 39–68) between 1990 and 2000[17]. Low birth weight remains a concern, due to its implications for long-term poor adult health[18,19].

Thailand had the highest annual rate of reduction in child mortality among 30 low- and middle-income countries between 1990 and 2006[20], and in 2006, Thailand had the second lowest level of child mortality (Table 7.1).

Accurately establishing the level of maternal mortality is much more problematic. Various estimates show a steep reduction between 1960 and 1990, followed by relative stagnation since 1990 (Figure 7.5)[21]. In Table 7.1, Thailand can be seen to have a relatively low rate in 2005, but not markedly low (110 per 100 000 live births), although the most recent estimates, for 2008, were 47[10] and 48[26] per 100 000 live births.

Table 7.1   Low- and middle-income countries ranked by average annual rate of reduction in under-5 mortality rate, 1990–2006

		Annual reduction under-5 mortality rate (1990–2006) (%)	Under-5 mortality rate 2006 (per 1000 live births)	Maternal mortality ratio 2005 (per 100 000 live births)
1	Thailand	8.5	8	110
2	Vietnam	7.1	17	150
3	Peru	7.1	25	240
4	Brazil	6.5	20	110
5	Indonesia	6.2	34	410
6	Syria	6.2	14	130
7	Egypt	6.0	35	130
8	Sri Lanka	5.6	13	58
9	Nepal	5.5	59	830
10	Morocco	5.5	37	240
11	El Salvador	5.5	25	170
12	Ecuador	5.4	24	210
13	Tunisia	5.1	23	100
14	Dominican Republic	5.0	29	150
15	Laos	4.9	75	660
16	Bangladesh	4.8	69	570
17	Honduras	4.8	27	280
18	Iran	4.7	34	140
19	Bolivia	4.5	61	290
20	Kazakhstan	4.5	29	140
21	Eritrea	4.3	74	450
22	Guatemala	4.3	41	290
23	Philippines	4.1	32	230
24	Turkmenistan	4.1	51	130
25	Haiti	4.0	80	670
26	Nicaragua	4.0	36	170
27	Paraguay	3.9	22	150
28	China	3.9	24	45
29	Cuba	3.9	7	45
30	Malawi	3.8	120	1100

Note: Table only includes countries with GNI US$ 5000 per capita or less and births ≥100 000/year.
Source: Data from reference 20.

The total fertility rate fell significantly from 6.3 births per woman in 1965, to below the replacement rate in 1994[27], and to 1.7 in 2003. In 2006, the average age of women at their first birth was 22.8 years, 24.0 in urban areas and 22.3 in rural areas[28]. However, the prevalence of teenage pregnancies has increased, from 11% in 1996 to 12% in 2000 and to 15.7% in 2009, leading to problems of preterm delivery, low birth weight and neonatal mortality[29,30].

Progress in maternal and child health indicators was confirmed by the experiences of several experts who participated in this study. All of the people who were interviewed agreed that Thailand has achieved good maternal and child health in a relatively low-cost manner. They had evidence from their experience to justify their statements.

> *Good health, yes. Thailand has already achieved MDG numbers four and five. We are moving towards MDG Plus.*
>
> *Policy-maker outside MOPH*

> *… The health of pregnant women is fairly good. When I go to the field, about 100% of pregnant women get antenatal care from mostly public health facilities; there is only one case I have ever seen of a woman who had no antenatal care due to personal reasons, because she was a teenage pregnant woman. Probably the comprehensive distribution of primary health care services to the most peripheral areas of the system (subdistrict level) is the key explanation as to how good maternal and child health were achieved.*
>
> *NGO representative*

In order to relate reductions in death rates to contributions of the health system, it is important to understand changes in the causes of child and infant deaths. Table 7.2 shows the top 20 causes of deaths among children under 5 years of age in 1996, 2000, 2005 and 2009. Mortality from lower respiratory tract infections, heart failure, septicaemia, communicable and parasitic diseases, and diarrhoea demonstrated a downward trend between 1996 and 2009, and have been addressed by adequate access to primary care services, public health interventions and maternal and child health services. Drowning as the sixth cause of child mortality was unchanged, at 0.52 and 0.54 in 1996 and 2009, respectively, similar to road traffic accidents. Mortality from low birth weight, other congenital anomalies, congenital heart diseases and conditions arising from the perinatal period showed an increasing trend, and were the main contributors to perinatal mortality.

Table 7.2   Top 20 causes of death of children under 5 years, per 1000 live births, 1996–2009

	1996	2000	2005	2009
No diagnosis	1.29	3.26	1.47	1.45
▼ Other ill-defined	1.12	0.53	0.19	0.18
▼ Lower respiratory tract infections	1.03	0.47	0.56	0.46
▼ Heart failure	0.99	0.10	0.00	0.00
▼ Septicaemia	0.59	0.80	0.38	0.30
▼ Other chronic respiratory diseases	0.52	0.32	0.19	0.20
◆ Drowning	0.52	0.76	0.65	0.54
▼ Other communicable and parasitic diseases	0.35	0.28	0.15	0.15
▼ Other cardiovascular disease	0.30	0.06	0.09	0.10
▲ Low birth weight	0.29	0.25	1.01	1.04
▼ Diarrhoea	0.26	0.25	0.16	0.09
◆ Road traffic accidents	0.24	0.32	0.20	0.19
▲ Other congenital anomalies	0.24	0.39	0.76	0.77
▼ Ill-defined heart disease	0.24	0.08	0.05	0.05
▲ Congenital heart disease	0.23	0.36	0.61	0.67
▼ Other neurological diseases	0.21	0.13	0.09	0.07
▼ Endocrine and metabolic disorders	0.20	0.22	0.07	0.05
▼ Other digestive diseases	0.18	0.17	0.12	0.10
▼ Ill-defined unintentional accidents	0.17	0.08	0.04	0.02
▼ Other unintentional injuries	0.17	0.19	0.18	0.14
▲ Other conditions arising in the perinatal period	0.16	0.91	2.24	2.02
Top 20 causes of death, per 1000 live births	9.30	9.93	9.23	8.62
All others, per 1000 live births	1.25	2.01	1.55	1.31
Under-5 mortality rate, per 1000 live births	10.55	11.93	10.77	9.94

Note: ▼: Decreasing trend; ▲: Increasing trend; ◆: No change.
Source: Data from reference 31.

■ What has Thailand done to improve health?

The analysis of how Thailand achieved good maternal and child health outcomes sought to link the improvements to a range of specific interventions that have been undertaken over the years. Table 7.3 lists 25 interventions that are effective in addressing nine major causes of under-5 mortality[a] and are generally viewed as critical for child survival[32], as well as desirable for the survival of mothers. Table 7.3 presents an assessment of current coverage levels based on interviews with a maternal and child health programme expert (a clinician in a teaching hospital). Most interventions have high coverage, except for exclusive breastfeeding at six months, which was 5.3% in 2006, and antenatal steroids to prevent premature labour, which is in the scaling-up phase. There were no policies regarding the use of zinc to prevent diarrhoea, or antibiotics for premature rupture of membranes.

All interventions were fully integrated into primary health care networks and were implemented through district health systems. A typical district health system consists of 10–12 health centres, each covering 5000 people, and a district hospital covering 50 000 people. District health systems integrate maternal health, covering antenatal care, pregnancy, childbirth and early neonatal care, and family planning; and child health programmes, including immunization and well-baby clinics[37].

Nurses and public health workers are the backbone of rural health systems; they are multipurpose and are well trained to serve the community in particular public health functions, such as health promotion services, preventive services, and other community-based health services such as school health and home visits. Some professional nurses have one-year post-service training as anaesthetic nurses and conduct local and general anaesthesia in district hospitals, including for caesarean sections and other obstetric emergencies.

Nurses in district hospitals also provide the first antenatal care visit, which requires laboratory screening with consultation backup by general doctors (not obstetricians) for high-risk pregnancies, such as women with diabetes, a history of preterm labour and hypertension. Subsequent antenatal care visits are mostly managed by health centres. Nurses in district hospitals are also trained to provide counselling for HIV/AIDS in pregnancy, offering advice about prevention of mother-to-child transmission. Nurses are responsible for normal uncomplicated deliveries, while complicated cases are referred to general doctors in district hospitals or to provincial hospitals where obstetricians are available.

---

[a] Diarrhoea, pneumonia, measles, malaria, HIV/AIDS, birth asphyxia, preterm delivery, neonatal tetanus and neonatal sepsis.

Table 7.3   Assessment of coverage of maternal and child survival
             interventions, 2010

Interventions	Coverage	Comments
I. PREVENTIVE		
Water, sanitation, hygiene	Universal	Universal coverage of safe water and clean sanitation achieved; 98% have access to safe water
Newborn temperature management	Universal	In-hospital case management for preterm newborns, incubators well equipped in all hospitals, including district, but not health centres
Tetanus toxoid	Universal	Integrated in antenatal care with high coverage
Nevirapine and replacement feeding	Universal	Triple ART (zidovudine, lamivudine, lopinavir) in PMTCT, high coverage as integrated with antenatal care, high level of vertical transmission prevention, PMTCT and breast milk substitutes up to 18 months of age are free of charge
Antenatal care	Universal	Very high coverage, with percentage of four visits increasing from 62% in 1988 to 82% in 2006. The national *Reproductive Health Survey* from 2006[28] reported 98.9% "ever antenatal care". Government health services are the main antenatal care provider, with 80.3% of total services
Antenatal steroids to prevent preterm delivery	At scaling-up phase	National policy recently launched and implemented, rapid scale-up observed[33]
Safe delivery	Universal	Coverage increased from 66% in 1986 to >80% in 1990 and almost 100% since 1995. In 2006, 92.4% of total births in public sector, 6.2% in private sector and 1.3% home deliveries (most in the southern Muslim provinces)[28]. Skilled birth attendants in 98.6% of total births in hospitals, according to the national *Reproductive Health Survey* 2009[34]
Exclusive breastfeeding	Very low	Immediate mother–newborn bonding and breast milk initiation; support six-month exclusive breastfeeding but coverage is very low. The 2006 Multi-Indicator Cluster Survey reported that only 5.3% of infants under 6 months were exclusively breastfed[8]

Table 7.3 (continued)

Interventions	Coverage	Comments
Measles and other EPI vaccines	Universal	Measles vaccine integrated in national EPI programme, although sporadic measles outbreaks from children >12 years, catch up campaign for measles not yet a policy. EPI is solely provided by public health sector, with very limited role of private sector. Vaccine-preventable diseases[35] captured by MOPH diseases surveillance system were reduced sharply in association with >90% EPI coverage in 1990s[36]. Mortality from these diseases was extremely low due to prompt detection and treatment
Haemophilus influenzae type B (Hib) vaccine	Not a major public health problem	Not implemented
Zinc	No policy	No clear policy
Antibiotics for premature rupture of membranes	No policy	There is no national guideline; implemented upon clinical judgment by individual physicians
Insecticide-treated materials	Not a major public health problem	Fully implemented in three provinces bordering Myanmar and Cambodia
Antimalarial intermittent treatment in pregnancy	Not a major public health problem	Not routinely practised
Complementary feeding	Cannot assess	Appropriate feeding advice in postnatal follow-up and well-baby clinics, no assessment on coverage
Vitamin A	Cannot assess	Combined in multivitamin in well-baby clinics
Family planning	Universal	CPR increased sharply from 14.7% in 1970, to 67.5% in 1987, 79.2% in 2003, and 81.1% in 2006. Rural–urban gap of CPR reduced until full equity was reached in 1984. The national *Reproductive Health Survey* 2006 reported CPR of 81.2% in urban and 80.9% in rural areas[28]. In 2006, health centres and district hospitals provided 62.6% of total family planning services. Private pharmacies have had an increasing role in recent years

Table 7.3 (continued)

Interventions	Coverage	Comments
II. TREATMENT		
Oral rehydration therapy	Universal	Full coverage, integrated at primary health care level, also support for home preparation
Antibiotics for pneumonia	Universal	Full coverage, integrated in health delivery systems + referral backup from health centre to district hospital, and from district to provincial hospitals
Antibiotics for sepsis	Universal	Available in district hospitals upward, high clinical competency in case management
Newborn resuscitation	Universal	Doctors well trained, core clinical competency in medical curriculum. Nurses responsible for delivery are also well trained
Antibiotics for dysentery	Universal	Appropriate antibiotics given on laboratory confirmation of diagnosis
Zinc	No policy	Not yet implemented
Antimalarial prophylaxis	Not a major public health problem	Not routinely practised
Vitamin A	Cannot assess	Combined in multivitamin in well-baby clinics

Notes: ART: Antiretroviral therapy; PMTCT: Prevention of mother-to-child transmission of HIV; EPI: Expanded Programme on Immunization; CPR: Contraceptive prevalence rate;

A recent assessment of the capacity of government hospitals to provide essential obstetric care found them to be satisfactory in term of accessibility, utilization and quality[38]. Policies to reduce maternal mortality through unsafe abortions have yet to be developed. This is in light of the conservative stance towards, and societal dilemmas posed by, the provision of safe abortion services to respond to the increasing prevalence of unplanned pregnancies[39,40]. Laboratory capacities for providing safe blood transfusion in most district hospitals are important backup services for obstetric emergencies.

Nurses and public health workers are major providers of family planning services, mainly through the distribution of birth control pills and condoms.

During the active family planning campaigns of the 1980s, professional nurses were trained to provide intrauterine devices to clients with outcomes comparable to those of doctors[40], but at lower cost and greater accessibility. District hospital doctors have competencies to provide vasectomy and permanent female family planning services. Vaccinations are given by staff in the public sector, in particular in health centres and district hospitals located close to where rural people live.

What has the health system contributed to health improvement?

This section describes the key trends in health system development that ensured universal coverage of maternal and child health interventions and guaranteed that the vital services described above could be made widely available. The focus is on (1) developments in health care delivery and the health workforce that ensured the availability and functioning of the supply side, and (2) health financing reforms that ensured financial access to health care on the demand side. Both supply- and demand-side interventions concertedly address physical and financial barriers to access to care by the population.

Figure 7.6 plots chronological changes in the under-5 mortality rate through five-year National Economic and Social Development Plans (NESDP). The panel below the curved line shows significant health infrastructure and human resources developments, whereas the panel above the curved line tracks the extension of financial risk protection to different target populations. The annual reduction in under-5 mortality was high between 1970 and 1990 and levelled off thereafter.

Developments in health care delivery and the health workforce

When the MOPH was established in Thailand in 1942, it owned only 15 provincial hospitals outside Bangkok providing medical services for the entire population. The development of the health system – including infrastructure, human resources and financing – was guided by the five-year National Health Plan, which is an integral component of the NESDP. Expansion and upgrading of health facilities took 25 years, from the first NESDP until full coverage at all district and subdistrict levels by 1990 in the sixth NESDP. The first to the third NESDPs laid a solid foundation by expanding the number of provincial hospitals, to at least one in every province, and the fourth to sixth NESDPs did the same for district hospitals. Provincial hospitals were expanded first, in order to provide referral backup to district hospitals.

Figure 7.6 **Under-5 mortality, development of human resources and infrastructure, and financial protection, 1970–2010**

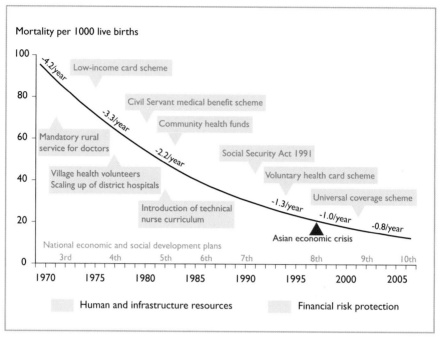

Source: Under-5 mortality data from reference 9.

Rapid scaling up of district hospitals began in 1977 and the next two decades witnessed a double-digit growth in the number of district hospitals (mostly with 10–60 beds) until every district had full coverage.

> *At the rapid scaling up of district hospitals during the fifth and sixth health plans, in Ubon province, six district hospitals were inaugurated each year; young doctors, nurses and other staff needed support but the Provincial Health Office was very stretched. Clinical, technical and administrative support from senior directors of neighbouring district hospitals was found to be very useful and practical. It was initiated based on a high spirit of commitment to rural health services.*
>
> *Researcher, MOPH*

This expansion of the district health system was critical. It laid a firm foundation for the future scaling up and equitable distribution of essential public health interventions and health services needed to achieve equitable and good maternal and child health outcomes.

Box 7.2 The history of government bonding of medical graduates

At the peak of the Vietnam War, American health care suffered from a lack of doctors as they were recruited to serve the war in Indochina. Thus, there was an exodus to the United States of a whole generation of Thailand's new medical graduates.

In 1967, having assessed the magnitude of loss and the lack of doctors serving rural areas, Thailand's Minister of Health, Phra Bamradnaradura, initiated a government bonding service policy for students in their first year of medicine. Opposition was minimized by making the policy prospective. Bonded students were required to serve three years in government health services. Students were initially allowed to opt out by paying a fine, but this was terminated a few years later because it benefited rich students. The first batch of bonded doctors graduated and started service in 1972.

The policy was fully supported by Professor Sood Sangwichian, former dean of the Faculty of Medicine at Siriraj Hospital. As he was one of the most charismatic leaders in medical education, the policy encountered no resistance from students and other faculties. Moreover, in 1967, students were in no mood to protest as the military government had recently suppressed their anti-American movement.

Excerpt from interview (retired MOPH policy-maker).

The adequate functioning of district health systems depended on the expansion of various cadres of health workers. One main achievement in human resources for health was mandatory public health service for all new medical graduates, which began in 1972 (Box 7.2). The government's bonding policy was considered to be legitimate, as medical and nursing education was heavily subsidized by tax-financed tertiary education. The bonding resulted in significantly increased numbers of doctors and nurses serving in rural district health services. Later, government bonding was extended to other cadres, such as pharmacists, dentists and other allied health professionals, including dental nurses, assistant pharmacists and laboratory technicians. Nursing students recruited from rural areas by the MOPH had fully funded four-year training in MOPH nursing colleges and had traditionally been able to serve their home town in MOPH health centres or district or provincial hospitals.

Historically, nursing faculties in universities under the Ministry of Education were unable to produce the number of nurses and midwives needed to meet demand for scaling up MOPH rural health services. In response to this challenge, in 1961, the MOPH established its own nurse and midwifery colleges, which were licensed and certified by the Thai Nurse and Midwifery Council.

Professional nurses were trained for four years and received bachelor degrees. In response to the rapid increase in the number of district hospitals, scaling up the production of nurses became a key policy goal. To do this, instead of nurses having four years of training, in 1982 a policy was introduced to produce a two-year trained diploma course for technical nurses. After a few years of mandatory rural services, these technical nurses completed an additional two years of post-service training, after which they were upgraded to professional nurses. The Nurse Council approved the technical nurse curriculum for a limited period of ten years, ensuring that all nurses ended up becoming professionally qualified.

To implement this policy, the MOPH benefited from its existing nursing colleges. There was no opposition from professional associations due to the undersupply of nurses. Producing more nurses eased the huge service loads in the public sector and had spillover benefits for the private health sector.

> *This policy got approval without resistance; the policy was welcomed by some universities (Siriraj, Khon Kaen and Prince Songkhla) and MOPH nursing colleges as was the policy on post-service upgrading to professional nurses.*
>
> *Expert in the Thai Nurse and Midwifery Council*

> *Nurses are the backbone of the health system, in particular, for primary health care and major maternal and child health service provision. Undeniably, it is the MOPH nursing colleges that produced these cadres of nurse personnel serving rural health systems, with universities having a limited role. We need to give credit to the predecessors in the MOPH who established nursing colleges and innovated these policies (particularly technical nurse production), and to nurse instructors and nurse fellows throughout the country.*
>
> *Retired MOPH policy-maker*

> *The production capacity of MOPH nursing colleges today is 70% of total annual national nurse production; while Ministry of Education produces 20% and private nurse colleges produce the rest, 10%, of the total.*
>
> *Expert in the Thai Nurse and Midwifery Council*

Figure 7.7 shows the benefits of the infrastructure and human resources policies in terms of improved population ratios covering the period from 1962 to 2007.

Figure 7.7   Health infrastructure and human resources trends in Thailand, 1962–2007

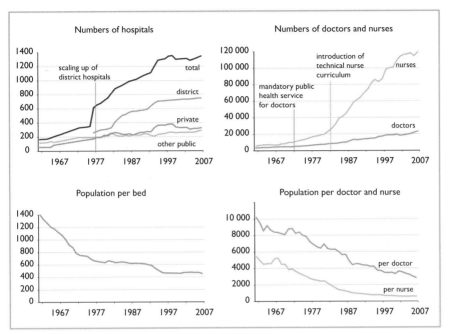

Source: Analysis using dataset from reference 42.

Interviewees agreed that health infrastructure and health workforce development significantly contributed to the success of maternal and child health services.

> The most important factor in the success of antenatal care was establishing health centres and district hospitals which covered all areas. It is not the private sector as advocated by many development partners. In the Thai context, it is the strength of public sector providers scattered around the country. I think extensive geographical coverage is a strong foundation for the health development of Thai people.
> *Current MOPH policy-maker*

> Health centres are the main contributor to the success of EPI [the Expanded Programme on Immunization]. It is the public health workers who lived in the staff house in the health centre or their own home in the village that provided these services. Undoubtedly, logistical support, and in particular, the cold chain, ensuring good quality vaccines from district hospital or district health offices, is also essential.
> *Retired MOPH policy-maker*

Almost all interviewees emphasized the importance of the expansion of health infrastructure to cover all districts of Thailand.

> *When I worked upcountry, it was clear that public health infrastructure was the most important … It was significantly developed during the era of rural development. The budget of provincial hospitals was shifted to rural areas, i.e. to build up the district hospitals.*
>
> *Retired MOPH policy-maker*

Over this period, there was constant turnover of governments and periodic economic crises (including the Asian economic crisis of 1997), but institutional continuity of senior officials in the MOPH, particularly in the Health Planning Division headed by the late Dr Damrong Boonyern[b] played a significant role, facilitated by the continuity provided by the five-year health planning process[43]. In addition, it should be stressed that the charismatic leaders who helped to steer the content of the National Health Plan came from rural areas and had experience working in rural health services. Thus, the content of the Plan was shaped by their conviction that favoured "good for the most" (benefits for the majority who were the rural poor) as opposed to "the best for a few" (the best for the urban elite). The continuity and engagement of young and old public health policy-makers ensured that this pro-rural ideology passed from generation to generation and that it remained the priority throughout four decades of health system development.

It is important to emphasize that these developments benefited from a supportive context. Peace and economic development were two other contributing factors for health infrastructure extension and human resource development. From 1965 to 1996, the Thai economy grew at a rate of 7.8% annually, with double-digit growth from 1986 to 1990. This sustained rapid economic growth allowed the government to pay off public debts and freed a large portion of the national budget for investment in the social sectors, including education and health. The proportion of the national budget devoted to public debt dropped from 24.7% in 1987 to 5% in 1997, and the education and health budgets rose from 18.1% and 4.1% in 1987, to 24.5% and 8% in 1998, respectively[44].

---

[b] Dr Damrong Boonyern, MD, DrPH (Tulane) had eight years of rural service experience in two provinces of the north-east region (1964–1972). He was head of the Policy, Planning and Research section of the Health Planning Division for eight years (1973–1981), then Director of the Health Planning Division for eight years (1981–1989), then deputy Director-General Department of Health for three years (1989–1992), Inspector General for two years (1992–1994), Director-General of the Communicable Diseases Control Department in 1994 and Director-General of the Department of Health from 1995 to 1997, when he retired.

The national five-year health development plans are funded mandates with adequate resources for programmes and activities to translate policy into real outcomes. These are not rhetorical statements delivered in the parliament or cabinet meetings.

Researcher in MOPH

Extension of financial risk protection

Expanding financial protection was another factor that led to improved health outcomes and access to services. In the early 1970s, user fees provided approximately half of the income of the district health services in Thailand, and the cost of obtaining health care was recognized to be an important cause of rural impoverishment. A policy on waiving user fees for low-income households was launched in 1975 as a tax-financed public welfare scheme; later, the scheme was extended to other vulnerable groups, such as the elderly, children under 12 years, and the disabled. Compulsory social health insurance under the Social Security Scheme was launched in 1991 for private-sector employees using tripartite payroll-tax contributions by employers, employees and the government. Beginning in 1984, the informal sector was able to purchase financial protection through a community-based health insurance scheme, financed by voluntary household contributions, which evolved into the publicly subsidized voluntary health insurance scheme in 1994, financed half by households and half by budget subsidies. Government employees were covered by a tax-financed non-contributory Civil Servant Medical Benefit Scheme.

This piecemeal, gradual extension of financial protection schemes had reached 70% of the total population by 2001. Coverage was not complete for all eligible groups due to the difficulties in administering fee exemptions for vulnerable households and incomplete take-up of public voluntary health insurance. In 2001, the government decided to simplify and universalize the arrangements by introducing universal health care coverage (known as UC). This was achieved in 2002 when the entire population was covered by one of the three insurance schemes: the existing social health insurance, the civil servant scheme or a new scheme for the remainder of the population[45].

A significant result of the extension of financial health protection was the reduction in both household out-of-pocket payments and catastrophic payments for health care among the poorest deciles, which further accelerated when the universal coverage scheme was launched in 2001 (Figure 7.8). This was achieved with relatively stable health expenditure as a percentage of GDP, although there was a significant shift in the shares of public and private expenditures. While the Asian economic crisis that started in July 1997 hit the economy hard for a few

Figure 7.8   Health expenditure trends in Thailand, 1994–2008

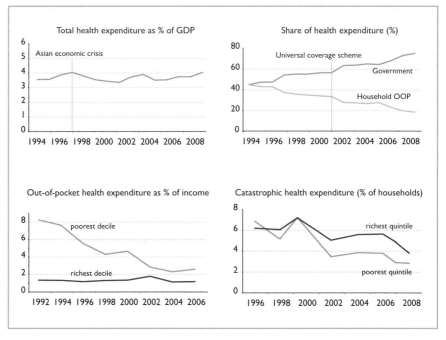

Source: Data from references 4 and 46.
Note: OOP: Out-of-pocket expenditure.

years, public spending on health was significantly protected and, indeed, universal coverage was introduced at the bottom of the slump in Thailand's GNI.

▇ How has Thailand achieved health system development?

This section explores why and how the policies that contributed to the development of the health system over the past four decades arose and were adopted. Who were the various actors involved in the policy processes, what was their power and position, and what were their motives?

Agenda setting: health has been given a high priority

Interviewees consistently argued that health received high priority in the national agenda, a point that was confirmed by the visibility of health plans in the NESDP process. Health has been included in policy statements by almost all

Thai Prime Ministers since 1942[47], and successive plans have introduced a number of key programmes such as the National Family Planning Programme in 1970, the national Expanded Programme on Immunization in 1977 and Safe Motherhood in 1998.

Prior to 1973, successive governments were dominated by military regimes, and after 1973, there was frequent political instability. Despite these difficulties, some health ministers appointed by military regimes were charismatic leaders who were also technocrats (civil servant administrators) with a strong public health or medical background and an equity orientation. Charismatic health ministers included Phra Bamradnaradura (1959–1969), Udom Posakrisana (1973–1975), Yongyouth Sajjavanich (1976–1978), Sem Pringpuangkeo (1980–1983), Pairoj Ningsanonda (1991–1992) and Mongkol Na Songkhla (2006–2008). For example, Minister Pairoj Ningsanonda, an ex-permanent secretary of the MOPH, passed a number of landmark laws including the Control of Tobacco Product Act 2535BE (1992), the Non-smoker Health Protection Act 2535BE (1992), the Health Systems Research Institute Act 2535BE (1992) and the Thailand Research Fund Act 2535BE (1992). The latter two contributed significantly to the strengthening of health system research and the generation of evidence for policy decisions. Minister Mongkol Na Songkhla fostered implementation of universal coverage by including renal replacement therapy for universal coverage scheme members. He also introduced a number of advanced laws, notably the National Health Act 2550BE (2007), which mandated an annual National Health Assembly to provide for grassroots participation in public policy development[48].

> *Whatever the MOPH does, it focuses on the poor or worse off and bene-*
> *fits the majority of the country, such as the rural sector where more than*
> *60% of the Thai population live and are the most poor and socially*
> *disadvantaged.*
>
> *Retired MOPH policy-maker*

In addition, various director-generals and leaders in the MOPH had overseas training as well as experience as provincial public health managers. These leaders influenced policy formulation or, through their policy networks, indirectly swayed the policy agenda in favour of rural health development. They did this over two to three decades, maintaining policy continuity and coherence. The 1986 Sasakawa Health Prize[49] awarded to Dr Amorn Nondasuta, the MOPH permanent secretary, further boosted national commitment towards rural primary care development. He was the pioneer of the voluntary health insurance scheme introduced in 1984 for the informal population, one of the key foundations for future universal coverage.

Box 7.3 The evolution of the Rural Doctors Society

The first wave of government-bonded doctors sent to district hospitals faced many administrative and logistical problems, such as inadequate equipment, lack of health staff, and a huge load of clinical care. To address this problem, the Rural Doctors Society was formed in 1978, coinciding with the Declaration of Alma-Ata. The ideology of the democratization movement of the early 1970s drove the Society's direction. Key principles were work for the betterment of Thai society, teamwork, and a holistic approach. The early mandates of the Society were developing district hospital management guidelines, journals, a newsletter and an annual conference. Four years later, the Rural Doctor Foundation was established and the annual Best Rural Doctor Award was granted to the most dedicated doctors in remote or underserved areas, conferring prestigious social recognition on rural doctors.

Since completion of the rural hospital network, the Society has played an active watch-dog role and has monitored corruption in the health system for the past two decades. Its exposure of a nationwide drug scandal in 1998 resulted in a jail sentence for the health minister[52].

Source: Reference 53.

Although critical support for health from strategic interest groups persisted over the period 1970–1996, the relative power of these interest groups was constantly evolving[50]. Between 1970 and 2000, political parties were not strong and most governments were coalitions. As a consequence, the bureaucratic elite or technocrats (military and civilian) played a significant role in policy formulation at the national level and in the translation of policy into effective implementation. However, the past two decades have seen a decline in the power of the bureaucratic elite and a related rise in the power of the economic elite, either directly or through their influence on political parties and government. With the landslide victory of the Thai Rak Thai party in 2001, the commercial economic elite started to play a significant role in setting the policy agenda: the so-called populist policies, advocating for the rights and interests of ordinary people in rural areas to obtain political advantages. This benefited health; in fact it was a political decision to put universal health care coverage on the election campaign agenda in 2001[51].

Other significant groups supporting the health agenda included the media, nongovernmental organizations (NGOs) and professional groups. Informal policy groups were also significant. The Rose Garden group, convened monthly for the last 20 years, is a classic informal policy group, closely linked with the Rural Doctors Society of Thailand (Box 7.3). Various policy agendas were generated from this think tank, such as universal health coverage and the anti-tobacco campaign, which led to two tobacco control acts[53].

Policy formulation: the role of technocrats and evidence

Although politicians determined and set elements of the health agenda, they had rapid turnover: specifically, there were 11 governments in the 19 years between 1969 and 1988. Therefore, technocrats were key players in policy formulation at national level and policy implementation at local levels. Between 1970 and 2000, technocrats with long-term institutional memory and exposure to rural health and public administration were promoted to high positions in the MOPH. They had strong direct and indirect influence in convincing politicians to endorse a number of key elements of the national health agenda.

> *Most MOPH policies (policy formulation, not setting the policy agenda) came from us, the health personnel on the ground, not the politicians. Many policies on health infrastructure and human resources development were initiated by us. When the politicians gave a policy the green light, the MOPH and health personnel at health facilities had to implement it until the targets and goals were reached.*
> *Retired MOPH policy-maker*

A number of success factors were synthesized from interviews and document reviews. Health personnel were culturally very well accepted by society, especially medical doctors, who usually received higher social recognition than other professions. In addition, they were recognized to be highly competent professionals and trusted by the communities.

> *We were really impressed by the medical doctors. They were the most able people in the country. Very high social and political recognition was given to the MOPH automatically. The MOPH was very active and the strongest players compared to other ministries. [The MOPH] led the team from various ministries to work together on rural development. The MOPH played the leading role in national policy development, e.g. rural development, such as for health education, hygiene and sanitation, 100% toilet coverage campaign, safe drinking water.*
> *Policy-maker outside MOPH*

Increasingly in Thailand, evidence is used to formulate policies, although strong individual and institutional capacity to generate evidence was only developed in the 2000s[54,55]. Prior to 2000, policy formulation was mostly based on experience and pilot testing.

> *It was not difficult to present new programmes to the MOPH policy-makers because normally we used evidence to support our thinking. We did not just think it up by ourselves. Normally, we had a mini-trial programme or pilot project to see the feasibility first. Academic work was strong from our side compared to other sectors.*
>
> *Retired MOPH policy-maker*

For example, the launch of the 1970 National Family Planning Policy was a result of the *Potaram* pilot to test community acceptability in 1963. The provider payment choice for social health insurance in 1990 between fee-for-service reimbursement and a capitation contract model was analysed and proposed by able technocrats, in particular, the reform champion the late Dr Sanguan Nittayaramphong.

> *The doctors or health workers at MOPH are generally good people. We quite believe in whatever programme they would implement. Usually, they are strong in technical matters. No doubt about their scientific knowledge and skill.*
>
> *NGO worker*

Although scientific evidence played a critical role in policy formulation relating to specific interventions, judgement, values and implementation capacity were influential as well. For example, an analysis of costs and benefits of the hepatitis B vaccination guided the decision to add the hepatitis B vaccine to the Extended Programme on Immunization[56]. However, the decision to adopt renal replacement therapy for universal coverage scheme members in 2007 set aside the evidence on cost-ineffectiveness[57] and the huge long-term budget implications[58], and prioritized evidence on the financial burden and impoverishment caused by payments for dialysis among affected households[59]. The decision to adopt universal antiretroviral therapy in 2003 was made before information on cost-effectiveness, and driven by:

- international advocates of antiretroviral therapy such as the WHO 3 by 5 Initiative;

- the civil society movement at country and international level; and

- most importantly, the capacity of the Government Pharmaceutical Organization to produce a low-cost (at US$ 300 per patient-year) generic combination of three medicines[60].

Meanwhile, the decision to adopt corticosteroid for treatment of preterm labour was based not only on published evidence from a multi-country trial involving Thai clinicians[61], but also on clinical competency and the health system's readiness to scale up rapidly[33].

Policy implementation: competency, participation and pragmatism

Health managers at provincial and district levels were capable of translating policies into successful programmes on the ground[62]. They were pragmatic and had the flexibility to adapt national policy to the local context (from interviews with a number of retired MOPH policy-makers). Managers had a broad scope of authority in managing financial and human resources according to the government and MOPH regulations. For example, all revenue generated from user charges was retained at local level. In some provinces, a common drug list used by district and provincial hospitals was formulated and purchases of medicines were pooled to obtain the best possible prices; this voluntary process did not require MOPH approval. These innovations were not possible without flexibility and implementation capacity at local level. Effective communication and feedback loops between implementers and policy-makers fostered the successful implementation of policy.

The concept of integration drove the introduction of new policies, avoiding national vertical programmes. For example, the prevention of mother-to-child transmission of HIV programme was integrated with antenatal care at district level, and nurses responsible for antenatal care were given the additional task of the prevention programme. Pilots were customarily used to test, assess and adjust new programmes prior to nationwide scaling up, as in the case of family planning and the national Expanded Programme on Immunization.

> *The MOPH leaders are practical and they simplify things and make it easy for implementation to suit local context. A standard blueprint of different sizes of district hospitals made maintenance easy and future plans for expansion were well thought out from the drafting of the blueprint.*
>
> *Academic in a teaching hospital*
> *who previously worked as a physician in a district hospital*

Reliance on domestic resources for health system development with independence from donors was another major contributing factor for sustainable programme implementation. Different governments demonstrated financial commitment to the health sector, as noted above.

Health programmes have been well received by villagers and communities. No resistance was observed, and publicity and community awareness – for example, of the need for family planning because of poverty related to large families – minimized demand-side barriers (from interview with a retired physician at district hospital). There has been very high compliance with family planning services and immunization schedules, as well as confidence in the quality and safety of the free vaccination programme. Public trust and confidence have gradually been built into the district health delivery systems.

In summary, the development of the health delivery system and other health programmes were endorsed by governments at the highest level, driven by able technocrats, and well accepted by society and villagers. Effective implementation with limited resources, in addition to the strong motivation of all stakeholders to improve society, made the policies successful.

The intrinsic factors: role models and their inspiration

From various interviews, a key message emerged that intrinsic factors relating to authoritative individuals played a critical role in setting a standard of high commitment and motivation in order to bring health to the rural poor. This was reflected by their lifetime of hard work, dedication and sacrifice.

> *Professor Sem Pringpuangkeo is our 'grandfather'... as director of Chiangrai Prachanukhror[c] hospital, he introduced user charges without official approval to mobilize local resources to expand service capacity in light of the meagre government budget. He was investigated by the finance ministry for not abiding by the rules, but finally high-level policy-makers understood the real situation and an official user charge policy emerged... His lifelong contribution to health development in Thailand is enormous.*
>
> *Retired MOPH policy-maker*

In addition, Dr Boonyong Wongrakmit's lifelong contribution to health in the rural northern mountainous province of Nan was recognized by His Majesty King Bhumibol Adulyadej in 1968. He was awarded a Royal Privy grant to upgrade the infrastructure of Nan provincial hospital during the royal visit to the hospital by the King and Queen of Thailand (from interview with a retired physician at a provincial hospital). Twenty years after his retirement, Dr Boonyong Wongrakmit still plays an active role in the civil society health movement. Such doctors are highly regarded and are heroic leaders for the younger generations.

---

[c] Prachanukhror is a combination of two words: *pracha* means people or public, and *anukhror* means sponsor or support. Chiangrai Prachanukhror means the Chiangrai hospital, which is financially sponsored by the people through user charges.

Financial incentives, although important, had less influence than social recognition (from a number of interviews with retired MOPH policy-makers, retired physicians at district and provincial hospitals, and a health officer at a provincial level).

> *A medical doctor always gets high recognition from villagers. Even if he is a new graduate he would be greeted by older villagers and he would be invited to be a chairperson of many important events in the district, e.g. funerals, sports day and the New Year festival. This high social recognition is naturally given to medical doctors and other health personnel. When one gets high recognition, he or she should preserve it as much as possible by paying back to the society.*
>
> *Academic in a teaching hospital*

The most important reason, cited frequently by many interviewees to explain the dedication of public doctors, is that the MOPH health personnel are civil servants who work for the King. Therefore, it is the highest honour "to serve the country for the King and Royal Family".

A key role model was Prince Mahidol Na Songkhla, the father of the present King Bhumibol, who trained in public health in the early years of the 20th century. He untiringly promoted public health and medical care in Thailand through his work with the Rockefeller Foundation in establishing medical colleges in Thailand. He is revered as the father of modern medicine in Thailand.

■ What have other sectors contributed?

A number of other sectors and developments also contributed to improving the health of the Thai population, including economic growth and poverty reduction, education, social equity and inclusion policies, and public infrastructure.

Economic growth and poverty reduction

Rapid economic growth (Figure 7.2) was associated with significant poverty reduction, as indicated by a fall in poverty incidence from 49.7% of the rural Thai population in 1988 to 10.7% in 2007 (Figure 7.9). The rural–urban gap has been reduced although it is still large, with the urban population much less affected by the economic crisis of 1997 than the rural sector.

Despite the reduction in the incidence of poverty, income distribution has been very slow to change. It took almost 25 years to reduce Thailand's Gini index

Figure 7.9 Poverty incidence, selected years, 1988–2007

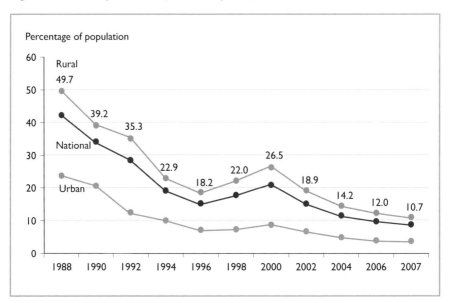

Source: Data from reference 63.

from 45.2 in 1981 to 42.5 in 2004. It has never been on Thailand's political agenda to introduce land and inheritance tax, a major policy instrument for income redistribution.

Education

Thailand started the period under examination with relatively high levels of literacy. These further improved and gender disparities decreased and even disappeared with respect to youth literacy (Table 7.4)[11]. In 2002, universal basic education was extended to compulsory secondary education.

Social equity and inclusion

The Gender-related Development Index (GDI) measures inequalities between women and men: it is simply the Human Development Index (HDI) adjusted downward for gender inequality. The greater the gender disparity in basic human development, the lower a country's GDI relative to its HDI. Thailand's GDI value is 99.9% of its HDI value. Out of the 155 countries having both HDI and GDI values, only 14 countries have a better ratio than Thailand's.

Table 7.4   National adult (15+) and youth (15–24) literacy rate, 1980, 2000 and
2005

	Adult literacy, >15 years (%)				Youth literacy, 15–24 years (%)			
	Both	Male	Female	Gender parity	Both	Male	Female	Gender parity
1980	88.0	92.2	83.9	0.91	96.9	97.6	96.2	0.99
2000	92.6	94.9	90.5	0.95	98.0	98.1	97.8	1.00
2005	93.5	95.6	91.5	0.96	98.1	98.2	97.9	1.00

Source: Data from reference 11.

The Gender Empowerment Measure (GEM) reveals whether women take an active part in economic and political life, tracking gender inequality in opportunities in selected areas, including the share of seats in parliament held by women and the gender disparity in earned income, reflecting economic independence. In contrast to the GDI, Thailand does not perform well on the GEM, ranking 76th out of 109 countries in the GEM and indicating a large scope for improvement regarding women's engagement in economic and political life. Female labour force participation is high, although a gender gap persists. In 2008, 81% of men, but only 65.9% of women, aged 15 years or older participated in the labour market.

Public infrastructure

Economic growth enabled substantial government investment in infrastructure, such as provincial and district feeder roads and communication. For example, the percentage of paved roads increased from 50% of the total roads in 1990 to almost 100% in 2000. This not only supported the distribution of agricultural products and generated income for rural populations, but it also facilitated access to health and education services. Various health and welfare surveys reported improved access to health services by rural populations, in particular during the 1990s. Moreover, increased household income facilitated investment in safe water and sanitation, better shelter and healthier cooking fuels (replacing charcoal with natural gas), improved diets and higher nutritional status.

The percentage of the population with access to improved water sources increased from 91% in 1990 to more than 98% by 2008[5], with a preferential growth of coverage in rural areas. Access to safe water significantly contributed to personal hygiene, food safety and a reduction in gastrointestinal diseases. At the same time, the percentage of the population covered by mobile and fixed-line telephones increased significantly in the 2000s, from less than 20% in 2000 to 100% in 2008.

■ Lessons learned and future challenges

Relative to countries with similar income levels, Thailand has achieved significant health improvements at relatively low cost in terms of total health expenditure per capita and percentage of GDP devoted to health. Health gains have been achieved in conjunction with reductions in the rich–poor health inequity gap, although there are continuing challenges of geographical inequity.

These achievements have been possible because, over a 40-year period, critical maternal and child health interventions addressing the key causes of mortality and morbidity were made widely available, achieving high coverage of the rural population. These interventions were predominantly provided through the public primary care and district health infrastructure, which was substantially and deliberately expanded over the same period, with concomitant investment in human resources and adequate financial resource allocation to make primary health care a reality. District health systems, including subdistrict health centres and district hospitals, function as strategic hubs, translating national health plans into effective programmes on the ground.

Later, action was taken to limit the financial barriers to accessing care, through a range of financing schemes for specific population groups, such as low-income households, the informal sector, civil servants and private-sector employees. These fragmented schemes were succeeded by the 2001 reform, which ensured universal coverage for the entire population. Consistent improvements in financial protection have clearly led to reduced levels of both catastrophic health expenditure and health impoverishment[13].

In addition, there were developments in other sectors, which wider evidence indicates would have contributed to health improvements. Among others, economic growth and poverty reduction, an increased level of adult literacy, a diminished gender literacy gap and a high level of female literacy contributed to health gains.

These health and wider development gains were underpinned by the implementation of a series of five-year National Health Plans and NESDPs over a 45-year period (1960–2006). These Plans provided consistent and sustained support for a range of interacting health and development policies, focusing on rural development between the 1970s and 1990s.

The consistent development and implementation of these sets of policies was made possible by pro-poor, pro-rural ideology covering not only health but also other key sectors such as education, agriculture, employment, transportation and public infrastructure. Commitment to health was not rhetoric, but reflected actual allocations assisted by favourable economic growth. The consistent increase in public expenditure on health resulted in the reduction in household out-of-pocket payments for health to the level of the Organisation for Economic Co-operation and Development average in 2008.

The consistent pro-poor line of health policy reflected a particular national focus on equitable health and health development, the role of strong policy networks favouring rural areas and a strong and stable technocratic base (despite highly unstable politics). This included use of evidence and experience in policy formulation, strong implementation capacity and a pragmatic, learning approach to policy implementation. Finally, the value base of policy-makers in the MOPH and leading role models in the medical profession demonstrating lifelong commitment to improving the health of the poorest were a vital influence, underpinned by the motivation of the Royal Family and its support to health.

With improvements in child health secured, current challenges are in improving adult health, and especially reducing adult mortality[64] and morbidity from traffic injuries, HIV/AIDS and chronic noncommunicable diseases. A burden of disease study revealed that the top five causes of total mortality among men were HIV/AIDS, cerebrovascular diseases, accidents and injuries, liver cancer and chronic obstructive pulmonary diseases. Similarly, among women, HIV/AIDS ranks second and cerebrovascular diseases ranks first. Multisectoral action is required to address risk factors such as tobacco and alcohol use, changing diets and poor law enforcement, which contributes to traffic injuries; the future challenges are daunting. While sustaining mother and child health outcome achievements, there is need for a major policy review on how Thailand controls risk factors contributing to adult mortality. Policy-makers are aware of the emerging challenges; major programmes addressing the social determinants of chronic noncommunicable diseases have been launched.

ACKNOWLEDGMENTS

We wish to thank all those interviewed for their frank views and experiences on the historical development of the health system in Thailand. Findings indicated untiring contributions by public health workers throughout the country, technocrats who influenced policy formulation and various leaders in the MOPH who were highly committed to contributing to the health development of the country.

The National Statistical Office, which generates evidence from household surveys and routine administrative datasets maintained by relevant departments of the MOPH and other ministries, provided indispensable support. Thanks to all colleagues in the International Health Policy Programme who were involved in supporting this work. Without them, this chapter would not have been possible.

We enjoyed working with other members of the London School of Hygiene & Tropical Medicine who steered this work, as well as colleagues from four other countries – Bangladesh, Ethiopia, Tamil Nadu (India) and Kyrgyzstan. Thanks to Lesong Conteh who visited Thailand and provided technical support on qualitative analysis using NVivo.

REFERENCES

1. United Nations. *MDG-Plus: a case study of Thailand.* New York: United Nations Development Programme; not dated (http://www.undp.org/mdg/goodpractices/Thailand-casestudy.pdf, accessed 4 January 2010).

2. Waage F et al. The Millennium Development Goals: a cross-sectoral analysis and principles for goal setting after 2015: Lancet and London International Development Centre Commission. *Lancet* 2010; 376(9745):991–1023.

3. WHO. *World health statistics* [online database]. Geneva: World Health Organization; 2010 (http://www.who.int/whosis/whostat/en/index.html, accessed 7 June 2010).

4. Thai working group on National Health Account. *The report on 1994–2008 National Health Expenditure.* Nonthaburi: International Health Policy Program, Ministry of Public Health; 2010 (http://www.ihppthaigov.net/nha/thai_nha_1994-2008.xls, accessed 20 February 2010).

5. World Bank. *World development indicators* [online database]. Washington DC: World Bank; 2011 (http://data.worldbank.org/country/thailand, accessed 17 July 2011).

6. Thailand National Statistical Office. *Population and housing survey 2000*. Bangkok: National Statistical Office; 2001.

7. WHO. *National health accounts, country health information*. Geneva: World Health Organization; 2011 (http://www.who.int/countries/tha/en/index.html, accessed 17 June 2011).

8. Thailand National Statistical Office. *Thailand multiple indicator cluster survey (MICS) December 2005 – February 2006, final report*. Bangkok: National Statistical Office; 2006 (http://www.unicef.org/thailand/resources_356.html, accessed 7 June 2010).

9. Institute for Health Metrics and Evaluation. *Infant and child mortality estimates by country 1970–2010*. Seattle: Institute for Health Metrics and Evaluation; 2010 (http://www.healthmetricsandevaluation.org/record/infant-and-child-mortality-estimates-country-1970-2010, accessed 7 June 2010).

10. Hogan MC, et al. Maternal mortality for 181 countries, 1980–2008: a systematic analysis of progress towards Millennium Development Goal 5. *Lancet* 2010; 375(9726):1609–23.

11. UNESCO . *National literacy rates for youth (15–24) and adults* (15+) [online database]. Montreal: UNESCO Institute for Statistics; 2010 (http://stats.uis.unesco/TableViewer/tableView.aspx?ReportID=210, accessed 18 April 2010).

12. Limwattananon S, Tangcharoensathien V, Prakongsai P. Catastrophic and poverty impacts of health payments: results from national household surveys in Thailand. *Bulletin of the World Health Organization* 2007; 85(8):600–6.

13. Prakongsai P, Limwattananon S, Tangcharoensathien V. The equity impact of the universal coverage policy : lessons from Thailand. In: Chernichovsky D, Hanson K, eds. *Innovations in health system finance in developing and transitional economies*. London: Emerald Group; 2009:57–81.

14. Bundhamcharoen K et al., eds. *Burden of disease and injuries in Thailand: priority setting for policy*. Bangkok: Thai Working Group on Burden of Disease and Injuries, Ministry of Public Health; 2002.

15. Thailand National Statistical Office. *Expectation of life at birth from the 1995–1996 and 2005–2006. Survey of population change* [online database]. Bangkok: Thailand National Statistical Office; 2007 (http://web.nso.go.th/eng/en/stat/popchang/popchg00.htm, accessed 18 April 2010).

16. Bureau of Policy and Strategy. *Thailand health profile 2001–2004*. Bangkok: Ministry of Public Health; 2008 (http://www.moph.go.th/ops/thp/index.php?option=com_content&task=view&id=7&Itemid=2, accessed 18 April 2010).

17. Vapattanawong P et al. Reductions in child mortality levels and inequalities in Thailand: analysis of two censuses. *Lancet* 2007; 369:850–5.

18. Barker DJP. Maternal nutrition, fetal nutrition, and disease in later life. *Nutrition* 1997; 13:807–13.

19. Morley R. Fetal origins of adult disease. *Seminars in Fetal and Neonatal Medicine* 2006; 11:73–8.

20. Rohde J et al. 30 years after Alma-Ata: has primary health care worked in countries? *Lancet* 2008; 372:950–61.

21. WHO. *Maternal mortality in 2005.* [Estimates developed by WHO, UNICEF, UNFPA and the World Bank.] Geneva: World Health Organization; 2007 (http://www.who.int/whosis/mme_2005.pdf, accessed 19 April 2010).

22. Ministry of Public Health. *Maternal deaths 1960–2006* [online database]. Nonthaburi: Ministry of Public Health, Bureau of Policy and Strategy; 2010 (http://bps.ops.moph.go.th/Mather.html, accessed 19 April 2010).

23. Ministry of Public Health. *Maternal mortality ratio 1990–2006* [online database]. Nonthaburi: Bureau of Health Promotion, Ministry of Public Health; 2008 (http://www.anamai.moph.go.th/main.php?filename=Statistics, accessed 19 April 2010).

24. Kanchana S, Amornvichet P, Kulruek N. *Reproductive age mortality study (RAMOS) in 1995–1997 in Thailand. Thai report.* Nonthaburi: Bureau of Health, Ministry of Public Health; 1999 (www.hiso.or.th/hiso/picture/reportHealth/pro2 -chapter1(4).doc, accessed 19 April 2010).

25. Chandoevwit W et al. Using multiple data for calculating the maternal mortality ratio in Thailand. *TDRI Quarterly Review* 2007; 22(3):13–19 (http://www.tdri. or.th/library/quarterly/text/s07_2.pdf, accessed 19 April 2010).

26. WHO. *Trends in maternal mortality: 1990 to 2008.* Geneva: World Health Organization, 2010.

27. Prachuabmoh V, Mithranon P. Below-replacement fertility in Thailand and its policy implications. *Journal of Population Research* 2003; 20:35–50.

28. National Statistical Office. *The Fourth Reproductive Health Survey.* Bangkok: Ministry of Information, Communication and Technology; 2006.

29. Chen XK et al. Teenage pregnancy and adverse birth outcomes: a large population based retrospective cohort study. *International Journal of Epidemiology* 2007; 36:368–73.

30. Ohlsson A, Shah P. *Determinants and prevention of low birth weight: a synopsis of the evidence.* Alberta: Institute of Health Economics; 2008.

31. Thai Working Group on Burden of Disease. *Unpublished report on causes of death of children under 5 years, 1996–2009.* Nonthaburi; International Health Policy Program, Ministry of Public Health; 2010 (retrieved data from Civil Registration Office, Ministry of Interior, Thailand).

32. Jones G et al. How many child deaths can we prevent this year? *Lancet* 2003; 362: 65–71.

33. Saengwaree P, Liabsuetrakul T. Changing physician's practice on antenatal corticosteroids in preterm birth. *Journal of the Medical Association of Thailand* 2005; 88:307–13.

34. Thailand National Statistical Office. *Reproductive health survey 2009.* Bangkok: Ministry of Information, Communication and Technology; 2010.

35. Bureau of Epidemiology. *National diseases surveillance report.* Nonthaburi: Ministry of Public Health; various years.

36. Bureau of General Communicable Diseases. *Thai report on EPI coverage applying thirty cluster sampling surveys in 1990.* Nonthaburi: Department of Disease Control, Ministry of Public Health; 1990. (http://thaigcd.ddc.moph.go.th/download//EPI/20090201-Survey51-1.pdf, access 7 June 2010).

37. Lawn J et al. Why are 4 million newborn babies dying each year? *Lancet* 2004; 364:399–401.

38. Liabsuetrakul T et al. Emergency obstetric care in the southernmost provinces of Thailand. *International Journal for Quality in Health Care* 2007; 19(4):250–6.

39. Warakamin S, Boonthai N, Tangcharoensathien V. Induced abortion in Thailand: current situation in public hospitals and legal perspectives. *Reproductive Health Matters* 2004; 12:147–56.

40. Boonthai N et al. Improving access to safe termination of pregnancy in Thailand: an analysis of policy developments from 1999 to 2006. In: Whittaker A, ed. *Abortion in Asia: local dilemmas, global politics.* New York: Berghahn Books; 2010:221–39.

41. Tangcharoensathien V et al. Intrauterine contraceptive devices: comparing health centre and district hospital costs in Thailand. *Health Policy and Planning* 1990; 5:177–81.

42. Bureau of Policy and Strategy. *Data of health resources, 1994–2009.* Nonthaburi: Ministry of Public Health (http://moc.moph.go.th/Resource/index.php, accessed on 17 April 2010).

43. Sala C, Wongpiyachon S, It-tisan P. *Thai report on special interview of Dr Damrong Boonyern – a doctor and national public health planning expert.* Nonthaburi: Ministry of Public Health; 1997 (http://advisor.anamai.moph.go.th /211/21109.html, accessed 7 June 2010).

44. Wibulpolprasert S, Thaiprayoon S. Thailand: "good practice" in expanding health care coverage lessons from the Thai health care reforms. In: Gottret P, Schieber G, Waters H, eds. *Good practices in health financing: lessons from reforms in low and middle-income countries.* Washington, DC: World Bank; 2008:355–83.

45. Tangcharoensathien V et al. From targeting to universality: lessons from the health system in Thailand. In: Townsend P, ed. *Building decent societies: rethinking the role of social security in development.* Basingstoke: Palgrave Macmillan; 2009:301–21.

46. Thailand National Statistical Office. *Database of socio-economic survey 1996–2008.* Bangkok: National Statistical Office; 2010. (data retrieved directly from the National Statistical Office, Thailand, 20 November 2010).

47. Jindawatana A, Wibulpolprasert S. *The first Thai National Health Assembly 1988.* Bangkok: Ministry of Public Health; 1988.

48. Rasanathan K et al. Innovation and participation for healthy public policy: the first National Health Assembly in Thailand. *Health Expectations* 2011; doi: 10.1111/j.1369-7625.2010.00656.

49. WHO. *Recipients of the Sasakawa Health Prize.* Geneva: World Health Organization; 2010 (http://www.who.int/governance/awards/sasakawa/sasakawa _winners/en/index.html, accessed 8 June 2010).

50. Green A. Reforming the health sector in Thailand: the role of policy actors on the policy stage. *International Journal of Health Planning and Management* 2000; 15:39–59.

51. Pitayarangsarit S. *The introduction of the universal coverage of health care policy in Thailand: policy responses.* [Doctoral thesis]. London: London School of Hygiene & Tropical Medicine, University of London; 2004.

52. Cameron S. Corruption in Ministry of Public Health, Thailand. In: Transparency International. *Global Corruption Report 2006.* London: Pluto Press; 2005 (http://www.transparency.org/publications/gcr/gcr_2006#download, accessed 8 June 2010).

53. Wibulpolprasert S et al. *Twenty-five years of rural doctor movement in Thailand.* Bangkok: Srangsue; 2003.

54. Pitayarangsarit S, Tangcharoensathien V. Sustaining capacity in health policy and systems research in Thailand. *Bulletin of the World Health Organization* 2009; 87:72–4.

55. Pitayarangsarit S, Tangcharoensathien V. Capacity development for health policy and systems research: experience and lessons from Thailand. In: Green G, Bennett S, eds. *Sound choices: enhancing capacity for evidence-informed health policy.* Geneva: World Health Organization; 2007:147–66.

56. Munira SL, Fritzen S. What influences government adoption of vaccines in developing countries? A policy process analysis. *Social Science & Medicine* 2007; 65:1751–64.

57. Teerawattananon Y, Mugford M, Tangcharoensathien V. Economic evaluation of palliative management versus peritoneal dialysis and haemo-dialysis for end-stage renal disease: evidence for coverage decisions in Thailand. *Value in Health* 2007; 10:61–72.

58. Kasemsup V, Prakongsai P, Tangcharoensathien V. Budget impact analysis of a policy on universal access to RRT under universal coverage in Thailand. *Journal of the Nephrology Society of Thailand* 2006; 12:136–48.

59. Prakongsai P et al. The implications of benefit package design: the impact on poor Thai households of excluding renal replacement therapy. *Journal of International Development* 2009; 21:291–308.

60. Tantivess S. *Universal access to antiretroviral therapy in Thailand: an analysis of the policy process* [doctoral thesis]. London: London School of Hygiene & Tropical Medicine, University of London; 2006.

61. Pattanittum P et al. Use of antenatal corticosteroids prior to preterm birth in four South East Asian countries within the SEA-ORCHID project. *BMC Pregnancy and Childbirth* 2008, 8:47.

62. Russell S, Bennett S, Mills S. Reforming the health sector: towards a healthy new public management. *Journal of International Development* 1999; 11:767–75.

63. National Economic and Social Development Board. *Thai report on poverty mitigation and income distribution.* Bangkok: Division of Data Analysis for Development, National Economic and Social Development; 2009 (http://www.nesdb.go.th/econSocial/macro/macroeconomic/dev3.html, accessed 17 April 2010).

64. Rajaratnam JK et al. Worldwide mortality in men and women aged 15–59 years from 1970 to 2010: a systematic analysis. *Lancet* 2010; 375(9727):1704–20.

Costa Rica

Kerala

Sri Lanka

Chapter 8

GOOD HEALTH AT LOW COST REVISITED

Further insights from China, Costa Rica,
Kerala and Sri Lanka 25 years later

Benjamin Palafox

LSHTM

■ Introduction

In Chapter 1, we saw how China, Costa Rica, Kerala and Sri Lanka, the four low-income case studies profiled in the original *Good health at low cost* report from 1985, had achieved remarkable health gains by the early 1980s. Although they attained these gains in different ways, there were some important similarities that offered crucial evidence in support of the principles advocated at the Alma-Ata conference in 1978 and provided insight into ways that might reduce infant, child and maternal mortality.

From the health system perspective, key factors that emerged were long-term (and above average) *investment in financial and human resources* for health, especially in primary care; *strong political commitment* to good health for the whole population; a high degree of *community involvement*; and *equity of access and use*. In addition, each country had enacted policies *beyond the health system*, implementing wide-ranging policies which addressed many different determinants of health, with a particular emphasis on expansion of education, especially for girls[1].

The case studies also demonstrated the value of integrating services both horizontally and vertically, ensuring the inclusion of prevention within essential primary care and the necessary linkages between primary care and the rest of the health system. In Kerala and Sri Lanka, the expansion of essential primary health services, with a focus on maternal and child health, was considered critical for the reduction of both child and maternal mortality. Results were attributed to an emphasis on integrated service provision models that improved access to antenatal and postnatal care, and dramatically increased rates of institutional delivery and use of skilled birth attendants. The care of young children was boosted by measures to improve rates of immunization and effective management of communicable disease. Costa Rica's early reforms strengthened primary care (with a focus on family planning) and improved access to higher levels of care, extending coverage of immunization, and improving nutrition and sanitation. China also saw improvements in maternal and child health. As well as implementing maternal and child health interventions like those in the other countries, it engaged in a series of nationwide campaigns to control the vectors of communicable diseases, improve sanitation and increase access to clean water. A key feature of the Chinese approach was the involvement of barefoot doctors, a cadre of village health workers working to improve health within their communities.

By the early 1980s, after years of implementing these policies, China, Costa Rica, Kerala and Sri Lanka had achieved life expectancy approaching that of some high-income countries. However, with this came an epidemiological transition that rapidly increased the burden of chronic and other noncommunicable conditions, introducing a new set of challenges for health policy-makers. Adapting health systems to these new realities has been complicated by a number of important contextual changes since the mid-1980s, including uneven economic growth, political and economic crises, changing international trade flows, the emergence of new technology, and migration, all of which conspired to widen inequalities in wealth and, consequently, health. With relatively low per capita expenditure on health, how could they sustain progress already made, further reduce inequities in health and cope with the higher health care costs associated with an ageing population and changing lifestyles? Can these countries still be regarded as models of population health improvement by other developing countries?

In this chapter, we revisit the four original case studies and ask how each country has fared since 1985. We review the progress countries have made in improving infant and maternal mortality (as key indicators of health system performance), describe the main changes to their health systems and broad sociopolitical contexts, and examine the possible mechanisms through which these changes may have influenced population health. (Box 8.1 outlines the search strategy and data sources used to conduct this desk review, and Chapter 2 gives additional details on the conceptual framework, research approach and analytical methods.) We conclude by seeking lessons that can be learned from their experiences.

■ China

In 1978, Deng Xiaoping initiated wide-ranging economic reforms that swept away many elements of the centrally planned Chinese economy established by Mao Zedong. The introduction of free markets ushered in a process of rapid transition that set the country on track to become an economic powerhouse. In less than a decade, the country's economic base shifted away from agriculture to industrial production, with much of its output sold abroad. Since 1985, it has maintained a remarkable rate of economic growth of nearly 10% a year[2]. This achievement reflected many factors, but one of the most important was the establishment of special economic zones that allowed foreign investors to take advantage of low labour costs and favourable tax regimes. This facilitated the explosion of industrial manufacturing and fuelled the labour market in these zones and in urban areas in general. As a result, migration from rural to urban areas has increased the size of China's cities to meet the new labour demands, although more than half of its 1.3 billion people still live in rural areas.

Box 8.1 Desk review search strategy and data sources

We conducted a review of published, peer-reviewed literature using the PubMed and EconLit bibliographic databases. Relevant sources were searched first using both standardized terms and keywords based on the outcomes of interest (e.g. infant, child and maternal mortality). The results were then combined with searches based on relevant determinants of health. Health systems determinants were informed by the WHO Health Systems building blocks of service delivery, health workforce, information, medical products and technologies, financing, leadership. Non-health systems determinants were related to public expenditure, economic policy, rule of law, water and sanitation, education policy, social security, gender policy, public administration for public provisioning; plus structural factors (e.g. system of government, media, food supply, etc.), situational factors (e.g. elections, conflict, natural disasters, migration, etc.), cultural factors (e.g. religious values, accepted forms of hierarchy, awareness of rights, trust in institutions, etc.) and international or exogenous factors (e.g. foreign aid, international trade agreements, influence of civil society organizations, etc.) likely to influence policy. The results were then combined and limited to those pertaining to the four case countries for the years 1985–2009. Titles and abstracts of the remaining sources were screened for relevance and a review of bibliographies was conducted among selected documents to identify additional sources. This was supplemented with key informant interviews of national and international experts familiar with the case study contexts, and with a search of relevant grey literature since 1985. For this, we used similar keywords to search various document repositories such as the Eldis and British Library for Development Studies websites, and also those of multilateral organizations, such as WHO and the World Bank.

China's ascendancy in the global economy has been matched by progress in other areas. Since the late 1970s, it has managed to slow population growth to between 0.5% and 1.6% per year, and by 2008, the total fertility rate had fallen to 1.78 births per woman[2]. This is partially the result of the one-child policy introduced at the same time as the economic reforms. China has improved other key development indicators, particularly literacy, poverty and basic education. These developments were mirrored in health gains: between 1985 and 2008, overall life expectancy rose from 66.9 to 73.1 years, while vaccination coverage against diphtheria, pertussis and tetanus (DPT) among children under two years of age increased from 78% to 97% (Table 8.1).

The period from the 1950s to the early 1980s has been regarded as China's watershed period for health, when enormous gains were achieved. Life expectancy

Table 8.1   Selected development indicators, China vs. middle-income countries

Indicator	China		Middle-income countries[a]	
	1985	2008	1985	2008
Vaccination, DPT (% of children aged 12–23 months)	78	97[b]	47	81
Primary school completion rate, total (% of relevant age group)	n/a	96.0	n/a	92.3
Poverty gap at $2 a day (purchasing power parity) (%)	47.3[c]	12.2[d]	n/a	10.7[e]
Literacy rate, adult total (% of people aged 15 and above)	65.5[f]	93.7	n/a	82.7
Fertility rate, total (births per woman)	2.64	1.78	3.68	2.43
Life expectancy at birth, total (years)	66.9	73.1	62.7	68.5

Source: Data from reference 2.

Notes: n/a: Not available; DPT: Three doses, diphtheria, pertussis and tetanus; [a] Based on World Bank income grouping; [b] Value is for 2009; [c] Value is for 1984; [d] Value is for 2005; [e] Value is for upper-middle-income countries, as defined by the World Bank (for comparison, the value for lower-middle-income countries is 54.1%); [f] Value is for 1982.

increased across the entire country. After this period, China continued to experience health gains in some areas, most notably in maternal mortality, where a dramatic fourfold reduction has been achieved since 1980, reaching 40 per 100 000 live births in 2008[3]. However, in other areas, particularly child mortality, China has not performed as well[4]. Following China's impressive gains in infant mortality described in the original *Good health at low cost*, progress halted for nearly a decade, remaining at approximately 40 deaths per 1000 live births, until resuming a downward trend during the late 1990s. By 2008, this indicator had stabilized at a rate of approximately 15 deaths per 1000[5,6] (Figure 8.1).

The slower progress in infant mortality has been attributed to growing health inequalities, linked to the sweeping changes in the economy. There were winners and losers, with the winners concentrated in the areas undergoing the greatest

Figure 8.1   Infant and maternal mortality, China, 1970–2009

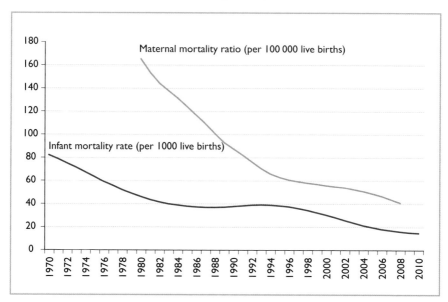

Sources: Data from references 3, 5 and 6.

economic reform[7,8]. A 2009 review of health and health care since economic liberalization found deepening inequalities between urban and rural areas, and among income groups[9]. For example, Shanghai, China's leading commercial centre, saw an improvement in life expectancy of four years between 1981 and 2000, to 78 years; while in Gansu, one of China's poorest provinces, the improvement was of only 1.4 years over the same period. Consequently, by 2000, a 13-year gap in life expectancy had opened up between the two regions; and when plotted against provincial GDP, a clear gradient in life expectancy was apparent[10]. Similar patterns were observed with infant mortality rates in rural areas. Rates were nearly five times higher in the poorest counties than in the wealthiest ones. These were also mirrored in under-5 mortality. Between 1996 and 2004, a sixfold difference emerged between the highest and lowest socio-economic quintiles, with a fall of 50% among wealthy rural populations compared with only 16% among the least wealthy groups[10].

The original *Good health at low cost* report linked China's remarkable health gains with its relatively well-developed social welfare system. In rural areas, where most Chinese people lived at the time, the commune played a central role. It owned the land and managed its use. It also administered the Rural Cooperative Medical Care System (RCMCS), a system that provided members of the community with a basic form of health protection. Basic curative, preventive

Figure 8.2   Timeline of key events influencing health, China, 1975–2010

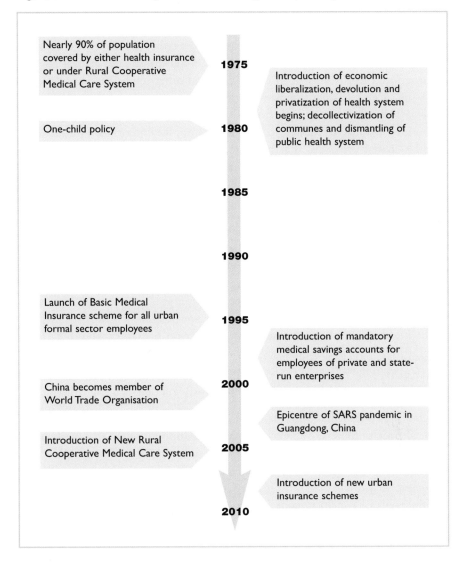

Nearly 90% of population covered by either health insurance or under Rural Cooperative Medical Care System

1975

Introduction of economic liberalization, devolution and privatization of health system begins; decollectivization of communes and dismantling of public health system

One-child policy

1980

1985

1990

Launch of Basic Medical Insurance scheme for all urban formal sector employees

1995

Introduction of mandatory medical savings accounts for employees of private and state-run enterprises

China becomes member of World Trade Organisation

2000

Epicentre of SARS pandemic in Guangdong, China

Introduction of New Rural Cooperative Medical Care System

2005

Introduction of new urban insurance schemes

2010

and public health services were largely delivered through health centres owned by the commune and operated by barefoot doctors[11]. By the 1970s, 90% of the population had health coverage, either from the RCMCS in the rural areas or from different state-owned enterprises in the cities (Figure 8.2).

Health status in rural areas continued to improve immediately following the privatization of agricultural production; this has been attributed to improvements in agricultural productivity that increased not only household income in rural areas but also nutrition[7,8]. However, these gains were short lived as the spread of economic liberalization left much of the rural population uninsured. Although many of those involved initially welcomed privatization of agricultural land previously owned by the communes, the process destroyed the economic basis upon which the RCMCS had operated[12]. Simultaneously, the central government reduced its investment in health care and other public services. Between 1978 and 1999, its share of national health care spending fell from 32% to 15%[12]. The areas it withdrew from were taken over by provincial and local authorities, who were required to fund them from local taxation. This favoured wealthy coastal provinces that had stronger tax bases over less wealthy rural provinces, and laid the basis for major and growing disparities between investment in urban and rural health care[12].

These overall reductions in funding had many negative consequences for the quality and affordability of local public health services. Out-of-pocket expenditure began to rise as health facilities relied increasingly on the sale of services to generate sufficient operating revenue, which was exacerbated by ill-conceived incentives, such as a salary bonus scheme that linked the size of the bonus to overall facility revenues[12,13]. Over the period of reform, income and the relative cost of treatment became increasingly important predictors of infant mortality as the health system began to rely more heavily on private expenditures[14]. By 2003, private expenditure reached 63% of total health spending, and 92% of private spending was out of pocket; however, by 2007, the proportion of spending from private contributions had declined to 55%[2].

Much of this decline has been the result of increasing government investment in the health sector made possible by the massive economic growth that has boosted government revenues. China's ageing population, the increasing prevalence of catastrophic health care costs, the severe acute respiratory syndrome (SARS) pandemic that originated in southern China, and the rising demand for rural health services have since made health a top government priority. One of the most significant developments has been the New Rural Cooperative Medical Care System (NRCMCS), introduced in 2005. While similar in spirit to its predecessor, which had become defunct by the late 1970s, this new programme is voluntary and the pooled risk fund is fed by members' contributions and by subsidies from central and local government. It works at the county level (much larger than the old communes) and focuses on protecting members from catastrophic medical expenses related to inpatient care (where the original RCMCS provided basic curative and preventive services).

In urban areas, formally employed residents have benefited from schemes implemented since 1995, such as the Basic Medical Insurance package and mandatory medical savings accounts. However, these benefits excluded dependents, and large groups of urban residents, particularly economic migrants from rural areas, were left mostly unprotected. To address this gap, the government began to scale up its Urban Resident Basic Medical Insurance scheme in 2008. The voluntary programme enrolls entire households, to target children, the elderly, the disabled and other non-working urban residents. Like the NRCMCS, the scheme is funded by contributions and also by premium subsidies from the government.

The government has also attempted to reduce the cost of care by encouraging the use of lower-level facilities, although perceptions of poor-quality service at these lower levels still remain a barrier. In response, government funds are being invested in new primary, preventive and rehabilitative centres and in renovating older village clinics and township health centres. Funds are also being used for training, advertising health facilities and improving community participation in the health system. The NRCMCS includes representatives of the farmers and village committees served by the programme and the new scheme is under county-level management, making it more accountable and closer to those who access the benefits of the programme (Bloom G, personal communication, 2010).

At this early stage, definitive evidence of the impact of these reforms on health and service utilization is not yet available. A review of some recent studies indicates that adverse selection may be a problem with the new insurance schemes, skewing enrolment towards those already unwell[9]. Another review of pilot studies of these insurance schemes has shown only moderate protection from catastrophic spending and limited protection for the poorest beneficiaries, as out-of-pocket spending remains a problem[15]. This has not, however, discouraged the Chinese Government, which has targeted universal health insurance coverage as a priority[12]. With nearly 90% of rural residents covered by the NRCMCS (accounting for 815 million people), and 65% of urban residents covered by the corresponding urban scheme by 2008[16], this target appears to be well within reach.

■ Costa Rica

Costa Rica has long been recognized as one of the most politically and economically stable countries in Latin America. Since 1985, there has been steady annual growth in GDP, often as high as 8 to 9%[2,17]. Despite having a per capita GDP that is merely average for an upper-middle-income country (US$ 6564 in 2008)[2,17], this small nation of fewer than five million people has consistently been among the top Latin American countries in terms of the Human

Table 8.2   Selected development indicators, Costa Rica vs. Panama

Indicator	Costa Rica		Panama[a]	
	1985	2008	1985	2008
Vaccination, DPT (% of children aged 12–23 months)	90	86[b]	73	82
Primary school completion rate, total (% of relevant age group)	77.3	92.9	82.4	n/a
Poverty gap at US$2 a day (purchasing power parity) (%)	8.6[c]	1.3[d]	13.1[e]	7.06[f]
Literacy rate, adult total (% of people aged 15 and above)	92[g]	96	88[h]	94
Fertility rate, total (births per woman)	3.46	1.96	3.34	2.55
Life expectancy at birth, total (years)	74.6	78.9	71.4	75.7

Source: Data from reference 2.

Notes: n/a: Not available; DPT: Three doses, diphtheria, pertussis and tetanus; [a] Selected as suitable comparator due to similar location, population, total GDP and GDP per capita; [b] Value is for 2009; [c] Value is for 1986; [d] Value is for 2007; [e] Value is for 1991; [f] Value is for 2006; [g] Value is for 1984; [h] Value is for 1980.

Development Index (HDI), a multidimensional measure of social and economic development that combines indicators of life expectancy, educational attainment and income: ranking 62 in the world and sixth among Latin American countries in 2010[18]. While many development indicators were already quite good in 1985, most have continued to improve since then and have even surpassed other countries in the region with comparable income levels, such as Panama (shown with Costa Rica in Table 8.2). For example, by 2008, the adult literacy rate was 96%, less than 2% of the population was living below the international poverty threshold of US$2 (adjusted for purchasing power parity) per day, more than 95% of the population had access to improved water and sanitation, and the total fertility rate was 1.96 births per woman[2].

Costa Rica has also maintained its impressive performance with respect to the health indicators documented in the original *Good health at low cost*, surpassing

Figure 8.3   Infant and maternal mortality, Costa Rica, 1970–2009

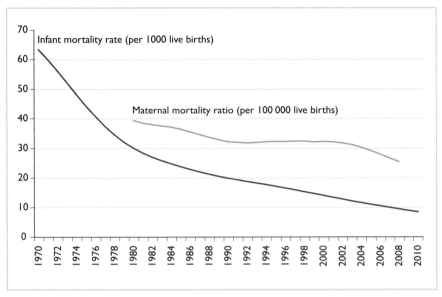

Sources: Data from references 3, 5 and 6.

all other countries of the same income level within the region. In 2008, life expectancy of 81.4 years for women and 76.6 years for men was second only to Canada in the western hemisphere[2]; the probability of maternal death was estimated to be approximately 25 per 100 000 live births; and infant mortality had declined steadily and is now estimated to be approximately 9.6 per 1000 live births, representing a sevenfold reduction over a three-decade span[3,5,6] (Figure 8.3).

This continued improvement is attributed to Costa Rica's long history of investment in social welfare, perhaps best represented by the Costa Rican Social Security Fund (CCSS), which was one of the first publicly administered social insurance models introduced in the region during the early 1940s. In addition to administering the national pension and other social security programmes, this autonomous public body also delivers most medical services free at the point of delivery, providing a comprehensive package of medical insurance benefits. The bulk of primary care is delivered through health centres and clinics that provide outpatient services, family and community medical services, and health promotion and prevention programmes, referring patients to higher levels of care as required. While the private sector is small in Costa Rica, public facilities may refer patients to the private sector when they are overloaded, or patients may choose to see a private physician to avoid long waiting times[17]. To address some issues of insufficient capacity in the public sector, the CCSS also contracts out some services to private entities, mainly to health cooperatives for primary services in urban areas, but also to private laboratories for diagnostics. In addition to overseeing and regulating the health system, the Ministry of Health shares responsibility for public health service delivery with the CCSS.

Total health expenditure as a proportion of GDP has remained consistent at approximately 8% (slightly higher than the average of approximately 7% for developing countries in Latin America and the Caribbean)[2]. In 2007, 27% of this expenditure was private, 85% of which covered out-of-pocket payments for ambulatory care in the private sector (Rosero-Bixby L, personal communication, 2010)[19]. Two thirds of the 73% public health expenditure was from the CCSS, making it the country's most important source of health financing[2,19]. As an independent public institution, the CCSS is financed primarily by contributions from employers (9.25% of payroll) and workers (5.5% of wages). Following worker protection legislation introduced in 2000, the self-employed are required to contribute 4.75% of their reported income, and the poor are covered by several subsidized schemes[19]. By 2006, 88% of the population was covered by the CCSS and 93% of the population had adequate access to primary care services[19].

Health system reforms since 1985

In addition to the factors already noted in the original *Good health at low cost* volume, including sustained public health expenditures, political stability and commitment, clear national consensus on the role of the health system and popular support for the CCSS[17,20–22], several reforms that were implemented from 1994 onwards further strengthened the Costa Rican health system and have been linked with improved health outcomes (Figure 8.4). These reforms, which followed the vision for the health system set out in the 1970s, have been associated with reductions of 8% and 2% in child and adult mortality rates, respectively[20], and fall into two main categories: further extending coverage and quality of primary care, focusing on underserved areas; and further improving the management, financing and delivery of medical services under the CCSS.

Achieving universal access to primary care, particularly in underserved rural areas, was greatly facilitated by the introduction of the EBAIS community clinics (*Equipos Básicos de Atención Integral en Salud*). Each clinic is responsible for a geographical area that covers approximately 4000 people and offers a full range of primary care, health promotion and preventive services. Where necessary, the EBAIS is mobile. At a minimum, EBAIS clinics are staffed by a doctor, a nurse and a technician, who are supported by personnel from the higher-level

Figure 8.4   Timeline of key events influencing health, Costa Rica, 1985–2010

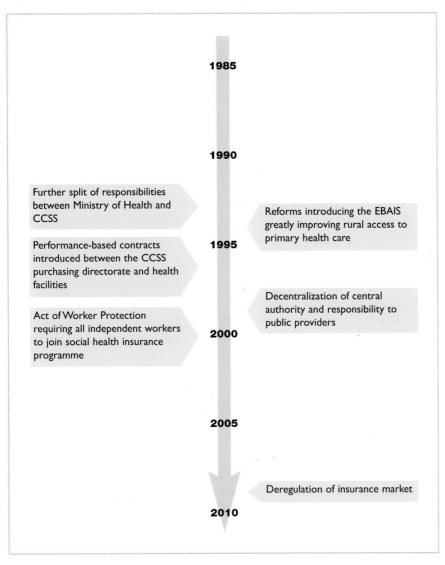

administrative grouping (known as the health area) to which the EBAIS belongs. These can include laboratory technicians, social workers, dentists, nutritionists, pharmacists and medical records specialists[23]. During the first stage of implementation, 232 EBAIS were established in 1995, with priority given to the most underserved communities. By 2004, there were a total of 855 EBAIS across the country[19].

The literature is characterized by broad consensus on the favourable impact that expansion of primary care has had on improving equitable access in Costa Rica. Prior to 1994, access to primary care was restricted to approximately 25% of the population. One analysis found that in the areas where reforms were implemented after 1995, the percentage of the population with adequate access to health services had risen from 64% to 79% by 2000[20], while the national rate of health coverage rose to 69% over the same period. Today, coverage is nearly universal[17,19,23,24]. Data presented in the original *Good health at low cost* showed that, between 1972 and 1980, 41% of the decline in infant mortality could be attributed to primary care interventions, while an additional 32% was due to improvements in secondary care. Socioeconomic progress and declining fertility rates explained the remaining decline[25]. In 1991, further analysis supported these original conclusions[26]. Although there is little evidence directly linking continued health gains in Costa Rica since 1985 to continued improvements in primary care access, the country's previous experience suggests that it may be continuing to play a part.

While the EBAIS greatly enhanced the physical reach of the CCSS, other important reforms implemented since the 1990s have focused on the organization's administrative structure. One such reform was the creation of a purchasing division within the CCSS, further separating the financing, purchasing and service provision functions of the organization. This allowed for improvements in quality and efficiency, such as the shifting away from a historical budgeting approach to resource allocation towards one intended to enhance production, user satisfaction and clinical practice, based on performance management contracts between the newly created purchasing division and service providers[17,27].

Another important reform during this period was the 1998 Law on Decentralization[28], which aimed to improve health system responsiveness by means of administrative decentralization of the CCSS. One of the mechanisms supporting this transfer of power was the creation of democratically elected community health boards to supervise the delivery of local services. This broadened community participation as local decision-makers became involved in setting priorities and performance targets for health[17,19].

However, the financial sustainability and equity of Costa Rica's state-driven model remain pressing issues as the cost of financing the health system continues to increase with the ageing population and the changing burden of disease. Despite the large operating revenues provided through member contributions, the government continues to commit substantial portions of its annual budget to health. For example, more than a fifth of total government expenditure went to health between 2003 and 2007[2]. As the success of the health system is dependent on the principle of solidarity to maintain high participation rates in the scheme across all population groups and enhance the progressive character of the overall system, low rates of affiliation (52%) among the economically active population and the high prevalence of contribution evasion among employers and workers alike threaten financial sustainability[19]. Until recently, the government of Costa Rica resisted the introduction of private insurance, largely because it did not believe it was in the citizens' best interest and because it feared that, once introduced, foreign corporations would quickly dominate the entire insurance market[27]. From this perspective, the deregulation of the health insurance market in 2009 to allow private medical insurance creates an obvious risk to equity, with scope for wealthy and healthy patients to opt out of publicly funded care, so undermining popular support for the CCSS. Costa Rica's experience will undoubtedly continue to yield further insight into best practices in health financing.

Kerala

For most of the 20th century, the economy of this southern Indian state lagged behind much of the rest of the country. Between 1970 and 1987, Kerala's annual growth in net domestic product was an average of 1.9%, nearly half of the all-India figure. But post-1987, the state's economy grew at a rate of 5.8% per year, and by 2000, its per capita income was 20% higher than the all-India figure[29]. This growth has largely been driven by the service sector, related to transportation, trade, hotels, restaurants and telecommunications, rather than the more conventional production of commodities. The increasing demand for these services has been linked to the increase in disposable income and ownership of assets such as homes, vehicles and appliances, which were supported largely by the huge influx of remittances from Keralites who since the 1970s have migrated to work in other parts of India and in the Gulf States[30].

Underlying Kerala's remarkable change in economic growth was the state government's long political commitment to investment in social welfare and equality, as characterized by the development of universal access to education, strong labour organization and popular movements promoting dialogue among castes. Since its formation in 1956, Kerala has consistently ranked higher on the HDI than all other states in India. By 2005, Kerala had nearly achieved universal elementary education and had attained a gender ratio of 1.058 females to every male: identical to that in Europe and North America, but quite different from many other parts of India where selective female abortion is widespread[29]. Gaps in human development also continue to close across gender and social groups. Census data

Table 8.3   Selected development indicators, Kerala vs. all India

Indicator	Kerala		India	
	1992–1993	2005–2006	1992–1993	2005–2006
Vaccination, DPT (% of children aged 12–23 months)	n/a	84.0	46.9	55.3
School attendance (% of children 6–10 years)	94.8	98.4	68.4	82.9
Literate persons (% of total population aged 15–49)	89.8[a]	93.5[b]	52.2[a]	63.4[b]
Undernutrition prevalence, weight for age (% of children under 5 years)	28.5[c]	22.9	53.4[c]	42.5
Fertility rate, total (births per woman)	2.0	1.9	3.4	2.7

Sources: Data for 1992–1993 from reference 32, unless stated otherwise; Data for 2005–2006 from references 33 and 34.

Notes: n/a: Not available; DPT: Three doses, diphtheria, pertussis and tetanus; [a] Values are for 1991 and data from reference 29; [b] Values are derived from combining weighted national estimates for women and men; [c] Values are for children under 4 years.

from 1961 to 1991 show that the literacy gap between the general and rural scheduled caste populations (representing those on Kerala's social margins) has consistently narrowed. The same data also show that the state's growth in literacy was higher than in all other Indian states, with the greatest relative gains among women. The availability of schools and good road networks, typical outputs of the state government's past investments, were identified as key factors in explaining the observed gains in literacy[31] (Table 8.3).

This continued performance on development indicators is also mirrored in Kerala's improving population health, better than all other Indian states. In 1980, overall life expectancy at birth was 66 years[35], and by 1995, it had risen to 70.4 years for males and 75.9 years for females compared with Punjab, which during the same period had the next-best life expectancy across India, at 66.7 years for males and 68.8 years for females[29]. Infant mortality experienced a dramatic decline and more than halved from 1981 to 2005–2006, when it was estimated at approximately 15 deaths per 1000 live births (Table 8.4). By

Table 8.4   Infant and maternal mortality, Kerala, 1981 to 2005–2006

Health indicator	1981[36]	1992–3[32]	1998–9[37]	2005–6[33]
Infant mortality rate (per 1000 live births)	39.1	23.8	16.3	15.3
Maternal mortality ratio (per 100 000 live births)	n/a	n/a	n/a	95[36]

Sources: References 32, 33, 36, 37.

Note: n/a: Not available.

comparison, Maharashtra, the state with the second-lowest infant mortality rate, experienced 48 per 1000 live births in 2000[29]. It is also remarkable that infant mortality rates in Kerala show almost no difference between rural and urban areas, unlike the rest of the country where a large gap persists[29]. While reliable time series data do not exist for maternal mortality in Kerala, in 2006, it was estimated to be 95 deaths per 100 000 live births, approximately one third of the estimated rate for India as a whole[38].

Despite its low mortality overall, Kerala now has some of the highest rates of noncommunicable disease mortality and morbidity in the country[39,40]. A recent study of adult mortality patterns within a rural community showed that coronary heart disease has now overtaken communicable diseases to become the leading cause of death in the state, and that the burden of coronary heart disease deaths now exceeds that of industrialized countries[41]. The prevalence of obesity is also rapidly increasing, and Kerala has the second highest rate of obesity among women of all states in India (21% with body mass index of 25+, while the national average is 11%)[29]. Trends in alcohol consumption are also a cause for concern because, although the overall Indian average is low, consumption in Kerala is the highest in the country, at more than double the all-India average[29,42].

Health system changes since 1985

Kerala's current health system is composed of parallel public and private sectors. While traditional medicine is important in the state's health system, the share of modern (that is, allopathic or western) health services is highest in Kerala among all Indian states[43]. The public sector has a well-developed network of health facilities (a legacy of Kerala's prior investment in social welfare), with nearly 200 hospitals and more than 1000 primary health facilities, each staffed with a doctor providing a full range of treatment and prevention services (for example, vaccinations and family planning)[44]. As elsewhere in India, private sector growth increased dramatically in the early 1980s and quickly surpassed that in the public sector (Figure 8.5). For example, between 1986 and 1996, the number of private sector beds rose by 40%, from 49 000 to 67 500, while the number of beds in public facilities grew by only 5.5% over the same period, from 36 000 to 38 000[45]. But despite varying degrees of service quality[46], a lack of regulation[47] and concerns of supplier-induced demand[48], the private sector now handles most of the caseload in the state and has also surpassed the public sector in other areas, including the availability of advanced diagnostics, such as magnetic resonance imaging. However, unlike Sri Lanka, where private-sector outpatient services tend to complement the hospital-dominated public sector, the private sector in Kerala offers a mix of services that are in direct competition with the public sector.

The shift from the public to private sector was facilitated by a number of developments. Fiscal crisis in the 1970s and in the 1990s led to the introduction of poorly implemented cost-recovery mechanisms (i.e. user fees) that generated insufficient operating revenues. The fiscal crisis also decreased health budgets, and funds earmarked for health were increasingly used to meet salaries. Between 1985 and 2003, the share of health in the state revenue budget fell from 7.7% to 5.4%[49]. Shortages of medicines and other consumables decreased the quality of public-sector services and negatively impacted upon popular confidence in the government-funded health system, encouraging patients to seek private health care. Increased purchasing power among poorer groups (brought about by increasing incomes across all socioeconomic groups and decreasing fertility rates) further fuelled the already high demand for modern health services, so much so that by the mid-1980s health service use – both among low- and high-income groups – was already shifting towards the private sector.

These factors have compounded over the years and the effect is clearly seen in current patterns of health spending. Compared with all other Indian states, Kerala spends at least twice the annual amount per household, at nearly US$ 38 per capita in 2004–2005[a]; and 86.3% of this falls upon households as out-of-pocket spending. Public funds account for slightly less than 11% of total health expenditure, and are raised from both tax and non-tax revenues at national and state level, with a small proportion also generated from user fees[49]. Funds from the central government are allocated to states to implement national

---

[a] Historical exchange rate of US$ 1 to 44.94 Indian rupees was used, averaged over the fiscal year from 1 April 2004 to 31 March 2005. Exchange rate obtained from http://www.oanda.com/currency/historical-rates.

Figure 8.5 Timeline of key events influencing health, Kerala, 1955–2010

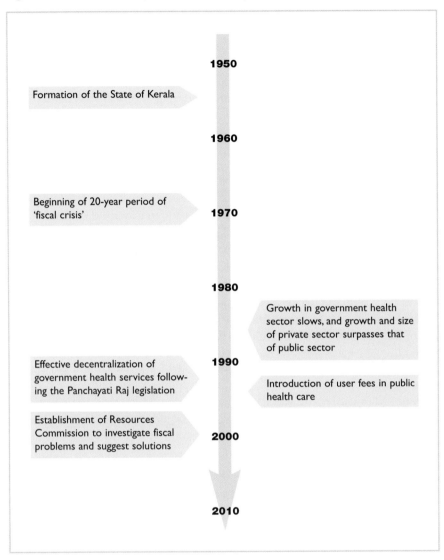

programmes, while programmes delivered by local governments (*panchayats*) are financed by transfers from the state government.

Not surprisingly, the reliance on household spending has had adverse implications for poor and marginalized groups. One study that looked at household spending on health across income groups showed that the poor spent 40% of their income on health care in 1996, while the rich spent only 2.4%. Compared with what they were spending ten years previously, this represents a 450% increase in out-of-pocket expenditure among poor households compared with an increase of 12% for rich households[50]. A more recent study of inpatient health expenditure in rural Kerala showed private spending to be significantly male biased, as greater amounts tended to be spent on the hospitalization of men (about US$ 129) compared with women (about US$ 93)[51]. Access in rural areas is further threatened by the persistent underfunding of primary care, and public sector shortages of doctors and essential commodities, such as drugs, result in the rural poor shifting to private health care at a much higher cost[52]. As in other settings, health inequities are closely linked to such inequalities in access.

The decentralization reforms introduced with the Panchayati Raj legislation[53,54] in the mid-1990s transferred much of the decision-making related to social welfare from the central government to the state and local (*panchayat*) levels. These are considered to be the most likely reforms to address the inequities in health that have emerged and have persisted since the 1980s. Theoretically, decentralization of responsibility to the *panchayat* level was intended to make public services, including the health system, more responsive to the communities being served through greater involvement of the community in decision-making processes[55]. However, the full impact of these reforms on the health sector has yet to be realized.

One evaluation suggested that decentralization had not yet brought any significant change to the health sector[56]. The analysis showed that *panchayats* in Kerala had, in fact, allocated a lower level of resources to health than what had been allocated by the state government prior to decentralization. This was largely due to the absence of sufficient support, innovation and technical expertise at the local level to compete effectively for limited *panchayat* funds. In addition, a directive issued by the State Planning Board barred spending of *panchayat* funds for the purchase of medicines or the maintenance of health facilities, thus compounding the public-sector quality issues[56].

Despite its many years of steady economic growth, greater fiscal pressure may also arise as state government revenues continue to be eroded by remittances from foreign workers from which income taxes are not obtained. This is coupled with the continuing shift away from the primary sector towards the tertiary sector (i.e. the state economy now relies heavily on retail sales, from which it is also difficult to extract tax revenues) (Acharya A, personal communication, 2010). An ongoing challenge for the government will be to ensure that the state's economic prosperity is effectively translated into public goods and used to address key health issues, such as obesity and chronic disease, and to tackle the widening inequities that affect access to health services.

■ Sri Lanka

Despite nearly three decades of civil war, Sri Lanka has performed well economically for many years, experiencing steady growth in GDP since 1985, with peak annual growth of 8% in 2006. In addition, with an estimated per capita GDP of US$ 2013 in 2008, this country of 20 million people has the highest per capita income in south Asia[2]. While its economy historically relied on agricultural commodities, over the course of the last century, Sri Lanka has moved steadily towards an industrialized economy with the development of food processing, textiles, telecommunications and the finance sector. Also, there are now nearly 1.5 million Sri Lankan citizens working abroad, including many in the Gulf States and the Middle East. Remittances from these migrant workers, estimated to total US$ 2.9 billion in 2008, are an important source of foreign exchange and have contributed to rising household incomes[57].

In the first decade of this century, however, Sri Lanka has had to cope with a series of challenges. For example, in 2001, Sri Lanka experienced its first-ever recession, a period characterized by power shortages, budgetary problems and intensification of the civil strife that started in the early 1980s. The December 2004 tsunami devastated several areas along the southern and eastern coasts of Sri Lanka. A short time later, there was a resurgence of fighting in the ongoing civil war, continuing until May 2009, when government forces declared the conflict over. Since then, Sri Lanka has experienced a post-war economic boom; however, more than 300 000 people remain internally displaced as a result of the conflict[58], and despite being relatively low (5.9% in 2009), unemployment also persists, disproportionately affecting women and educated youth[57].

Since 1985, Sri Lanka has been able to maintain progress on a number of indicators related to human development, largely primed by its early commitment to social welfare. As a result, a number of these indicators have significantly improved, while others, such as poverty and undernutrition, persist. Table 8.5 shows key changes, and compares them with India's.

Key indicators on population health outcomes have also generally improved since 1985. Total life expectancy in 2008 reached 74 years[2]; infant mortality has experienced a threefold reduction to approximately 10 per 1000 live births, and maternal mortality is currently estimated to be 30 per 100 000 live births, less than half compared with that two decades earlier[3,5,6]. However, as is clear from Figure 8.6, the pre-1985 downward trajectory in both of these mortality indicators was not maintained. Indeed, at times during the post-1985 period, rates of infant and maternal mortality increased before returning to their downward trajectory. Furthermore, these health gains have not been equally distributed

Table 8.5   Selected development indicators, Sri Lanka vs. India

Indicator	Sri Lanka		India[a]	
	1985	2008	1985	2008
Vaccination, DPT (% of children aged 12–23 months)	70	97[b]	18	66
Primary school completion rate, total (% of relevant age group)	83.0	98.4	n/a	93.6[c]
Poverty gap at $2 a day (purchasing power parity) (%)	16.1	11.9	36.7[d]	30.4[e]
Literacy rate, adult total (% of people aged 15 and above)	86.8[f]	90.6	40.8[f]	62.8[g]
Undenutrition prevalence, weight for age (% of children under 5 years)	29.3[h]	21.1[i]	n/a	43.5[g]
Fertility rate, total (births per woman)	2.92	2.33	4.32	2.74
Life expectancy at birth, total (years)	69.0	74.1	56.9	63.7

Source: Data from reference 2.

Notes: n/a: Not available; DPT: Three doses, diphtheria, pertussis and tetanus; [a] Selected as suitable comparator due to similar location and World Bank income group; [b] Value is for 2009; [c] Value is for 2007; [d] Value is for 2002; [e] Value is for 2005; [f] Value is for 1981; [g] Value is for 2006; [h] Value is for 1987; [i] Value is for 2007.

throughout the population, and some groups even experienced worsening health during this period. Life expectancy for women in 2008 (78 years) was eight years longer than that of men[2]; significantly higher mortality overall was reported among tea, rubber and coconut plantation workers (although some decline has been observed more recently)[59]; and there is higher maternal mortality in the northern and eastern districts affected by conflict. For example, in 1995–1996, the maternal mortality ratio in these districts was 3.5 times higher than that of the entire country, most likely due to poorer access to health services, education, nutrition, water and sanitation[60].

Figure 8.6   Infant and maternal mortality, Sri Lanka, 1970–2009

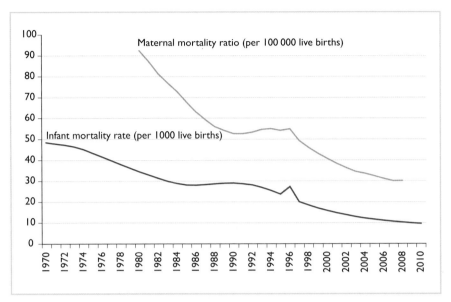

Sources: Data from references 3, 5 and 6.

The health system and its performance since 1985

As in other social sectors, the foundation for Sri Lanka's current health system was laid prior to 1960 and no major structural changes have occurred since then (Figure 8.7). Today, the overall health system is composed of parallel public and private sectors. The comprehensive public system is financed and operated by the Ministry of Health in Colombo and eight provincial departments of health, and almost all care from preventive services to specialist tertiary care is free at the point of delivery. Units run by medical officers provide most preventive and public health services through teams of health workers[59]. Having grown steadily since the 1960s, the private sector is also very prominent and focuses mainly on outpatient care, but there is also a small private hospital sector concentrated in the capital[59]. Much private sector activity is actually provided by government medical officers working during their off-duty hours. This practice allows these public servants to supplement their relatively meagre government wages and promotes the retention of health professionals in the public service. As such, the overall outpatient load is shared between the public and private sectors, while the public sector provides more than 95% of inpatient care[59].

Figure 8.7 Timeline of key events influencing health, Sri Lanka, 1960–2010

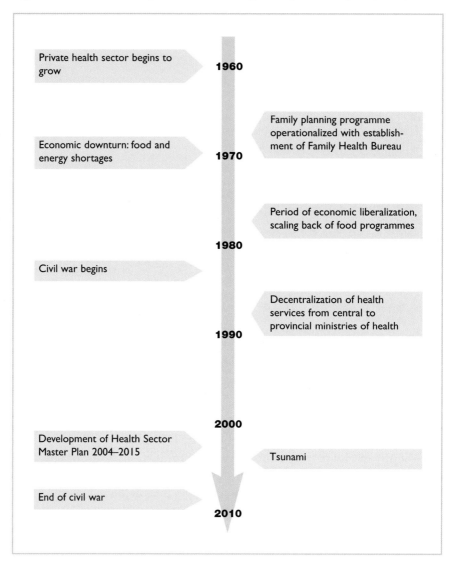

Good access to health services is likely to explain at least some of the country's overall health performance. After decades of government investment in hospital infrastructure, most Sri Lankans live within 3 km of a public facility[59], and since 2000, there has been an average of three hospital beds per 1000 people (compared with the average of two beds per 1000 people in middle income countries)[2]. Another legacy of this early investment is the low overall spending on health: in 2007, total health expenditure was estimated to be 4.2% of GDP, slightly lower than other countries at the same income level[2]. However, just 47% of this expenditure is now public (constituting 8.5% of total government expenditure), leaving more than half of health spending financed privately, 86% of which comes out of pocket, as private health insurance coverage is low[2]. Increasing private expenditure is the main driver of increasing health expenditure overall. The majority of public funding goes towards the provision of in-patient services, while the bulk of private funding is spent on outpatient care[59]. These public–private divisions in provision and spending have imparted to Sri Lanka's overall health system several interesting performance characteristics, most notably with respect to equity and quality.

Good geographic access and lack of financial barriers to public facilities combine with several aspects of health financing to produce a relatively equitable health system in Sri Lanka. First, public health spending is relatively progressive, reflecting the role of direct taxation. The ability of the rich (who would typically contribute more but use services less) to opt out of the public system has tended to leave public outpatient care dominated by the poor[61], resulting in the poorest quintile benefiting from 27% of public spending in this sector, compared with 11% for the richest quintile in 2003–2004[59]. However, because of the tendency to use the public system for inpatient care across all income groups, government spending for this type of care is more evenly distributed (18% for the poorest quintile versus 16% for the richest, although this takes no account of the much greater health needs of the poor)[59].

The high use of public sector inpatient care by all groups provides some protection from catastrophic health expenses by limiting out-of-pocket payments. One study that looked at the incidence of such expenses across a number of Asian countries showed that only a very small percentage of Sri Lankan households were affected, which was much better than in many other low- and middle-income countries[62]. High utilization of inpatient services in the public sector is maintained by a perception of good quality based on the widely held view that public hospitals have the best staff and equipment to deal with serious conditions[61,63]. In outpatient clinics, on the other hand, perceived low quality of public sector services persuades richer patients to pay for private care[59].

It has been argued that the high standard of training received by practitioners in the public sector has helped to create and maintain quality in the private sector, since, as a consequence of dual practice, most doctors are drawn from the public sector and are believed to apply the same practice standards in both sectors. One study conducted in 2001 estimated that between 50% and 70% of the private sector caseload was being seen by doctors regularly employed in the public sector[64]. This means that although use of the private sector has grown it has not involved the expansion of unqualified, informal providers, which characterize this sector in many other developing countries[60]. Furthermore, because most private practitioners are drawn from public cadres working within the same area, both patients and providers already know which private providers offer a high standard of care (Russell S, personal communication, 2010). There are, of course, well-known disadvantages arising from dual practice, including the incentive to exert more effort in the more lucrative private sector or even to stimulate private demand by underperforming in public practice[65].

Overall, Sri Lankans place a great deal of confidence in their health system – both public and private sectors – because of the quality care, ease of access and level of risk protection it provides. Nevertheless, decreasing levels of government health investment have affected hospital care, which could drive greater numbers of patients to seek care in the private sector. For example, between 1987 and 2004, the percentage of patients who sought modern care from the private sector (including clinics, hospitals and pharmacies) increased by nearly 8%, to reach 45.1%, while recent analysis of the impact of government health spending indicates a shifting of benefit from the poor to the urban better-off[59]. It is recognized that the continued shift of patients out of the public system may destabilize the health system by undermining popular support for government health services[59]. With the recent end of the longstanding civil war, an opportunity has arisen for the 12–14% of total government expenditure previously spent on the military to be redistributed across other national priorities[2].

■ Concluding remarks: Further insights after 25 years?

The original *Good health at low cost* in 1985 concluded with three recommendations for other developing countries seeking to improve population health. Countries should work first to ensure *equitable access* to public health services and health care; second, to provide *universally accessible education*; and third, to guarantee *adequate nutrition* to all levels of society. Taken together with other important features identified from the case studies, including universal franchise, promotion of social and economic equality, and development of public infrastructure, these are all products of what has been defined as the 'support-led security' approach to development[66]. A sustained long-term commitment to this approach by each of the governments studied aided the formation of a virtuous cycle of human development that served to build popular trust and confidence in the state's ability to provide for its citizens' needs, leading governments to be more responsive and accountable to these needs.

From examining how China, Costa Rica, Kerala and Sri Lanka have fared 25 years later, it is evident that the benefits of these virtuous cycles continue to compound and have contributed to the impressive health gains observed since 1985. While the original lessons clearly continue to be relevant today, revisiting these case studies in light of the many contextual changes that have occurred since 1985 has generated new lessons on how health systems can respond to meet the challenges that are posed not only by increasing burdens of chronic disease and ageing populations but also by changing economic and social realities, such as migration, values and the ever increasing number of actors involved in health.

Echoing the first recommendation from the original *Good health at low cost*, ensuring access to modern health services remains crucial to improving population health. But in contrast to the early stages of health system development where the aim was to provide a basic level of care to the entire population, *this priority has broadened to encompass higher levels of care and preventive services* in order to adapt to changing health needs. One of the guiding principles of this expansion is guaranteeing that it happens in an equitable way to counterbalance the effects of changing economic conditions and demographic trends that continually work to widen health inequalities.

Second, achieving equity of access was also shown to be dependent on the acceptability of the care being provided – a concept that has evolved beyond the cultural acceptability as defined by Alma-Ata in 1978 to *also include values driven by increasing consumer awareness*. In several of the case studies, the role that differences in real and perceived quality played was clear in shifting utilization away from readily available care towards more expensive care in either the private sector or in urban areas. Quality was also seen to be important in maintaining popular confidence in publicly funded health services and public institutions. This confidence is a key factor in keeping health as a political priority and ensuring the financial sustainability of the health system.

Both of these lessons underscore the third emerging theme from the case studies: that *governments continue to play a central role* in developing health systems. It is interesting to note that the motivation for the original *Good health at low cost* volume was partially a reaction to the privatization discourse that dominated the politics of the 1980s, and that updating these case studies has once again highlighted the importance of continued government leadership in developing accessible and responsive health systems. While there is no one-size-fits-all model for such participation, the case studies have clearly shown that governments have a variety of tools at their disposal to help to build and maintain equitable access and quality care. Direct provision of health services through public-sector facilities was an important avenue to ensure equitable access in each of the case studies. The case studies also described several mechanisms by which government involvement influenced the quality of care (e.g. direct investment, regulation, efficiency interventions). But with tightening budgets and the unavoidable increases in private-sector participation and out-of-pocket expenditures, perhaps where government involvement can have the greatest impact is through the design, implementation and regulation of financial protection mechanisms that are appropriate for the context, sustainable and pro-poor.

ACKNOWLEDGEMENTS

I would like to thank Gerald Bloom (Institute of Development Studies, University of Sussex), Arnab Acharya (London School of Hygiene & Tropical Medicine), Steven Russell (School of International Development, University of East Anglia), Luis Rosero-Bixby (Centro Centroamericano de Población, Universidad de Costa Rica), and Kent Ranson (World Health Organization) for their contribution to this work. I would also like thank Dina Balabanova, Gill Walt, Anne Mills and Martin McKee, all from the London School of Hygiene & Tropical Medicine, and Joanne McManus for their guidance and helpful suggestions.

REFERENCES

1. Halstead SB, Walsh JL, Warren KS, eds. *Good health at low cost.* New York: Rockefeller Foundation; 1985.

2. World Bank. *World development indicators* [online]. 2009 (http://ddp-ext.world bank.org/ext/DDPQQ/member.do?method=getMembers&userid=1&queryId=, accessed 30 May 2010).

3. Hogan MC et al. Maternal mortality for 181 countries, 1980–2008: a systematic analysis of progress towards Millennium Development Goal 5. *Lancet* 2010; 375(9726):1609–23.

4. Wagstaff A et al. *Reforming China's rural health system.* Washington, DC: World Bank; 2009.

5. Rajaratnam JK et al. Neonatal, postneonatal, childhood, and under-5 mortality for 187 countries, 1970–2010: a systematic analysis of progress towards Millennium Development Goal 4. *Lancet* 2010; 375(9730):1988–2008.

6. IHME. *Datasets*. Seattle, WA: Institute for Health Metrics & Evaluation, Department of Global Health, University of Washington; 2010 (http://www.healthmetricsandevaluation.org/resources/datasets.html, accessed 21 May 2010).

7. Banister J, Zhang X. China, economic development and mortality decline. *World Development* 2005; 33(1):21–41.

8. Audibert M, Mathonnat J, Chen Y. *Does external openness influence the infant mortality rates? An econometric investigation for the Chinese provinces.* Clermont-Ferrand: Centre d'Etudes et de Recherches sur le Développement International; 1999 (CERDI Working Paper: 1998311998).

9. Wagstaff A et al. China's health system and its reform: a review of recent studies. *Health Economics* 2009; 18(Special Issue):S7–23.

10. Tang S et al. Tackling the challenges to health equity in China. *Lancet* 2008; 372(9648):1493–501.

11. Sidel VW. The barefoot doctors of the People's Republic of China. *New England Journal of Medicine* 1972; 286(24):1292–300.

12. Blumenthal D, Hsiao W. Privatization and its discontents: the evolving Chinese health care system. *New England Journal of Medicine* 2005; 353(11):1165–70.

13. West LA, Wong CPW. Fiscal decentralization and growing regional disparities in rural China: some evidence in the provision of social services. *Oxford Review of Economic Policy* 1995; 11(4):70–84.

14. Grigoriou C, Guillaumont P. *Child mortality under Chinese reforms.* Clermont-Ferrand: Centre d'Etudes et de Recherches sur le Développement International; 2004 (CERDI Working Paper: 2004102004).

15. Sun X et al. Catastrophic medical payment and financial protection in rural China: evidence from the New Cooperative Medical Scheme in Shandong Province. *Health Economics* 2009; 18(1):103–19.

16. Qingyue M, Shenglan T. *Universal coverage of health care in China: challenges and opportunities.* Geneva: World Health Organization; 2010.

17. Unger JP et al. Costa Rica: achievements of a heterodox health policy. *American Journal of Public Health* 2008; 98(4):636–43.

18. UNDP. *Human development reports* [online]. New York: United Nations Development Programme; 2010 (http://hdr.undp.org/en/, accessed 4 January 2011).

19. Cercone J, Pacheco Jimenez J. Costa Rica: "good practice" in expanding health care coverage – lessons from reforms in low- and middle-income countries. In: Gottret P, Schieber GJ, Waters HR, eds. *Good practices in health financing: lessons from reforms in low- and middle-income countries.* Washington, DC: World Bank; 2008:183–226.

20. Rosero-Bixby L. [Assessing the impact of health sector reform in Costa Rica through a quasi-experimental study.] [In Spanish] *Revista Panamericana de Salud Pública* 2004; 15(2):94–103.

21. McGuire JW. *Politics, policy, and mortality decline in Costa Rica.* Middletown, CT: Wesleyan University; 2007.

22. deBertodano I. The Costa Rican health system: low cost, high value. *Bulletin of the World Health Organization* 2003; 81(8):626–27.

23. Clark MA. Reinforcing a public system: health sector reform in Costa Rica. In: Kaufman RR, Nelson JM, eds. *Crucial needs, weak incentives: social sector reform, democratization, and globalization in Latin America.* Baltimore, MD: Johns Hopkins University Press; 2004:189–216.

24. Kruk ME et al. The contribution of primary care to health and health systems in low- and middle-income countries: a critical review of major primary care initiatives. *Social Science & Medicine* 2010; 70(6):904–11.

25. Rosero-Bixby L. Infant mortality decline in Costa Rica. In: Halstead SB, Walsh JL, Warren KS, eds. *Good health at low cost.* New York: Rockefeller Foundation; 1985:125–38.

26 Rosero-Bixby L. Socioeconomic development, health interventions and mortality decline in Costa Rica. *Scandinavian Journal of Social Medicine.* Supplement 1991; 46:33–42.

27. Homedes N, Ugalde A. Why neoliberal health reforms have failed in Latin America. *Health Policy* 2005; 71(1):83–96.

28. Costa Rica. Decentralization of hospitals and clinics (GLIN ID 87021). *La Gaceta, Diario Oficial,* December 1998

29. Centre for Development Studies. *Human Development Report 2005.* Thiruvananthapuram: State Planning Board, Government of Kerala; 2006.

30. Pushpangadan K. *Remittances, consumption and economic growth in Kerala: 1980–2000.* Trivendrum: Centre for Development Studies; 2003.

31. Narayanamoorthy A, Kamble BN. Trends and determinants of rural literacy among scheduled caste population: a state level analysis. *Journal of Educational Planning and Administration* 2003; 17(1):35–52.

32. International Institute for Population Sciences. *National family health survey (MCH and family planning), 1992–93: India.* Bombay: International Institute for Population Sciences; 1995.

33. International Institute for Population Sciences and Macro International. *National family health survey, 2005–06: India, Volume I.* Mumbai: International Institute for Population Sciences; 2007.

34. International Institute for Population Sciences and Macro International. *National family health survey, India, 2005–06: Kerala.* Mumbai: International Institute for Population Sciences; 2008.

35. Krishnan T. Health statistics in Kerala State, India. In: Halstead SB, Walsh JL, Warren KS, eds. *Good health at low cost.* New York: Rockefeller Foundation; 1985:39–46.

36. Directorate of Economics and Statistics, Government of Kerala. *Annual reports on sample registration.* Thiruvananthapuram: Government of Kerala; 1981.

37. International Institute for Population Sciences and ORC Macro. *National family health survey (NFHS-2), 1998–99: India.* Mumbai: International Institute for Population Sciences; 2000.

38. National Rural Health Mission. *Kerala State file* [online]. Mumbai: Ministry of Health & Family Welfare, Government of India; 2010 (http://www.mohfw.nic.in/NRHM/State%20Files/kerala.htm, accessed 1 June 2010).

39. Kumar BG. Low mortality and high morbidity in Kerala reconsidered. *Population and Development Review* 1993; 19(1):103–21.

40. Narayana D. High health achievements and good access to health care at great cost: the emerging Kerala situation. In: Haddad S, Barı E, Narayana D, eds. *Safeguarding the health sector in times of macroeconomic instability: policy lessons for low- and middle-income countries.* Trenton: Africa World Press/IDRC; 2008.

41. Soman CR et al. All-cause mortality and cardiovascular mortality in Kerala State of India: results from a 5-year follow-up of 161 942 rural community dwelling adults. *Asia-Pacific Journal of Public Health 2010*; May 10 [Epub ahead of print].

42. WHO. *Global status report on alcohol 2004.* Geneva: World Health Organization, Department of Mental Health and Substance Abuse; 2004.

43. Panikar P. *Health transition in Kerala.* Thiruvananthapuram: Kerala Research Programme on Local Level Development, Centre for Development Studies; 1999.

44. Sato H. Social security and well-being in a low-income economy: an appraisal of the Kerala experience. *Developing Economies* 2004; 42(2):288–304.

45. Kutty VR. Historical analysis of the development of health care facilities in Kerala State, India. *Health Policy and Planning* 2000; 15(1):103–9.

46. Levesque JF et al. Outpatient care utilization in urban Kerala, India. *Health Policy and Planning* 2006; 21(4):289–301.

47. Nabae K. The health care system in Kerala: its past accomplishments and new challenges. *Journal of the National Institute of Public Health* 2003; 52(2):140–5.

48. Dilip TR. Utilization of inpatient care from private hospitals: trends emerging from Kerala, India. *Health Policy and Planning* 2010; 25(5):437–46.

49. Rao KS et al. *Financing of health in India (Section IV)*. New Delhi: National Commission on Macroeconomics and Health, Ministry of Health & Family Welfare, Government of India; 2005.

50. Kunhikannan T, Aravindan K. *Changes in the health status of Kerala 1987–1997*. Thiruvananthapuram: Kerala Research Programme on Local Level Development, Centre for Development Studies; 2000.

51. Ashokan A, Ibrahim P. Inpatient health care expenditure: some new evidences from rural Kerala. *Indian Journal of Economics and Business* 2008; 7(2):297–307.

52. Nair VM. Health in South Asia: future of Kerala depends on its willingness to learn from past. *British Medical Journal* 2004; 328(7454):1497.

53. Constitutional (73rd Amendment) Act (1992).

54. Kerala Panchayt Raj Act (13/1994) (1994).

55. Drèze J, Sen A. *India: economic development and social opportunity*. Oxford: Clarendon Press; 1995.

56. Varatharajan D, Thankappan R, Jayapalan S. Assessing the performance of primary health centres under decentralized government in Kerala, India. *Health Policy and Planning* 2004; 19(1):41–51.

57. US Department of State. *Background note: Sri Lanka*. Washington, DC: Department of State; 2010 (http://www.state.gov/r/pa/ei/bgn/5249.htm, accessed 12 July 2010).

58. Amnesty International. *Sri Lanka's displaced face uncertain future as government begins to unlock the camps*. Updated 11 September 2009 (http://www.amnesty.org/en/news-and-updates/news/sri-lanka-displaced-uncertain-future-government-unlock-camps-20090911, accessed 7 July 2010).

59. Rannan-Eliya RP, Sikurajapathy L. Sri Lanka: "good practice" in expanding health care coverage. In: Gottret P, Schieber GJ, Waters HR, editors. *Good practices in health financing: lessons from reforms in low- and middle-income countries*. Washington, DC: World Bank; 2008:311–54.

60. McNay K, Keith R, Penrose A. *Bucking the trend: how Sri Lanka has achieved good health at low cost – challenges and policy lessons for the 21st century.* London: Save the Children; 2004.

61. Russell S, Gilson L. Are health services protecting the livelihoods of the urban poor in Sri Lanka? Findings from two low-income areas of Colombo. *Social Science & Medicine* 2006; 63(7):1732–44.

62. van Doorslaer E et al. Catastrophic payments for health care in Asia. *Health Economics* 2007; 16(11):1159–84.

63. Russell S. Treatment-seeking behaviour in urban Sri Lanka: trusting the state, trusting private providers. *Social Science & Medicine* 2005; 61(7):1396–407.

64. Rannan-Eliya R et al. *Equity in financing and delivery of health services in Bangladesh, Nepal and Sri Lanka.* Colombo: Institute of Policy Studies; 2001.

65. Ferrinho P et al. Dual practice in the health sector: review of the evidence. *Human Resources for Health* 2004; 2(1):14.

66. Drèze J, Sen A. *Hunger and public action.* Oxford: Clarendon Press; 1989.

Chapter 9

THE CONTRIBUTION OF HEALTH SYSTEMS TO GOOD HEALTH

Dina Balabanova[1], Lesong Conteh[2] and Martin McKee[1]

1 LSHTM, 2 Imperial College London

■ Introduction

This chapter examines the role of the health care system in improving health outcomes in the study countries, with a focus on maternal and child health. Chapter 1 illustrated the substantial increase in the potential for health care to save lives and prevent disability since the publication of the original *Good health at low cost* report in 1985. What do these changes imply for how health systems should be organized?

The approach taken throughout this volume is based loosely on the health system building blocks set out by the WHO[1]. In each country we seek to identify:

- health interventions that can be linked to specific health gains;
- developments within the health system that supported the effective delivery of these interventions; and
- contextual factors that explain how and why these developments were possible.

The approach was comparative, employing an iterative process to identify common themes before exploring areas of convergence and divergence among countries. While the focus is primarily on the five study countries, where appropriate, we have placed countries in the context of their neighbours or countries with comparative settings. Thus, this chapter draws primarily on the case studies set out in the preceding chapters, supplemented by evidence from other published sources.

We were able to identify eight broad sets of issues that seemed to be associated with the achievement of 'good health at low' cost across the countries studied. They mapped on to the building blocks and included:

- good governance;
- effective institutions and bureaucracies;
- scaling up the health workforce;
- efforts towards fair and sustainable financing;
- financial protection;
- innovative ways of securing health system inputs; and
- building resilience in the health system.

These will be considered in turn. Box 9.1 outlines key messages for success.

> **Box 9.1 Characteristics of successful health systems: key messages**
>
> A health system has been found to be successful when it:
>
> - has vision and long-term strategies;
>
> - takes into account the constraints imposed by path dependency;
>
> - builds consensus at societal level;
>
> - allows flexibility and autonomy in decision-making;
>
> - is resilient and learns from experiences, feeding back into the policy cycle;
>
> - receives support from the broader governance and socioeconomic context in country, and is in harmony with culture and population preferences;
>
> - achieves synergies among sectors and actors; and
>
> - demonstrates openness to dialogue and collaboration between public and private sectors, with effective government oversight.

■ Good governance

Governance is a key function underlying all the other health system building blocks[1]. Sometimes linked to the concepts of stewardship[2] and leadership, it comprises the arrangements through which the system operates, including how it sets and monitors its overall goals and how the various components of the system interact to achieve them. Research on the factors underlying success and failure in many different sectors has identified the importance of good governance as underlying social development[3]. The original *Good health at low cost* report was among the first sources that reinforced the importance of governance, with the role of the government seen as central in increasingly pluralistic health systems. There is a rich literature on the conceptual and normative aspects of governance[4,5], but here we explore how good governance, in practice, can promote better health.

Government leadership and vision

In each of the countries, we could identify the importance of *effective leadership, based on clear political vision*. This vision was typically set out in a national plan or strategy that was feasible and that set realistic goals. For example, within five years after independence from the USSR, Kyrgyzstan has developed and endorsed a comprehensive reform programme (*Manas*) that paved the way for subsequent coherent reforms. This plan facilitated the creation of an early Sector-Wide Approach (SWAp); indeed, this remains the only example of such an approach in the former USSR[6]. This made it possible for Kyrgyzstan to develop the most comprehensive health sector development programme of any former Soviet republic, subsequently enabling it to attract extensive financial and technical support from a range of donors. In contrast, after independence in 1991, the central Asian countries that lacked a comprehensive plan ended up implementing disjointed and fragmented reforms. For example Tajikistan began to prepare a National Health Strategy in 2009, 18 years after independence, and much wealthier Kazakhstan only began to formulate a plan in 2011.

Our research reveals how this plan has retained support from successive Kyrgyz Governments, providing an agreed and consistent set of priorities and facilitating sustained donor support. Despite the presence of multiple stakeholders, government ownership was strong. Commentators in Kyrgyzstan see their country as a leader in the region, applauding its sense of national ownership and clarity of vision.

The Ethiopian Government also seized the initiative in coordinating the activities of donors and other development partners. This is exemplified by the Health Extension Programme, which is credited with enabling essential health services to reach remote communities and combating major communicable diseases[7,8] While many countries have succeeded in developing primary care programmes, the Ethiopian Government had the vision and leadership required to mobilize and coordinate the substantial resources from many different donors that were needed to deliver this ambitious programme. Our Ethiopian partners saw the Health Extension Programme as only one manifestation of a number of effective development policies in the country.

Leadership was also apparent in Ethiopia's broader engagement in international and regional partnerships. In November 2009, it was the first country in the region to sign a national agreement, a compact with development partners, based on a comprehensive Health Sector Development Programme. This set out the principles of reform, and quantified the scale and nature of the aid being sought. Although not legally binding, it clearly established the desired direction of travel. Ethiopia has aimed assiduously to increase not only the magnitude of development assistance for health in the period 2009–2015 but also its predictability, as well as to ensure that the activities of donors were coordinated with the intentions of the government. All of these activities were underpinned by a clear focus on progress towards the Millennium Development Goals (MDGs).

The Ethiopian Compact is considered to be the most comprehensive approach to donor coordination in this region, all the more remarkable as it was achieved within only one year of signing the Global International Health Partnership Compact. In some ways, it represented a continuation of the work of the Ethiopian Minister of Health, who had played an active role in the International Health Partnership (IHP) process and other initiatives, catalysing support for great donor harmonization and mobilization of resources within the region (Dr Tewodros Adhanom. Speech given at the IHP+ launch meeting. Ethiopia, 2008).

Although it is too early to know whether the IHP will influence health, the process by which it was taken forward demonstrates the ability of the Ethiopian Government to show leadership throughout the process. Here it is possible to draw parallels with Kyrgyzstan, as both countries have emerged as key regional players, attracting others eager to learn from their experiences to regional work-shops and training events. As in Kyrgyzstan, there is a perceived receptive environment to regional collaboration, with support for the process from national officials.

In Tamil Nadu, the considerable achievement in maternal and neonatal health, compared with many of its neighbours in India and elsewhere in South-east Asia, has been attributed to a mix of strong political commitment to health, irrespective of the party in power, and a paradigm shift in public health policy. These factors are considered to have created a health system that is now able to deliver much more effective and equitable care. There is currently much improved access to high-quality antenatal care, emergency obstetric care and institutional delivery. Broader governance also affected health through inter-sectoral policies to improve literacy, reduce age at first marriage and increase public awareness of family planning and good nutrition.

All country studies demonstrated how *political elites considered improving population health a priority*. This facilitated the mobilization of financial and human resources and supported the creation of political will at local level. Thus, the importance of health was established in the 1972 Bangladesh Constitution. The right to health care was also enshrined in the constitution enacted in Kyrgyzstan following independence, echoing a universal provision in the previous Soviet Constitution, although with some user payments in practice. In Thailand, bureaucratic elites played a significant role in driving the public health agenda between 1970 and 2000. The Thai political discourse focused on the need to provide effective services for the poor as a first step in expanding them to others. This contrasted with the situation in many other low- and middle-income countries where both mandatory and voluntary insurance tended to benefit the middle classes or elites the most, as the poor lacked political voice.

The reasons why these elites prioritized health varied. In some cases, it reflected a groundswell of pressure from community organizations or donors that permeated the political classes (e.g. Bangladesh). Elsewhere, the coincidence of interest by donors and political changes created windows of opportunity (e.g. Ethiopia, Kyrgyzstan). In Kyrgyzstan, independence from the USSR in 1991, the process of state building and drastic decline in funding and deterioration of the health system facilitated the rapid introduction of radical legal and policy changes that both strengthened governance arrangements and transformed health systems.

Achieving continuity and coherence of reform plans and strategies

Continuity emerged as a key contributor to success in the countries studied. As noted above, initial blueprints often helped to clarify the direction of subsequent reforms and provided a basis for monitoring their implementation. Crucially, the content of programmes could survive changes in their nomenclature; for example, the *Manas* and *Manas Taalimi* programmes in Kyrgyzstan covered a 15-year period, with the latter building explicitly on the former. These programmes survived three major political upheavals as well as a series of economic shocks; this continuity starkly contrasts with what happened in other former Soviet countries that experienced regime change. Kyrgyzstan's long-term approach also facilitated the process of learning lessons from pilot programmes, designed to inform the broader health strategy based on consensus. Thus, when programmes were rolled out nationally, there was already considerable experience of what was needed to ensure that they worked.

Continuity is also apparent in Thailand's progress towards universal coverage from the early 1990s onwards. Growing numbers of groups, defined on the basis of their occupational or socioeconomic status, were enrolled in financial protection schemes which were then merged, so that the whole population could be covered in 2002. This was accompanied by an expansion of networks of provincial and district health facilities, which ensured access to modern health care outside the main cities. One of the few constant elements in a period of frequent changes in Thai Government was the issuance of a continuing series of statements on the importance of health. Important roles were also played by the Thai National Health Assembly (see section below on Coordination of different actors) and the Royal Family.

Continuity can also be seen in the four consecutive Ethiopian Health Sector Development Plans, each spanning a five-year period and building on the experiences of earlier plans. Thus, the current goal, which builds on the greatly increased coverage achieved during the last plan, is to improve the quality of services now being provided. The latest proposals envisage shifting some services from regional facilities to village level.

The importance of seizing windows of opportunity and sustaining action

Some of the greatest successes took advantage of *political windows of opportunity created by national and international events*. Health system development and commitment to improving health in Bangladesh were triggered by political independence in 1971. The new 1972 Constitution created a fertile environment for the emergence of voluntary and donor-led initiatives supplementing state initiatives and motivated by the same policy goals. In Ethiopia, the creation of a new government in 1994 enabled the development of a new health policy that could benefit from increases in external funding. In Kyrgyzstan, the *Manas* process was made possible by independence from the USSR in 1991, yet other countries in the same position failed to seize the initiative. Proactive leaders entered into negotiations with donors shortly after gaining independence, creating a receptive political climate that contrasted with the situation in neighbouring countries. Health system reform was seen as a flagship programme that could attract international attention to what was perceived as success in one of the poorest of the former Soviet republics, lacking the natural resources of some of its neighbours. Subsequent political events acted as drivers for further change, with the initially popular Tulip Revolution reaffirming a commitment towards democratization and strengthening donor commitment to public sector reform.

Careful sequencing of steps in reform emerges as an important prerequisite for success. This was apparent in the experience of the original *Good health at low cost* countries after 1985, where the sequencing of reforms was important to achieve success in scaling up services. A stepwise approach allowed for experimentation, demonstrated early progress that created momentum and garnered support for less-popular initiatives[9,10].

The role of sequencing is apparent in the high level of immunization coverage achieved in Tamil Nadu. This was the product of a long-term process in which a political priority given to maternal and child health extended to behavioural and cultural change among policy-makers and the general population, rather than to particular vertical programmes. This created fertile ground for other programmes, including birth control. The relative success of these programmes in Tamil Nadu and Kerala, as compared with the rest of India, was attributed to the fact that they were embedded within political and cultural change.

Research by others has identified Kyrgyzstan, alongside the Republic of

Moldova, as the two most successful reformers in the former USSR. Both successfully transformed the financing of their health sectors, despite experiencing some of the worst economic conditions in the region[11]. The factors identified by the authors as contributing to their success support our findings. These include the importance of sequencing and the coherence of reform: establishing clear policy objectives at the outset, taking advantage of political opportunities, and developing plans that are feasible and realistic. Furthermore, governments and donors in both countries prioritized the development of capacity to monitor and evaluate the reform process, making it possible to create feedback loops and learn lessons as reforms proceeded.

Responding to population needs

Effective health system governance requires adequate responses to diverse population needs. This includes providing services that are appropriate given the burden of disease, but also responding to the expectations of the population. All countries included in the original report sought to improve access to care among underserved populations, particularly poor and rural communities, although public sector investment was not always able to match expectations, contributing to the rapid growth of the private sector to fill the gap[12,13].

The importance of responding to population needs was a recurring theme in each country, highlighting the need for *systems operating at district level that can reach rural, isolated and marginalized populations.* This was most clearly seen in Thailand, Bangladesh and Ethiopia, all of which face major challenges because of their large size and diverse population groups.

Since the early 1960s, Thailand's health plans demonstrate a commitment to extending services to underserved rural populations through the expansion of infrastructure and human resources, facilitated by economic growth and bureaucratic stability. This was underpinned by a commitment to pursue "good for the most" as opposed to "the best for a few" (see Chapter 7).

In Ethiopia, the introduction of the Health Extension Programme was an explicit attempt by the government to take much needed services to households in rural and remote areas.

Tackling corruption and ensuring accountability

We expected that measures to combat corruption would emerge strongly in our case studies, but they did not. There were, however, some examples of targeted efforts in some of the countries. For example, In Kyrgyzstan, soon after independence, there was a large-scale investment in building accountability and transparency, linked to patient rights. Early initiatives by the World Bank and other donors to improve governance and increase the accountability of public administration, budgeting and expenditure, led to the Public Financial Management project (2002–2007) funded by Department for International Development, United Kingdom. This has been given credit for improvements within the health system and other sectors at all levels. Related initiatives included creating complaints channels, such as confidential telephone numbers where citizens could make anonymous complaints about being refused access or asked to pay in health facilities. Since 2000, over 300 complaints have been received annually, with actions taken, showing considerable public trust in the possibility for redress. Opportunities to meet senior staff working in ministries and key public offices have increased, through published contact details. In each facility, key health indicators are on display (monthly and yearly), are presented in an accessible manner and show how each facility compares with other similar ones.

The economic crisis that hit Thailand in 1997 led to concerns about rising pharmaceutical costs, with public hospitals especially at risk. Since 2004, the Thai Ministry of Health has developed and implemented an ambitious Good Governance for Medicines programme, jointly with the WHO and involving agencies beyond the health sector, such as the Food and Drug Administration of Thailand and research institutions[14]. This has strengthened accountability in the procurement of pharmaceuticals, promoting rational drug use and cost containment, and reducing inefficiencies through pooled purchasing schemes at provincial level, which lowers costs and improves quality. The Rural Doctors Society, which represents doctors working in rural areas, was active in exposing the scale of corruption in the pharmaceutical sector, as well as encouraging prosecutions. Various policy initiatives were taken nationally to increase awareness of prices and to reduce corruption and unethical practices. These included amendments to legislation, the public provision of information on prices of drugs supplied to hospitals and publishing the minutes of national policy meetings. Overall, the programme is viewed as having improved transparency and as having generated momentum for better health sector governance overall. There were spin-offs from health to other sectors, as it equipped organizations in other sectors with tools to achieve common objectives, in this case reducing the financial burden on poor people.

▉ Effective institutions and bureaucracies

Stability of bureaucracies

The evidence gathered in the case studies suggests that *well-functioning mid-level bureaucracies that are stable over time* are important in translating strategies and plans formulated centrally into improved services and, ultimately, better health outcomes.

While individuals may come and go with political change, the existence of strong bureaucracies that retain an institutional memory of past reforms seems to be a major contributor to success. Success can be measured not only through the sustainability of specific reforms but also through underlying principles and values. While some of the countries have experienced a succession of changes in government, sometimes with significant political turmoil, the implementation of key reforms by mid-level bureaucracy has been largely unaffected, ensuring institutional memory.

This can be seen clearly in the way the reform process was sustained during a series of political crises in Thailand. Senior officials in the Thai Ministry of Public Health (MOPH) developed and implemented five-year health plans, drawing on previous plans and assessing what had already been achieved. Continuity among managers and planners ensured that principles and values underlying the reforms (equity, with increasing access to health care for all and an emphasis on rural health) were maintained in successive strategies. This was facilitated by knowledge transfer across generations of personnel and by recruiting staff with experience in rural areas to national bodies.

Kyrgyzstan has had two revolutions since independence, but the long-term reform programme remained largely unaffected. This is in contrast to countries elsewhere in the region that have also experienced major changes (such as Georgia), but which have implemented contradictory reforms that have radically changed direction. Continuity in Kyrgyzstan was facilitated by the country's early adoption of regulations that restricted the ability to hire and fire civil servants, thus reducing the politicization, and consequently turnover, of managerial and administrative staff in the public sector.

Regulatory and managerial capacity

Well-functioning health systems require strong regulatory and managerial capacity, especially where resources are scarce, and there are many examples of this in all the country case studies. In Kyrgyzstan, the government was able to rapidly enact changes in the legal and regulatory framework, speeding up the reform process, and enabling donor investment to be absorbed and targeted effectively. For example, the parliament passed three new laws within four years, providing the legal basis for mandatory health insurance, a process that took much longer in the other countries in the region. Indeed, even now, many of these countries lack an effective legal framework for health care delivery.

A key message from Tamil Nadu is that many of the interventions that led to success could not have been possible without a competent public health management cadre at the district level (unique in India) that was given sufficient power and space to manage services. This was further enhanced by an autonomous and stable district civil service that not only applied government policies to the local context but was able to contribute innovative ideas and suggestions at the state level, some of which were later institutionalized. Enhancing managerial capacity was supported by effective use of intelligence and evidence. Tamil Nadu developed a system of surveillance and audit of maternal deaths, aggregating information on maternal deaths in both the public and the private sector[a]. Reporting of deaths became mandatory, and this change was backed up by a programme of training for health workers. Reviews of deaths and near misses are carried out by district level officials working with legal representatives and involving family members. These reviews have identified systemic gaps and faults in the existing management procedures, leading to improvements in the delivery of care at district level. For example, changes include better availability of blood and enhanced training of health workers in blood transfusion; improved communication between health professionals and managers; and increased access to referral facilities. District-led initiatives have been scaled up, for example through the introduction of state-level standard protocols. This situation was very similar to Bangladesh's emphasis on creating effective regulatory mechanisms and autonomous managers at district level.

One way of assessing management capacity is to examine the use of intelligence to inform concrete actions. This was seen clearly in Kyrgyzstan, where all sectoral strategies have had strong monitoring and evaluation components, with clear links to management and policy processes. Crucially, there is recognition of the value of integrating monitoring and evaluation systems across government, with the country's Ministry of Labour and Social Protection developing a system to identify disadvantaged groups that will be linked to health insurance data. This is far beyond what is seen in the other central Asian countries. Similarly, Thailand has invested resources in the creation of an autonomous International Health Policy Programme within the MOPH, which can monitor and conduct

---

[a] Based on interviews with officials in Tamil Nadu, conducted by the country team.

evaluations that respond directly to the needs of policy-makers. One effect of the close link between researchers and policy-makers is the increasing frequency of surveys (annually) in Thailand to monitor universal coverage.

Implementing policies: institutional autonomy and flexibility

It is necessary for officials to have *sufficient power and discretion to implement reforms*. Thus, in Tamil Nadu, the Medical Services Corporation, an autonomous body managing drug procurement, has been able to bypass bureaucratic procedures to introduce innovative measures that improved availability of essential drugs and promoted rational drug use. A similar degree of flexibility was seen in many district health authorities, which were able to attract support from charitable bodies to implement immunization programmes and other primary care measures, insulated from often changing state-level political priorities.

Such officials, however, should have systems in place that allow them to *learn lessons*. In Kyrgyzstan, there is a formal process of piloting reform in one region, followed by evaluation and, if successful, scaling up nationally. Donor representatives report a culture of pragmatism in deciding whether reforms work or not, and taking action where needed. There were feedback loops informing development of new policies.

The example with maternal mortality surveillance given above illustrates how district officers in Tamil Nadu were given power to develop locally appropriate solutions to problems that emerged from maternal death reviews, and successful local strategies were replicated in other districts. Some of this experience was used at the level of the state to inform evidence-based practices[15]. This contrasts with the situation in Kerala, widely admired in the 1985 *Good health at low cost* report, where decentralization of decision-making following enactment of the Panchayati Raj legislation made it more difficult for those responsible for developing and implementing health reform at local level to translate new ideas into funded programmes, as they lacked the necessary support[16].

Creation of adequate capacity at local level has not always been straightforward, however. In Ethiopia, where the Ministry of Health had almost no presence outside the capital until the 1970s, efforts have focused on building up the regional tier[17]. In Bangladesh, authorities at the district level are instrumental in implementing government formulated policies and programmes, in delivery of emergency obstetric care (some through subdistricts, *upazilas*), and in contracting NGOs to provide services to underserved groups (rural and poor urban). The existence of strong managerial capacity at this level is seen as important as the contractual mechanisms are becoming increasingly sophisticated. However, there are significant variations in performance across districts.

Pluralism and managing engagement with the non-state sector

Since the original *Good health at low cost* report, there has been rapid growth of the private health care sector in China, Costa Rica, Kerala and Sri Lanka with considerable implications for how the health systems in these countries operate. However, the scale of change has varied. In Kerala, the private sector has become the dominant provider of care throughout the state, even for the poor; in contrast, in Costa Rica, the public sector is still the largest provider of care, although an increasing number of middle-class citizens are seeking private care, so far mostly paying out of pocket.

These changes are reflected to varying extents in the countries included in the present study, in particular in Tamil Nadu, Bangladesh and Thailand. These countries have a long history of vibrant private provision, delivering both western and traditional treatments. Some liberalization of the market can also be seen in Ethiopia and in Kyrgyzstan, albeit from a much lower initial level. The emergence of pluralistic health sectors has created a need to reconsider options for engagement with the non-state sector, ranging from coexistence to longer-term public–private partnerships. The countries studied have sought to implement a range of pragmatic solutions, with flexible models of collaboration that take account of local context.

In Tamil Nadu, 80% of outpatient treatment and 60% of inpatient care is now in the private sector. However, core maternal and child health services are still provided in the public sector. Examples of public–private engagement include joint awareness-raising campaigns and contracting out of services; for example, a government facility that does not have its own laboratory hires the services of reputable private laboratories procured through the independent Tamil Nadu Medical Services Corporation.

It should be noted that Tamil Nadu provides an example of responsiveness to public preferences. In response to popular demand, allopathic care is now provided alongside non-allopathic care within the public health system. Numerous public facilities have separate Siddha medicine wards and Ayurveda, Unani medicines are provided at primary care facilities.

Bangladesh has seen a major expansion of NGOs operating in the health sector. Indeed, it has some of the world's largest NGOs, such as the well-known BRAC, which traces its origins to the founding of an independent Bangladesh in 1972.

BRAC estimates that it reaches 110 million people by means of 64 000 village health workers. These huge NGOs have high levels of autonomy and flexibility, and have been able to play an important role in improving health, for example by preventing diarrhoeal deaths in children and by reaching out to marginalized populations living in isolated areas or suffering from stigma or lack of resources.

There are, however, some important negative consequences of the growth of the private sector. In Thailand, the rapidly expanding private sector is attracting health workers from the public sector. In Bangladesh and in Tamil Nadu, the growth in caesarean sections is much higher in the private than the public sector[18–20], and is an increasing source of concern.

Another issue is the blurring of boundaries between the public and private sectors on the demand side. Large private sectors in low-income settings are associated with high levels of private expenditure; in several of the countries, there are widespread out-of-pocket payments, both formal and informal. In Kyrgyzstan, informal payments represent over 50% of all out-of-pocket health expenditure, slightly above the average in the former Soviet countries[21], and have remained consistently high throughout the transition. In Bangladesh, out-of-pocket payments are high, but their consequences may be somewhat mitigated by social networks that can facilitate loans at community level.

Finally, another development, so far little evaluated, is the emergence of Tamil Nadu (specifically Chennai city) and Thailand as regional and even global centres for medical tourism. Analyses of the situation in South-east Asia highlight concern over risks of maldistribution and brain drain of health workers to serve such tourists rather than the local population[22].

Multisectoral focus

We found several examples of the importance of *coordinating action across sectors*, both in the original countries and the new ones. As discussed in the review of the original *Good health at low cost* countries, Costa Rica and Sri Lanka, which were able to strengthen intersectoral engagement and achieve coordinated action across public and private sectors, have fared better than China in terms of expanding access to health care.

Development and implementation of *comprehensive reform programmes* seeking to address multiple aspects of health system functioning, and providing a strategic framework for addressing broader determinants of health, provided continuity through different reform stages and the possibility to coordinate initiatives in different sectors.

Many of these multisectoral approaches aiming to promote social development have impacted on maternal and child mortality. In Bangladesh, for example, families who participate in microcredit programmes achieve better child survival[23,24]. Other approaches linked to better outcomes address female literacy, clean water and sanitation, as seen in the original countries.

It is easy to overlook the importance of basic infrastructure for health. In Bangladesh, a major expansion of road building and electricity supply has facilitated greater uptake of childhood immunization, and mobile phone networks support the work of community health workers throughout the country. In Thailand, the first modern health plan, in the 1960s, also benefited from the rapid expansion of electricity and highway construction. In Ethiopia's Poverty Eradication Strategy, health sits alongside other key developmental issues.

Coordination of different actors

The involvement of multiple actors in the policy process and their implementation was seen as beneficial in each country, consistent with evidence in the existing literature[25]. This was apparent in a number of ways. One was the *involvement of communities or their representatives in implementing effective interventions*. This went beyond simply seeking cooperation with particular programme beneficiaries, but involved working more widely with elected or informal community organizations to ensure that local health needs and patterns of utilization are reflected in service design and that communities are able to feed their views back to local and district level authorities. For example, Kyrgyzstan, uniquely in the former USSR, established village health committees staffed by volunteers who deal with a wide range of local issues, including public health, facilitating access to care and health education.

In Bangladesh, the important role played by community organizations in improving access to maternal and child care is well known, including both those whose primary focus is health and those engaged in microfinance[23]. However, they have been less successful in influencing policy at national level. This reflects a limited capacity and the few formal opportunities for lobbying at national level, the lack of politically active consumers or patient organizations, and the lack of national public debate about health care.

In Thailand, health assemblies have been convened since 1988 as fora in which to build consensus around core public health issues. These assemblies have received high-level support, especially from successive prime ministers and from Princess Mahachakri Sirindhorm. They involve 550 participants from different government agencies, NGOs and professional organizations[26]. This is just one manifestation of Thailand's strong tradition of participatory policy-making.

True participation has, however, been limited in many places. In Bangladesh, despite the existence of formal consultative processes under government leadership, informed by evidence and involving diverse stakeholders, donors, scientists, the media and the Bangladesh Medical Association, key policy decisions are often opaque and are not actually made collaboratively.

There are many examples of *synergy between governments and donors* in policy formulation, agenda setting and implementation. In Kyrgyzstan, successive governments and ministers of health collaborated with donors in setting priorities, aligning strategies and allocating resources within the frameworks of SWAps and national health programmes. This consensus-based policy-making, joint action (especially among managerial staff) and willingness to reconcile different interests may have been crucial in achieving success. Similarly, strong government ownership combined with active engagement with donors within SWAps was seen in Ethiopia. Coordination between governments and donors in Bangladesh received momentum with the 1998 SWAp, which aggregated 120 health initiatives, dramatically reducing fragmentation and improving management.

Success in *engagement between governments and NGOs* has been mixed across the study countries. In Bangladesh, NGOs have worked successfully alongside and as an extension of government initiatives. For example, an NGO–government partnership has trained and supported household visits by health assistants and family welfare assistants; this is seen as instrumental in the success of health and family planning programmes. In Kyrgyzstan, engagement and coordination with civil society was seen as problematic due to the perceived weaknesses of civil society organizations. The relationship between the Ethiopian Government and NGOs has been chequered. While there was much government interest in fostering strong partnerships with international donors, there was much less interest in working with domestic civil society organizations, which were not consulted on some important issues. An evaluation of the International Health Partnership implementation, for example, found "government-centric focus" and lack of civil society participation in the development of Ethiopia's Country Compact[27]. This has since been disputed by the Ethiopian Minister of Health, who attributed the lack of involvement by civil society organizations in the compact development process to their limited capacity (Dr Tewodros Adhanom. Speech at the IHP+ launch meeting. Ethiopia, 2008). The civil society law "Proclamation for the Registration and Regulation of Charities and Societies" adopted in January 2009 has attracted criticism from donors and civil society for restricting the role of foreign-funded NGOs beyond service provision and, in particular, for blocking them from foreign funding for the promotion of democratic rights, gender equality and accountability of law enforcement agencies. However, the European Union has continued to provide grants to Ethiopian civil society organizations (€1.6 million over a six-year period from 2006 to 2011) for work on governance, female empowerment and conflict resolution.

Another area of commonality among all countries was proactive *partnerships between health systems and the media* that have fostered change. This link has contributed to the dissemination of public health messages and increased awareness of entitlement to effective interventions, particularly among disadvantaged groups. The media has also played a role in influencing beliefs about health related issues; in Tamil Nadu, the media was used in campaigns to promote AIDS control and played an important role in fertility transition, specifically through promoting small family size. The Behaviour Change Communication programme in Bangladesh involved community health workers and managers working closely with educators, NGOs and local journalists, building on each others' skills to engender change. The programme is highly regarded.

In some countries, such as Thailand and Bangladesh, the media also provided a mechanism for accountability, facilitating a public forum to discuss the rationale for reform. It also created linkages among different tiers of the system, enabling local issues to be raised by advocacy organizations nationally, with the resulting high profile contributing to policy change. In these ways, the media has served as a catalyst for change.

■ Scaling up the health workforce

Innovative approaches to human resource generation

The innovative responses to scarce human resources emerges as a key issue in each country, typically by means of original country-specific solutions or approaches adapted from international experience.

Each country has designed and implemented a mix of traditional and innovative *strategies to overcome staff and skill shortages.* Extending access to well-trained health workers, especially in primary health care, was linked to better health outcomes in the original *Good health at low cost* report. Examples varied from the Chinese barefoot doctors to teams of health professionals, including a doctor, nurse and technician, working in remote areas of Costa Rica[10].

The case studies were also able to identify initiatives at all levels of service provision, from initial training to deployment and continuing professional development, and from community health workers to specialized medical doctors. In Thailand, expanding human resources was seen as a cornerstone of improving coverage. In Kyrgyzstan, a new Family Medicine Training Centre within the existing State Medical Institute of Retraining and Postgraduate Education has been created and there has been an expansion of capacity to train family practitioners, drawing on government and donor support.

Bangladesh made a major investment in capacity for emergency obstetric care in the public sector, with new facilities and trained staff deployed in rural areas. However, this indirectly led to a massive growth of the private sector, with providers engaged in dual practice or leaving the public sector to run their own private maternity hospitals. The percentage of live births in public facilities only increased from 6.1 to 7.1% between 2004 and 2007; however, those in private health facilities increased from 3.2% to 7.6% during the same period. Sixty eight per cent of caesarean sections (a proxy indicator of women's access to skilled care for complicated deliveries) take place in the private sector[28].

Overall, more Bangladeshi women do have access to emergency obstetric care. Nevertheless, fewer than 2% of deliveries by mothers in the poorest two quintiles are by caesarean section, indicating considerable unmet need for emergency obstetric care.

The Ethiopian Health Extension Programme is perhaps the most ambitious effort in sub-Saharan Africa to scale up the provision of essential primary health care and address geographical imbalances in the deployment of health workers between rural and urban areas. Health extension workers are community workers who are paid a salary by the government. There are two workers in each village health post and they deliver a package of essential primary care interventions. Nearly 34 000 health extension workers have been trained and sent to rural areas since the scheme began, reaching almost two thirds of the population by 2007[29,30]. The programme has achieved significant success in extending services for tuberculosis, HIV and maternal and child health as well as for building links among the different tiers of the health system[31]. The programme has also helped to increase immunization rates and prevent malaria through the distribution of insecticide-treated bednets. Nevertheless, its effect on utilization of key maternal and child services (for example, seeking treatment for diarrhoea and cough in children) has been mixed, perhaps because the services are still relatively limited in scope and quality[29].

A key issue facing all of these countries is retention of staff. The Ethiopian Health Extension Programme recruited workers from local communities and enrolled them in the civil service, providing them with stable employment, training and career development opportunities[8]. In Thailand, successive health plans have implemented a variety of strategies to enhance retention. These include compulsory posting of medical graduates to rural areas, training of village health communicators and village health volunteers, introducing new types of public health worker, and training of public health nurses. The decision to conduct medical training in Thai is credited with making it more difficult for medical graduates to migrate, in contrast to the situation in the Philippines, for example.

In Tamil Nadu, the Multipurpose Workers Scheme has been operational since the early 1980s, supporting a new system of primary care in rural areas. Nearly 60 training schools were opened to train multipurpose workers. In Tamil Nadu, they were officially renamed as village health nurses. The nurses are based at health subcentres, each of which serves an average of 5000 people, providing home visits, antenatal and postnatal care, vaccinations and contraception. The village health nurse initiative has been scaled up rapidly, facilitating improved access to essential services. It has also strengthened the integration of primary care with the rest of the health system, building bridges in particular with maternal and child health services. At the same time, the scope of primary care has increased steadily. These measures have been linked to evidence of increased antenatal visits and institutional deliveries in rural areas.

Innovative use of health workers

While the original report included a few examples of the innovative use of health workers, this was a key theme emerging from the current study. Several countries have sought to create a mix of skills that is more appropriate for the local disease burden. This has also enabled health workers to implement vertical programmes in a flexible manner, maximizing the potential impact on access to services.

Examples include the health extension workers in Ethiopia, who deliver a package of primary care services and receive additional training to implement add-on programmes. In Kyrgyzstan, a cadre of trained general practitioners has been created and family group practices, working together with community health committees, are replacing the old polyclinics that were staffed by narrow specialists.

In Thailand and Tamil Nadu, community health workers and auxiliary staff visiting communities have been credited with a role in greater use of contraception and subsequent decreases in fertility. However, some have been more successful than others. In Bangladesh, although various types of para-professional were recruited locally and trained for work in district and subdistrict facilities, the improved outcomes were attributed to mid-level staff, such as health assistants (serving 6000 people on average) and family welfare assistants (female workers serving 5000 people on average in rural areas). As in India, home visits by the female family welfare assistants have been important, given cultural barriers limiting movement of women outside the home in rural areas. Their contribution to increasing the uptake of the measles vaccine, especially among the poorer groups, was highlighted in the 2010 Countdown report[32]. In both Tamil Nadu and Bangladesh, the tasks of all types of community health worker have been expanded gradually, sometimes as a consequence of shifting from vertical to integrated models of care. Thus, many of the older health assistants were smallpox vaccinators or malaria control workers during the 1960s and early 1970s, later providing more comprehensive primary care and even referrals.

Building on earlier policies is also apparent in relation to the decision of the government of Bangladesh to invest in a one-year basic training programme for about 16 000 village health workers each year, based on the Chinese model of barefoot doctors. After the original programme ended in 1982, many of those trained continue to work as local practitioners, termed *palli chikitsok* or village doctor[33,34] or as unlicensed providers. Although not subjected to formal evaluation, they have been credited by some observers with playing a role in the reduction of childhood mortality, in part by providing access to basic medical advice and low-cost pharmaceuticals[35–37].

Despite many achievements, however, progress still needs to be made. Several of the countries face a continued threat of brain drain, which can easily and rapidly reverse earlier advances. Currently, Ethiopia and Thailand are still facing problems in achieving adequate staffing levels in rural areas. Indeed, health workers in rural areas are often predominantly women, who also bear a high domestic burden[38]. In Kyrgyzstan, many doctors have moved to Russia and neighbouring oil-rich Kazakhstan after salaries there were raised.

■ Health system financing

Effective and efficient systems of health financing are critical if countries are to make sustained progress towards the health MDGs[39,40]. Somewhat remarkably, financing did not emerge from the interviews undertaken within this study as a major factor in the progress towards improving health in the countries studied. However, it was possible to elucidate the role of a range of financing arrangements in underpinning other elements of the health system and contributing to improved access and quality of care. It seems likely that those interviewed simply

Figure 9.1   Total expenditure on health per capita, (Int$), 2009

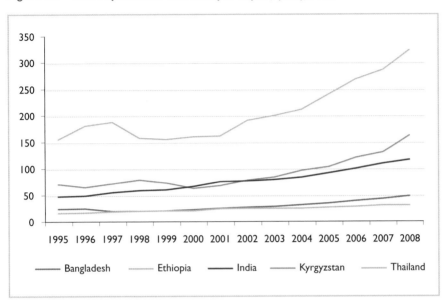

Source: Reference 41.

took the availability of finances as a given, with adequate sums necessary for the delivery of at least basic health care, while focusing on what was done within financial constraints.

Expenditure on health per capita, expressed in international dollars (2009) for each country, is shown in Figure 9.1. While all five countries have seen an increase in their expenditure on health since 1995, the rate of increase has varied. The greatest increase was in Thailand, while the smallest was in Ethiopia, although this seems surprising given the substantial and increasing donor support that Ethiopia has received in recent years (Figure 9.2).

Figure 9.3 shows that total health expenditure as a percentage of GDP has remained stable over the years. Only Kyrgyzstan has had any notable fluctuation, shown by a sharp drop in total health expenditure as a percentage of GDP in the late 1990s, followed by nearly a decade of recovery to previous levels. Absolute health spending, therefore, seems to have risen as a result of GDP growth in the study countries rather than marked proportional increases of national income. In other words, the documented health gains cannot be explained as a consequence of increased share of national income for health[43].

Figure 9.2   External resources on health as percentage of total health expenditure

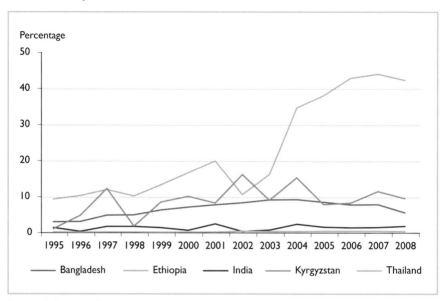

Source: Reference 41.

Figure 9.3   Total health expenditure as percentage of GDP

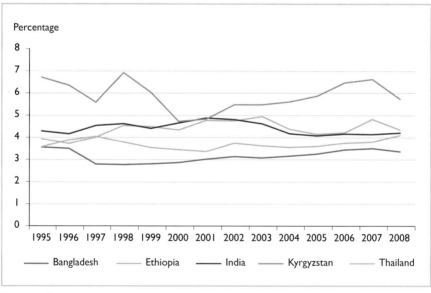

Source: Reference 41.

The next question is where do the funds come from and how sustainable are they? Here it is informative to look at Ethiopia. It has benefited greatly from increased development assistance as a consequence of geopolitical factors and greater budgetary transparency (Figure 9.3). An obvious concern is what will happen in the future. A recent study of countries worldwide found evidence that domestic funds were being crowded out by donor assistance[44]. In Ethiopia, development assistance for health rose by the equivalent of 1.2% of GDP between 2002 and 2006, while Ethiopian Government funding decreased by the equivalent of 1.4% of GDP. Given that three of the study countries receive significant contributions from donors for operating their health systems, they are vulnerable to changing global priorities.

Figure 9.4 shows the different proportions of government, out-of-pocket and other private expenditure that make up total health expenditure in all five countries. The shares of finance in the study countries have been relatively stable over time, with out-of-pocket expenditure remaining an important source. The

Figure 9.4   Changing sources of finance in the study countries

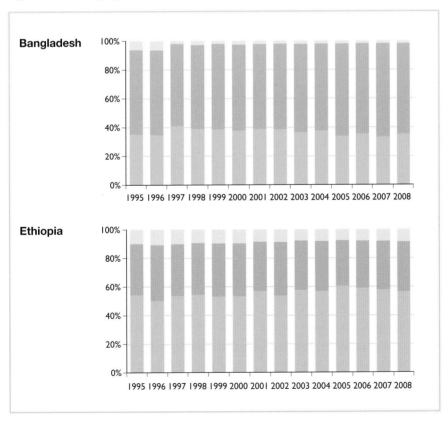

Figure 9.4 (continued)

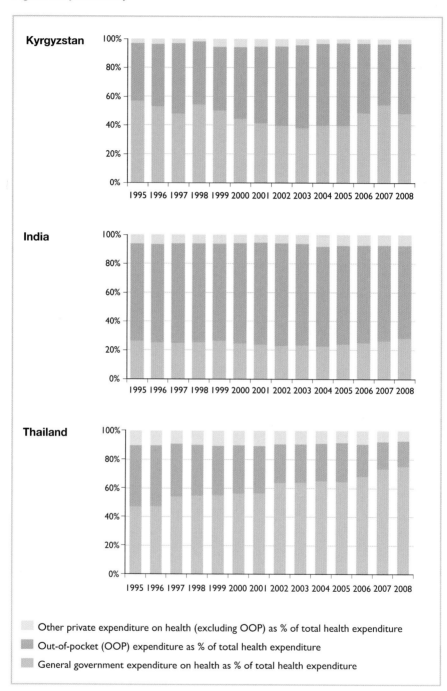

Other private expenditure on health (excluding OOP) as % of total health expenditure

Out-of-pocket (OOP) expenditure as % of total health expenditure

General government expenditure on health as % of total health expenditure

Source: Reference 41.

exception is Thailand, where the move to universal coverage from 2001 onwards has been associated with a steadily increasing proportion of health expenditure from government sources. Similarly, Costa Rica, which has achieved major expansions in essential services coverage, consistently spent more than a fifth of total government expenditure on health between 2003 and 2007 (Chapter 8). The Kyrgyz case study reports in more detail on efforts to reduce out-of-pocket payments, especially informal ones, which were initially unsuccessful but have recently started to show positive results according to survey data (Chapter 5).

■ Financial protection

All countries in both the original and current study sought to improve afford-ability as a means of improving access to health care by all socioeconomic groups. This recognizes that the financial burden of seeking health care has detrimental effects on vulnerable households through unexpected and often catastrophic out-of-pocket payments[42,45].

In China, the central government invested effort in developing new health insur-ance schemes (the New Rural Cooperative Medical Care System and the expanded Urban Residents Medical Insurance scheme)[46]. In Costa Rica, health insurance coverage has steadily expanded and is now virtually universal[9]. There have been some examples of backsliding: Costa Rica and Sri Lanka considered allowing the rich to opt out of coverage even though this would reduce the sums in the risk pool (Rosero-Bixby L, personal communication (Costa Rica), 2010) and [47], but the threat to the principle of universality was recognized. In Kerala, however, the rise of the private sector has reduced access by the poor and threat-ened their financial protection[48].

All countries in the present study implemented measures to increase financial protection. Ethiopia has seen recent moves to develop a system of Social Health Insurance for employees in the formal sector, as well as a system of community health insurance. Both Thailand and Kyrgyzstan have achieved virtual universal coverage, but elsewhere policies have not always achieved their desired effects; some population groups remain without coverage and very substantial out-of-pocket payments persist. In Thailand, the process began long ago by providing free care for low-income groups, followed by employment-based prepayment schemes that were gradually expanded to cover smaller firms. In Kyrgyzstan, universal coverage was achieved by means of a system of mixed financing (social insurance, tax, and co-payments). Those in work pay a payroll tax, while the government pays premiums for those unable to contribute. Yet, the Kyrgyz health system is still heavily dependent on out-of-pocket spending and government subsidies, with the added burden of informal payments, despite initiatives to tackle them.

The depth of coverage (benefits package) is important as well as the breadth of coverage. What is included in the benefit package reflects a range of considerations. In Thailand, the decision to include renal replacement therapy was designed to avert the risk of catastrophic expenditure associated with dialysis. The early adoption of antiretroviral therapy reflected the ability of the Thai Government Pharmaceutical Organization to produce a low-cost, generic combination of three key medicines.

In Kyrgyzstan, the State Guarantee Benefit Package has been revised annually to take account of available funds. Elsewhere, packages are not regularly revised even when, as in Bangladesh, there is substantial evidence of a shifting burden of disease, with noncommunicable diseases gaining increasing importance.

The degree to which financial protection is threatened by out-of-pocket payments reflects differing dynamics in different countries. Limited private sector development in Ethiopia coupled with low levels of informal payments and low level of service utilization, means that out-of-pocket expenditure is much lower than in Tamil Nadu and Bangladesh, both of which have vibrant private sectors. In Bangladesh, the three major suppliers of health care in the non-state sector are NGOs, formal and informal private sector providers and providers of traditional medicines requiring out-of-pocket payments. Kyrgyzstan provides a complex picture, with the introduction of an insurance scheme in a context of informal payments and gifts given at the point of use, a practice that was widespread across the former Soviet republics.

The problem of informal payments has been tackled in Kyrgyzstan by introducing formal co-payments for certain types of care in 2001, the first initiative of this kind in the region. A secondary goal was to enhance the managerial and financial autonomy of health facilities that could benefit from the collected revenue (Chapter 5). There is now evidence that there has been a reduction in informal payments over a six-year period, particularly for medicines, medical supplies and food. However, it was not possible to examine in detail the consequences of out-of-pocket payments on access to care. Their impact may be mitigated by families and social networks and, in some cases, people can plan for them (as with childbirth).

Despite a long-term reliance on high out-of-pocket payments in Bangladesh, large sections of the population are, in principle, exempt from payment. For example, in primary care facilities, there is no charge for people of any age for services related to HIV/AIDS, tuberculosis, malaria, acute watery diarrhoea and related illnesses, or for assisted and emergency delivery and immunization. Poor people can also receive medication for free if they show evidence of entitlement. Although the evidence is inconclusive[49–51], it has been argued that the widespread microcredit schemes may have helped to alleviate some of the burden on the households and may have enhanced women's autonomy in decision-making and access to health care, thus contributing to health improvements of mothers and children[52].

In Thailand, along with good quality public provision, relatively low levels of out-of-pocket payment reflect the success of the universal coverage policy. In Costa Rica, a third of health expenditure in 2007 was private, mainly consisting of out-of-pocket payments for ambulatory care in the private sector; access to public health care has mostly remained free at the point of use[53].

Given increasing interest in demand-side financing – despite the inconclusive evidence supporting it[54] – only Bangladesh had employed a financial incentive programme. In Bangladesh, a maternal voucher scheme was piloted in 2007, with the aim of increasing skilled attendance at birth, coupled with better ante- and postnatal care. Although it has not been subject to a formal evaluation, it has been received enthusiastically by health providers and beneficiaries[55].

■ Innovative ways of securing health system inputs

Improvements in drug supply systems were identified in all countries. In Tamil Nadu, computerized systems in pharmaceutical warehouses strengthened the operations of the supply chain and improved drug management. This had a knock-on effect on the private pharmaceutical market, which no longer had a local monopoly of the supply of certain products, so prices fell.

In Bangladesh, a pioneering drug policy launched in 1978 established a flourishing pharmaceutical sector that brought affordable antibiotics and other essential medicines within the reach of providers throughout the country. Bangladesh also became a pioneer in *low cost innovations* to treat common illnesses, such as oral rehydration solution (ORS) and zinc; delivery of ORS through community workers removed diarrhoea from being the leading cause of child death. Seeking to extend health system capacity, Tamil Nadu engaged in public–private partnerships, either with autonomous NGOs implementing disease-specific programmes (for example, tuberculosis, HIV/AIDS and blindness), or with private hospitals receiving subsidies to deliver specific services for which there were shortages in the public sector (for example, cataract operations and specialist maternal care). These flexible arrangements have been instrumental in achieving significant health gains through enhanced access to essential treatments.

In central Asia, Kyrgyzstan has been a pioneer in implementing a *new system of paying providers* that explicitly sought to shape how services were delivered[56]. Its key features were amalgamation of formerly fragmented risk pools into a single fund, developing mechanisms for strategic purchasing, and increasing provider autonomy[11]. Its introduction was complicated, as some facilities were paid according to outcomes, while others were still paid according to their inherited infrastructure and number of staff. Nonetheless, the payment system allowed Kyrgyzstan to reduce its excessive and inefficient inherited hospital capacity and to link hospital budgets to performance[11], a success that has eluded its neighbours. This has allowed hospitals to release funds used for maintenance of facilities to improve patient care.

In Costa Rica and China, management contracts include performance targets linked to different types of incentive. In Yunnan's Maternal and Child Health Programme, these were linked to managerial retention and promotion, while in Costa Rica, 10% of a facility's budget was withheld against achievement of targets for treatment and preventive services[10].

In Ethiopia, contracts with the private sector to train health personnel have lead to much-needed expansion of human resource capacity, both clinical and managerial.

Efforts to reorient services towards primary care are seen in all study countries. The original *Good health at low cost* report emphasized how achievement of significant health gains involved good access to primary health care, backed up, where necessary, by referrals to specialist facilities. These trends have continued; in China, the Health VIII programme has allocated substantial funds to rehabilitate existing community health facilities (which were traditionally the cornerstone of the health system)[57].

The experiences reviewed in the new countries support this message, emphasizing the importance of *effective primary care, backed up by ease of referral services to higher tiers*, a message consistent with a wealth of experience elsewhere[58]. This process is becoming increasingly important in light of emerging demographic and economic challenges. This is still work in progress, as in Bangladesh, where the process began in the 1970s with family planning as a vertical programme with separate management, staff training and models of delivery. This only gradually changed in the 1990s, when family planning was integrated into a comprehensive national reproductive health programme (with family welfare assistants and health assistants beginning to provide broader primary maternal and child health services). These workers also support prevention as a core part of health care and not simply an optional add on. For example, Bangladesh has managed to increase immunization coverage from about 2% in 1985 to the current level of over 75%[59], with even higher rates for some vaccines. In Thailand, immunization was a major feature of consecutive five-year plans, with specific strategies to implement it at district level according to the area and specific targets. In Tamil Nadu, access to primary health care has expanded, but institutionalizing appropriate referrals among the numerous available services is still to be achieved, which is a concern throughout India.

In situations where significant geographical and social barriers to services exist, measures to improve access to primary care have involved community-based activities or home visits in rural areas (Bangladesh and Tamil Nadu) or initiatives to deploy and retain primary health care personnel. Maintaining a basic but functioning primary care infrastructure, often supported by community efforts, has been emphasized in Tamil Nadu and Thailand.

■ Building resilience in the health system

One unexpected issue to emerge from our study was the importance of resilience of the health system to external shocks. Although this concept has long featured in areas such as engineering and defence, its importance is only now being recognized in the health sector, in part because of the growing awareness of the need to anticipate and prepare for extreme climatic, economic and political events[60]. Bangladesh, Thailand and Ethiopia have all experienced major natural disasters, and each has put in place systems to help to prepare for such events. Bangladesh has invested in disaster preparedness in anticipation of the regular floods and cyclones to which it is exposed, building appropriate infrastructure, raising awareness and establishing systems to coordinate emergency responses. The lessons learned have enabled it to succeed in responding to many droughts and seasonal flooding. Thailand has implemented early warning systems for tsunami. Ethiopia has improved its system for responding to droughts, although there are often limitations to preparedness – especially in extreme climatic events such as the current famine in East Africa. Inevitably there will be pressures on the health system as its own citizens and those from neighbouring countries are affected[61]. Notably, in all the countries, health services have been included in emergency planning.

The health systems in these countries have benefited from effective planning, coupled with strong leadership and institutional structures. They also have demonstrated a willingness to draw on resources beyond the health sector, as in Bangladesh where the government linked health policy with community-based insurance and microcredit programmes.

■ Conclusions

In this chapter, we have attempted to distil some lessons from the countries examined in the case studies, as well as from more recent progress in the countries included in the original *Good health at low cost* study. In doing so, we have faced many difficulties. Health systems are themselves complex, and they exist in a dynamic, changing environment. Although, as far as possible, we seek to describe the ways in which each of the systems in our five countries operate, drawing on as wide a range of evidence as possible, inevitably we can only begin to understand the many informal mechanisms, rules and assumptions that exist and which may be much more important than the formal systems in shaping the experiences of patients and health workers. A rare example of research that studies informal mechanisms is a study of the experiences of patients with diabetes and their health care providers in Kyrgyzstan[62]. We are also conscious of the limitations of the basic data available to us, whether financial (for example, the extent to which it captures informal transactions) or health related (for example, given the challenge of knowing whether terminology, such as the definition of a nurse, has the same meaning in different countries).

In drawing conclusions, we have been severely constrained by the scarcity of rigorous evaluations. For example, we were unable to identify any longitudinal studies whose findings could be given a causal interpretation and, even when we located observational studies, the study findings were subject to many caveats. Encouragingly, in recent years, there has been an increasing interest in undertaking impact evaluations to explicitly assess the changes (both intended and unintended) that can be attributed to a particular intervention, such as a programme or policy, which should make future policy evaluation more systematic and robust[63,64]. It is a clear indictment of policy-makers in the health sector, however, that apart from a handful of examples[65,66] they have subjected so few of their policies to proper evaluation over the past decades. Hence, we were almost entirely limited to deciding whether, all else considered, the associations between policies and outcomes were plausible. One way of doing this was to seek similar experiences in different countries, a process facilitated by the comparative case study methodology we adopted. However, this does mean that we are rarely able to attribute observed outcomes to particular policies with any degree of certainty.

Notwithstanding these limitations, the fact remains that these countries have had important success in improving the health outcomes of their populations, and have done so despite very limited financial resources. Furthermore, it is possible to discern some common features. One is the presence of good governance. This encompasses leadership and vision by government, the ability to maintain continuity despite changes elsewhere, to seize windows of opportunity, to be responsive to population needs, and to be committed to accountability. While there is still much to do in these countries, there were many good examples of a vision being successfully translated into action.

Another is the presence of well-functioning institutions and bureaucracies that can provide some stability and institutional memory and that have adequate regulatory and managerial capacity. Given the growing complexity of the environment in which these institutions operate, they must also be flexible, with sufficient autonomy to adapt to changing circumstances, and also be able to work with the many actors inhabiting what is now often a very crowded health arena. Again, we were able to find many examples of institutions that had achieved these difficult tasks.

Health care is intrinsically labour intensive, demanding appropriately trained staff. All countries face a challenge in retention, reflecting an increasingly global market for their skills, but the problem is especially acute in remote rural areas. Nonetheless, the countries studied have developed strategies that begin to address this challenge.

Health care must be remunerated. This is always a challenge as it involves redistribution of resources from the rich and healthy to the poor and ill, a difficulty not confined to low- and middle-income countries. The five countries are at different stages on the journey towards universal coverage, with Thailand in the lead and Bangladesh and Tamil Nadu only beginning. Ethiopia has made considerable progress in a short time, while Kyrgyzstan has worked hard to find new ways to secure coverage in a very different environment from that of its past.

Our new study reinforces many of the messages that emerged from the original *Good health at low cost* report. These include the contribution of primary care, backed up by effective referral systems and the importance of strategic action supported by multiple stakeholders. However, it has also identified some new lessons, such as the importance of building resilience into the system, in recognition of the many dangers that can quickly appear. In addition, it is noteworthy that health successes were achieved despite high levels of out-of-pocket payment in several of the countries, indicating that these were perhaps more a threat to financial protection and increased poverty than to health gains. Finally, while we are unable to make concrete recommendations about what might work in particular circumstances, we do believe that this comparative analysis sets out some broad principles that are likely to be applicable elsewhere, and provides many specific ideas that are worthy of consideration by those seeking to improve the health of their populations.

REFERENCES

1. WHO. *Everybody's business: strengthening health systems to improve health outcomes. WHO's framework for action.* Geneva: World Health Organization; 2007.

2. WHO. *The world health report 2000. Health Systems: improving performance.* Geneva: World Health Organization; 2000.

3. DFID. *The politics of poverty: elites, citizens and states. Findings from ten years of DFID-funded research on governance and fragile states 2001–2010.* London: Department for International Development; 2010.

4. Brinkerhoff DW, Bossert TJ. *Health governance: concepts, experience, and programming options.* Bethesda, MD: Abt Associates; 2008.

5. Siddiqi S et al. Framework for assessing governance of the health system in developing countries: gateway to good governance. *Health Policy* 2009; 90(1):13–25.

6. Mirzoev T, Green, A, Newell J. Health SWAps and external aid: a case study from Tajikistan. *International Journal of Health Planning and Management* 2010; 25(3):270–86.

7. Datiko D, Lindtjørn, B. Health extension workers improve tuberculosis case detection and treatment success in southern Ethiopia: a community randomized trial. *PLoS One* 2009; 4(5):e5443.

8. Wakabi W. Extension workers drive Ethiopia's primary health care. *Lancet* 2008; 372(9642):880.

9. Cercone J, Pacheco Jimenez J. Costa Rica: "good practice" in expanding health care coverage – lessons from reforms in low- and middle-income countries. In: Gottret P, Schieber GJ, Waters HR, eds. *Good practices in health financing: lessons from reforms in low- and middle-income countries.* Washington DC: World Bank; 2008:183–226.

10. Clark MA. Reinforcing a public system: health sector reform in Costa Rica. In: Kaufman RR, Nelson JM, eds. *Crucial needs, weak incentives: social sector reform, democratization, and globalization in Latin America.* Baltimore, MD: Johns Hopkins University Press; 2004:189–216.

11. Kutzin J, Jakab M, Cashin C. Lessons from health financing reform in central and eastern Europe and the former Soviet Union. *Health Economics, Policy and Law* 2010; 5(2):135–47.

12. Kutty VR. Historical analysis of the development of health care facilities in Kerala State, India. *Health Policy and Planning* 2000; 15(1):103–9.

13. Rannan-Eliya RP, Sikurajapathy L. Sri Lanka: "good practice" in expanding health care coverage. In: Gottret P, Schieber GJ, Waters HR, eds. *Good practices in health financing: lessons from reforms in low- and middle-income countries.* Washington, DC: World Bank; 2008:311–54.

14. WHO. *Thailand a country case study: good governance and preventing corruption.* Geneva: World Health Organization; 2010 (http://www.who.int/features/2010/medicines_thailand/en/index.html, accessed 26 July 2011).

15. Human Rights Watch. *No tally of the anguish: accountability in maternal health care in India.* New York: Human Rights Watch; 2009.

16. Varatharajan D. Impact of fiscal crisis on public health services in Kerala. In: Prakash BA, ed. *Kerala's economic development: performance and problems in the post-liberalisation period.* Thousand Oaks, CA: Sage; 2004:335–55.

17. El-Sahartya S et al. *Improving health services in developing countries: improving health service delivery in Ethiopia. Country case study.* Washington, DC: World Bank; 2009.

18. International Institute of Population Sciences. *National family health survey-II, 1998–99.* Mumbai: International Institute of Population Sciences; 2000.

19. International Institute of Population Sciences. *National family health survey-III, 2005–06.* Mumbai: International Institute of Population Sciences; 2007.

20. NIPORT, Mitra and Associates, and Macro International. *Bangladesh demographic and health survey 2007.* Dhaka: National Institute of Population and Training, Mitra and Associates, and Macro International; 2009.

21. Balabanova D et al. Health service utilization in the former Soviet Union: evidence from eight countries. *Health Services Research* 2004; 39(6 Pt 2):1927–50.

22. Kanchanachitra C et al. Human resources for health in southeast Asia: shortages, distributional challenges, and international trade in health services. *Lancet* 2011; 377(9767):769–81.

23. Chowdhury M, Bhuiya, A. The wider impacts of BRAC poverty alleviation programme in Bangladesh. *Journal of International Development* 2004; 16(3):369–86.

24. Bhuiya A, Chowdhury M. Beneficial effects of a woman-focused development programme on child survival: evidence from rural Bangladesh. *Social Science & Medicine* 2002; 55(9):1553–60.

25. Rohde J et al. 30 years after Alma-Ata: has primary health care worked in countries? *Lancet* 2008; 372(9642):950–61.

26. Jindawatana A, Wibulpolpraset S. *The first Thai National Health Assembly.* Bangkok: Ministry of Public Health; 1988.

27. Conway S, Harmer A, Spicer N. *International Health Partnership: 2008 external review.* London: London School of Hygiene & Tropical Medicine; 2008.

28. NIPORT, Mitra and Associates, and ORC Macro. *Bangladesh Demographic and health survey 2004.* Dhaka: National Institute of Population Research and Training, Mitra and Associates and ORC Macro; 2005.

29. Admassie A, Abebaw, D, Woldemichael, A. *Impact evaluation of the Ethiopian Health Services Extension program: a non-experimental approach.* New Delhi: Global Development Network; 2009 (Working Paper No. 22).

30. UNICEF. *In rural Ethiopia, health extension workers bring care to new mothers.* New York: United Nations Children's Fund; 2010 (http://www.unicef.org/infoby country/ethiopia_55449.html, accessed 6 September 2011).

31. Assefa Y et al. Rapid scale-up of antiretroviral treatment in Ethiopia: successes and system-wide effects. *PLoS Med* 2009; 6(4):e1000056.

32. WHO/UNICEF. *Countdown to 2015 decade report (2000–2010). Taking stock of maternal, newborn and child survival.* Geneva: World Health Organization; 2010.

33. Bangladesh Health Watch. *The state of health in Bangladesh 2007. Health workforce in Bangladesh; who constitutes the health care system?* Dhaka: James P Grant School of Public Health; 2008.

34. Perry H. *Health for all in Bangladesh: lessons in primary health care for the twenty-first century.* Dhaka: University Press; 2000.

35. Mahmood SS et al. Are 'village doctors' in Bangladesh a curse or a blessing? *BMC International Health and Human Rights* 2010; 10(18).

36. Ahmed SM et al. Socioeconomic status overrides age and gender in determining health-seeking behaviour in rural Bangladesh. *Bulletin of the World Health Organization* 2005; 83(2):109–17.

37. Bhuiya A. Village health care providers in Matlab, Bangladesh: a study of their knowledge in the management of childhood diarrhoea. *Journal of Diarrhoeal Diseases Research* 1992; 10(2):10–15.

38. George A. *Human resources for health: a gender analysis.* Geneva: Women and Gender Equity, and Health Systems, Knowledge Networks (KNs) of the WHO Commission on the Social Determinants of Health; 2007 (Review Paper).

39. Fryatt R, Mills A. Taskforce on Innovative International Financing for Health Systems: showing the way forward. *Bulletin of the World Health Organization* 2010; 88(6):476–7.

40. Fryatt R, Mills A, Nordstrom A. Financing of health systems to achieve the health Millennium Development Goals in low-income countries. *Lancet* 2010; 375(9712):419–26.

41. WHO. *National health accounts* [online database] Geneva: World Health Organization; 2010 (http://www.who.int/nha/country/en/index.html, accessed 26 July 2011).

42. Gertler P, Gruber J. Insuring consumption against illness. *American Economic Review* 2002; 92(1):51–70.

43. Rajaratnam JK et al. Neonatal, postneonatal, childhood, and under-5 mortality for 187 countries, 1970–2010: a systematic analysis of progress towards Millennium Development Goal 4. *Lancet* 2010; 375(9730):1988–2008.

44. Ooms G et al. Crowding out: are relations between international health aid and government health funding too complex to be captured in averages only? *Lancet* 2010; 375(9723):1403–5.

45. Wagstaff A. The economic consequences of health shocks: evidence from Vietnam. *Journal of Health Economics* 2007; 26(1):82–100.

46. Wagstaff A et al. China's health system and its reform: a review of recent studies. *Health Economics* 2009; 18(S2):S7–23.

47. McNay K, Keith R, Penrose A. *Bucking the trend: how Sri Lanka has achieved good health at low cost – challenges and policy lessons for the 21st century.* London: Save the Children; 2004.

48. Levesque JF et al. Affording what's free and paying for choice: comparing the cost of public and private hospitalizations in urban Kerala. *International Journal of Health Planning and Management* 2007; 22(2):159–74.

49. Mohindra K, Haddad S, Narayana D. Can microcredit help improve the health of poor women? Some findings from a cross-sectional study in Kerala, India. *International Journal for Equity in Health* 2008; 7:2.

50. Gertler P, Levine DI, Moretti E. Do microfinance programs help families insure consumption against illness? *Health Economics* 2009;18(3):257–73.

51. Hamid S, Roberts J, Mosley P. Can micro health insurance reduce poverty? Evidence from Bangladesh. *Journal of Risk and Insurance* 2011; 78(1):57–82.

52. Pitt M, Khandker S, Cartwright J. Empowering women with micro finance: evidence from Bangladesh. *Economic Development and Cultural Change* 2006; 54(4):791–831.

53. WHO. *National health accounts country data: Costa Rica* [online database]. Geneva: World Health Organization; 2011 (http://www.who.int/nha/country/cri.pdf, accessed 26 July 2011).

54. Oxman A. Can paying for results help to achieve the Millennium Development Goals? A critical review of selected evaluations of results-based financing. *Journal of Evidence-based Medicine* 2009; 2(3):184–95.

55. Koehlmoos T et al. *Rapid assessment of demand side financing experience in Bangladesh.* Dhaka: International Centre for Diarrhoeal Diseases Research, Bangladesh; 2008 (ICDDR,B Working Paper No. 170).

56. Kutzin J et al. Bismarck meets Beveridge on the Silk Road: coordinating funding sources to create a universal health financing system in Kyrgyzstan. *Bulletin of the World Health Organization* 2009; 87(7):549–54.

57. Huntingdon D et al. *Improving maternal health: lessons from the basic health services project in China.* London: Department for International Development; 2008.

58. WHO. *World health report 2008. Primary health care – now more than ever.* Geneva: World Health Organisation; 2008.

59. Ministry of Health and Family Welfare. *Expanded Programme on Immunization (Bangladesh). Bangladesh EPI coverage evaluation survey, 2009.* Dhaka: Directorate General of Health Services, Ministry of Health and Family Welfare, Bangladesh; 2009.

60. Castleden M et al. Resilience thinking in health protection. *Journal of Public Health* 2011; 33(3):378–84.

61 World Food Programme. *Horn of Africa crisis* [website]. New York: United Nations World Food Programme (http://www.wfp.org/crisis/horn-of-africa, accessed 17 August 2011).

62. Hopkinson B et al. The human perspective on health care reform: coping with diabetes in Kyrgyzstan. *International Journal of Health Planning and Management* 2004; 19(1):43–61.

63. Gertler P et al. *Impact evaluation in practice.* Washington, DC: World Bank; 2011.

64. Mills A et al. What do we mean by rigorous health-systems research? *Lancet* 2008; 372(9649):1527–9.

65. King G et al. Public policy for the poor? A randomised assessment of the Mexican universal health insurance programme. *Lancet* 2009; 373(9673):1447–54.

66. Basinga P et al. Effect on maternal and child health services in Rwanda of payment to primary health-care providers for performance: an impact evaluation. *Lancet* 2011; 377(9775):1421–8.

Chapter 10

IMPROVING THE LIVES OF "HALF THE SKY"

How political, economic and social factors
affect the health of women and their children

Andrew Harmer

LSHTM

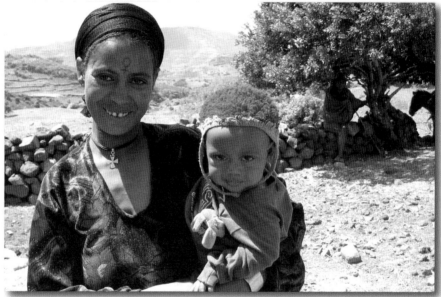

2005 Virginia Lamprecht, Courtesy of Photoshare

A community-based family planning distribution agent with her baby outside the health facility in Shallo, Ethiopia, where she reports and gets monthly updates. Plan International is implementing a family planning project in the area.

■ Key messages

- Strong and visionary political leadership has been essential in sustaining reform and championing the cause of improved health in the countries studied. This leadership is not restricted to politicians and includes senior civil servants, nongovernment elites and a variety of others who have provided inspiration.

- "Governance" is a complex construct that seems to be not especially well captured by existing indicators. However, the case studies do suggest a link between popular and informed engagement, especially of women, and improved health outcomes.

- Although the relationship between economic development and improvements in maternal and child health is complex and contested, it is apparent that improvements in physical infrastructure (such as transport and electronic communications) have improved access to services and raised awareness of what is possible.

- A link between empowerment of women and improvements in mother and child health is likely but the pathway is complex. While the evidence supports the conclusion that empowerment is a "neglected instrument for health", further work is required to understand better the virtuous cycle of gender equality and good health.

- Education emerges as a strong explanatory factor for better health in some of our country case studies. However, it remains unclear whether demand for education from an increasingly emboldened female constituency or an increase in the supply of education (more schools, better access) is the underlying driver of change.

- Civil society can, and does, play an important role in securing improved health outcomes for women and children, both through redressing inequality of access to services and through empowering women.

- Despite pro-poor policies and improvements in infrastructure, inequality continues to impede progress in mother and child health in each of the five case study countries, with many interventions and policies not benefiting the poorest groups.

■ Introduction

Although written a quarter of a century ago, there is much about today's political economy that would strike a chord with readers of the 1985 *Good health at low cost* study. Then, profound political change was just around the corner for what is now termed the former USSR; now the changes are taking place in countries in northern Africa and south-west Asia. Then, the world was only just recovering from one global economic recession and would be hit by another, two years later. Now, the world is again emerging from a global financial crisis yet so far has failed to address its fundamental causes, raising fears for the future. There have been seismic shifts too that distinguish, quite starkly, now from then. Politically, social-ist governments – flagged as having an important role in promoting good health in the 1985 report – have come under severe pressure from the forces of global capitalism. A bipolar world, dominated by the United States and the USSR, has given way to one that is multipolar, with China and India emerging as economic powerhouses; a resurgent European Union; and Brazil, South Africa, the Russian Federation and Nigeria waiting in the wings. Economies have become global since the first *Good health at low cost* study, heralding a new and interconnected world: words such as globalization or, indeed, global barely registered before in the health policy lexicon and yet today they shape how we perceive, and act upon, health problems worldwide. Technologically, we can now monitor epidemics globally, in real time, and utilize mobile technology for health interventions in ways that would defy the imagination of a 1980s' audience. In short, political, economic and social factors mattered to health then and matter just as much today, as this chapter seeks to demonstrate.

Patricia Rosenfield's contribution to the 1985 report was groundbreaking in its argument that a strong political commitment to good health was essential for countries seeking to strengthen their health systems[1]. Her analysis expressed a growing realization amongst the international health community that primary health care was more than just a technical intervention; it was also a springboard for holistic social, political and economic development. Therefore, education, universal franchise and land reform were viewed as integral components of an enlightened health policy. There is insufficient space here to explore the shift from comprehensive to selective primary health care but two points are striking when the 1985 report is compared with the analysis presented in this current study[2]. The first is that health systems remain under-resourced. By the end of the 1960s, it was evident that "teams with spray guns and vaccinating syringes" were insufficient to meet a society's most serious health needs[3]. Thirty years later, scholars were bemoaning the fact that new global responses to health through public–private partnerships were in danger of creating "islands of excellence" (specific health interventions) in "seas of underprovision" (health systems)[4]. Ten years further down the line and we are only now sufficiently appreciating the need for joined up thinking around disease-specific measures and health system strengthening[5,6]. Health systems are, therefore, back on the global health agenda and it is serendipitous that two Rockefeller Reports should bookend this shift in policy priorities.

The second point is that ideas about the importance of social determinants of health are enjoying a resurgence. Twenty years after the 1985 report, the WHO's Commission on Social Determinants of Health reinforced one of the study's key messages, arguing that poor health was not a natural state of affairs but the result of "a toxic combination of poor social policies and programmes, unfair economic arrangements, and bad politics" (p. 1)[7]. The importance of non-health factors (including literacy, social development and political leadership) as major predictors of health status has long been recognized[7–9]. For example, the impact of maternal education on child health was established in the 1980s, as demonstrated in a synthesis of evidence[10]. However, the extent to which non-health factors explain achievements in health is an area of research and policy that continues to excite broad interest[8,11–15]. The debate is particularly relevant to decisions on strategic investments designed to improve health, within the Millennium Development Goal (MDG) framework and beyond.

There is a wealth of literature seeking to answer the million-dollar question: which non-health factors contribute most to improved health outcomes? Perhaps unsurprisingly, different studies have reached different conclusions (Box 10.1). These studies have attached varying degrees of importance to non-health system versus health system factors. The ways in which these factors are conceptualized and form typologies clearly depend on the prevailing political and ideological climates, and different combinations of factors will be important in different settings. The case studies presented in this book identify those factors that were perceived as important in explaining achievements in health outcomes and intermediary indicators.

The purpose of this chapter is to present cross-cutting themes emerging from the experience of the study countries, while placing these in the context of other relevant work. The following analysis distinguishes three broad pathways to improving health outcomes: political, economic and social. As in most of the country chapters in this book, this chapter uses mother and child health as a tracer. It is accepted that progress in this area indicates a health system's strength to perform across the board. However, achievement of MDG4 and MDG5 has been problematic. As philanthropic and other donors finally begin to invest in the health of "half the sky" it is an appropriate moment to consider what effect non-health factors have on women's health as well as the health of their children[16].

Box 10.1 Non-health explanatory factors: two examples of typologies

1985: Rosenfield's five social and political contributions to good health[1]

Political and historical commitment to health as a social goal	Legislation
	Government expenditure on health
	Establishment of health facilities
	Historical and cultural influences
Social welfare orientation to development	Preventive orientation
	Support for basic necessities
	Educational programmes
	Land reform
Participation in the political process	Universal franchise and political engagement
	Extent of decentralization
	Community involvement
Equity-oriented services	Health, education and nutrition status of women, minorities, etc.
	Urban–rural coverage
	Income–asset distribution
Intersectoral linkages for health	Mechanisms to ensure linkage
	Incentives to ensure linkage
	Recognition that health is socially determined

2006: Croghan, Beatty & Ron: political, economic and social contexts for routes to better health[14]

Political context	Past colonial rule
	Stability of government
	Changes in government through violent and non-violent means
	Structure of government and political parties
	Leadership strength and stability
	Governance and corruption
Economic context	Per capita GDP
	Income inequality
	Foreign aid from bilateral and international development partners
	Management and integration of aid with existing internal resources
Social context	Basic and secondary education including but not limited to literacy
	Family planning policy
	Social integration and cohesion

■ Political pathways to good mother and child health

Rosenfield's original study put politics firmly on the map as an important explanatory factor of good health in low-income countries. The relevance of a government's political commitment to health remains as crucial today as it was in 1985. It has been repeatedly endorsed by WHO as a key factor in successful health reform, beginning with the push for primary health care in 1978 at Alma-Ata and in most subsequent *World Health Reports*. The political commitment to reform of mother and child health evident in each of our countries is all the more remarkable given their historically (and, for some, continuing) high levels of political instability. Indeed, as World Bank data show, a period of increasing political instability that began in the mid-1990s (Figure 10.1) also saw some improvement in the health of mothers and children. Is it possible to explain this apparent contradiction – political commitment and political instability? As our country chapters revealed, and as we explore further below, there is no one-size-fits-all response. Political pathways to good mother and child health are

Figure 10.1 Trend in perceived political stability in five countries

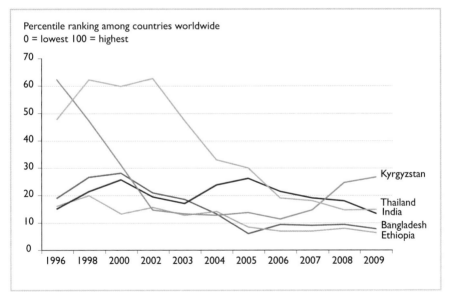

Source: Reference 17.

Note: The World Governance Indicators (WGI) are a set of aggregate indicators "based on several hundred individual underlying variables, taken from a wide variety of existing data sources"[18]. For a discussion of the methodology used see reference 18. The political stability indicator is a measure of perceptions of the likelihood that the government will be destabilized or overthrown by uncon-stitutional or violent means, including politically motivated violence and terrorism. The core data are derived from a wide range of surveys and from governmental and nongovernmental bodies.

complex, requiring an understanding not only of context but also of the plurality of actors engaged in the political process.

Exploring political commitment to health reform

Injudicious use of the phrase political commitment is an analytical accident waiting to happen and so we should be mindful of the difficulties it presents. For example, it tells us nothing about the length or intensity of the commitment and also raises the question why political commitment has led to good health in some countries but not in others[12]. Several scholars have attempted to define more precisely how political commitment can be translated to explain health priorities or progress to achieving various health goals[8,19].

In addition to its conceptual ambiguity, the evidence supporting political commitment as a key driver of good health outcomes has not been compelling. Researchers seeking to establish significant statistical correlations between political factors and improvements in child and maternal health have shown few positive results. Lykens et al. found no significant relationship between child survival and political and civil rights; Greco et al. argued that because donors tended to bypass political systems by giving aid directly to nongovernmental organizations, (NGOs) the politics of a country were less important than other factors; and Croghan et al. were unable to show a significant relationship between improved child health outcomes and either political will or positive social welfare orientation[14,15,20]. Consequently, if we are to present a narrative that gives politics a more prominent role in mother and child health than that afforded by previous studies we must accept that a degree of unpacking is required to understand how specific policy commitments translate into good health outcomes.

But health *is* political. In Bangladesh, health has long been perceived as a winning ticket to secure political advantage; the current government (2011) rose to power partly on the strength of its commitment to re-establishing community health clinics throughout rural Bangladesh. Implementing health reform can fatally damage political careers too, as the Bangladeshi political leader Ershad found in 1990 when he tried to introduce reforms to improve sanitation, nutrition and family planning services for poor people[21]. In Ethiopia, decentralization of decision-making – a fundamentally political decision – is identified in the country chapter as perhaps the single most important government decision to have improved mother and child health outcomes, but the process has been criticized for not being inclusive and was prone to capture by political elites.

In Tamil Nadu, shrewd politicians recognized the importance of new technologies for mother and child health and embraced them. For example, in the late 1990s the health secretary led a campaign against female feticide and used the media to generate public support for reform. In Bangladesh, politicians have made effective use of terrestrial and mobile technologies to cut through a tradition of mistrust of politics and deliver important health messages directly to its citizens. This contrasts with the experience in Kyrgyzstan, where public trust in government is much higher than in neighbouring countries (72% according to the World Bank's World Governance Indicators (WGI) database[17]). This helped the government to implement its radical *Manas* health reforms (described in Chapter 5). Innovation does not take place in a political vacuum either. In Tamil Nadu, leadership, vision and the commitment of senior bureaucrats were required to implement health reforms, as evidenced by support for policies regarding the surveillance of maternal deaths and establishing 24-hour emergency obstetric care[22].

Our country case studies also illustrate the important point that political leadership does not necessarily reside in government. For example, Thailand has had a rapid turnover of governments (11 in the 19 years between 1969 and 1988) and its technocrats have been key to maintaining policy formulation at national level and key policy implementation at local levels. However, it was the Thai royal family who motivated and supported annual public health conferences and galvanized public support for mandatory health policy reform. Thailand illustrates very clearly the multiple and overlapping political factors that have combined to explain effective implementation: consistent policy commitment by successive governments; the high profile of health in policy statements and plans since 1942; strong social recognition of the Ministry of Public Health; and, linked to this last point, strong motivation of all stakeholders to improve social development.

The contribution of multiple stakeholders – specifically the inclusion of civil society – in policy reform is not always evident in our case study countries. At various stages in their political histories, each country has experienced autocracy as well as democracy, and the people's voice has often been weak. Our study is not the first to reflect on the uncomfortable observation that autocratic governments can often be very effective in implementing desirable public health policies[12]. Bangladesh is a nascent democracy but its political decision-making remains largely top-down, bureaucratic and technocratic. It has a thriving civil society but its input on political life remains minimal – though this may not be the case in terms of its contribution to governance, as we explore later in the chapter. The newly emerging civil society in Kyrgyzstan remains relatively undeveloped and there are few examples of its influence on the policy process. In times of political, economic and social unrest, factors such as trust, allegiance to publicly respected figureheads and respect for civil society leaders helped to smooth the implementation of necessary health reforms in each of our countries.

Governing mother and child health

Governance is another term frequently associated with politics and government – though equally open to abuse. As Lawrence Finkelstein wryly observed: "we say governance because we don't really know what to call what is going on"[23]. Nevertheless, there *have* been international efforts to improve conceptual clarity and operationalize governance to a set of measurable indicators and indices. The MDGs are an obvious example, although it is salutary to recall early criticisms of their measurability as efforts to achieve them continue to falter in some regions[24,25]. National health systems are complex and rendered all the more so by their interaction with international and global health systems. Application of complexity theory to the field of public health is beginning to make some sense of these multiple interactions but development of meaningful measures of governance remains a work in progress[26].

The WGI express governance in terms of voice and accountability, political stability and absence of violence, government effectiveness, regulatory quality, rule of law and control of corruption[27]. While useful in providing a composite measure of a country's performance in governance, the WGI are not without their critics[28,29]. The WGI's authors have rebutted these criticisms, although debate will no doubt continue[30]. We utilize the WGI database in this chapter to draw attention to specific governance challenges while being mindful of its limitations. For example, as our case studies illustrate, advances in social factors such as gender and women's empowerment, education and civil society engagement have played key roles in improving health. Indeed, it is testament to the strength of these social drivers of change that they have been able to partially mitigate weak governance in some areas. Nevertheless, their contribution to systems of governance remains poorly understood. The WGI reduce civil society involvement in governance to little more than representation of minority views and it is likely that further refinement is required to capture fully civil society's complex governance role.

Controversy aside, when we apply the WGI to our countries, we find what previous studies of other developing countries have also found: that governance indicators are not strongly correlated to good mother and child health[14,15,20]. Indeed, only Ethiopia experienced a significant increase in any of the WGI noted above (Figure 10.2). To take one of the WGI indicators (control of corruption) as an illustration – although Ethiopia has worked hard to address corruption within government, there are few quantitative data to support the contention that this has resulted in better health outcomes. Similarly, corruption

Figure 10.2 Trend in ranking of control of corruption in five countries

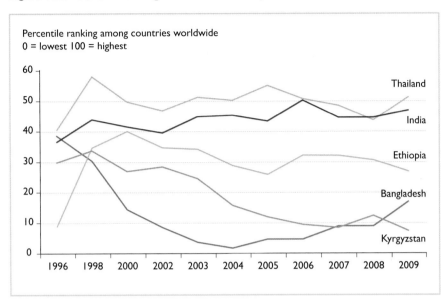

Percentile ranking among countries worldwide
0 = lowest 100 = highest

Thailand

India

Ethiopia

Bangladesh

Kyrgyzstan

Source: Reference 17.

Note: The WGI control of corruption indicator captures "perceptions of the extent to which public power is exercised for private gain, including both petty and grand forms of corruption, as well as 'capture' of the state by elites and private interests"[18].

in Kyrgyzstan has remained a significant problem. High levels of informal payments for inpatient care are reported in the country chapter, suggesting that a culture of illicit transactions and possible soliciting from staff persists despite efforts to reform. This is likely to reflect a wider occurrence of direct transactions between public service providers and clients beyond the health sector, reflecting culture but also possible insufficient trust in formal arrangements[31].

The key points that emerge from this overview of the political experiences of four countries and one southern Indian state are summarized below but it should be obvious that there is no one-size-fits-all blueprint for fledgling democracies to follow. Political factors such as country context, history, institutional strengths and weaknesses, social capital (the trust that a country's citizens place in their leaders and their willingness to 'chip in' to help push forward a health policy) all play their part. The next section of this chapter reviews the economic factors that feed into the mix.

Summary points

- Political pathways to improved mother and child health are complex and existing indicators struggle to capture this complexity.

- Political commitment is conceptually ambiguous and previous quantitative analyses suggest a weak correlation between political commitment and improved health. Nevertheless, strong leadership from government *and* nongovernment actors is a recurring motif in our country studies.

- While governments have changed frequently in our focus countries, strong political institutions committed to health reform have helped to overcome periods of political instability.

- Although WGI suggest that each of the countries studied performs poorly against a range of governance measures, understanding governance as a complex and adaptive system means thinking again about how to capture accurately what is going on. Civil society participation in mother and child health is a case in point. It has a role to play that is simply not captured through a crude measure of representation of minority views.

■ Economic pathways to good mother and child health

Worldwide, around nine million children die each year before their fifth birthday[32]. The vast majority of these deaths occur among children born in low- or middle-income countries and, within these countries, among children of more disadvantaged households and communities. While statistical data show an inverse correlation between increased income and the under-five mortality rate[33] and between GDP and the under-5 mortality rate[34], our five country case studies show that high per capita income is not a precondition for good child and health outcomes. Looking at different sets of developing countries, other studies have come to similar conclusions[14]. Indeed, the positive experiences recounted in the country chapters are in accord with a new wave of development analysis that focuses on the convergence of indicators such as health and education, rather than the divergence of economic indicators such as incomes and GDP (e.g. Kenny, 2011[35]). After all, the challenge is to understand how good mother and child health outcomes are possible *at low cost*.

There is an international dimension to the story. Since 2003, official development assistance for maternal, newborn and child health in all developing countries has increased by 105% (US$2632200 in 2003 to US$5395300 in 2008)[36]. This substantial increase in additional funding and support has meant more money for newborn. maternal and child health but has also encouraged efficiencies in the ways in which that money is spent by recipient governments[37]. Each of the five countries studied in this report received substantial funding from various donors in the 1980s and 1990s. Between 2003 and 2006, Bangladesh received a 233% increase in official development assistance for maternal, newborn and child health, while Ethiopia saw a 222% increase[20]. It is important to understand *how* donor funding might contribute directly to good health outcomes and Ethiopia provides a good case. As noted earlier in this chapter, the main factor that ensured successful implementation of devolution in Ethiopia was financial support from multilateral donors. In addition, support from the World Bank meant that Ethiopia's health sector continued to receive funding when the Ethiopian Government diverted resources to help to fund its 1999–2001 border dispute with Eritrea. However, as a 2010 study has shown, increased development assistance for health has resulted in a decrease in total government spending on the health sector in countries heavily dependent on external financial assistance[38]. This effect is especially marked in those countries subject to the strict conditionality associated with loans from the International Monetary Fund[39].

Clearly, the pathways by which poverty and prosperity affect health and mortality are complex. Recent years have seen advances in our understanding, particularly through studies undertaken by the Commission on Social Determinants of Health and its collaborators and networks[7,40]. At the national level, our country studies suggest positive mother and child health outcomes are linked not only to improvements in infrastructure (transport, water and sanitation) but also to equitable distribution of access to health care. These are explored in more detail below.

Developing infrastructures

Of the five countries, Thailand's policies seem to reflect the most explicit understanding of the benefits of non-health investment and the need to target health policies towards the poorer population. Increased investment in rural electrification in Thailand seems to have had a significant impact on fertility rates[41]. The pathways are complex but the link between electrification and knowledge of health issues – through increased access to technologies such as television – is now well documented[42]. The Thai Government's additional spending on research to improve agricultural productivity has also had an impact on rural poverty reduction and rural education[43], while the economic growth that Bangladesh has experienced in the past decade has led indirectly to improved health by providing the capital to improve the country's transport infrastructure.

Figure 10.3 Access to improved water source in rural areas, by country

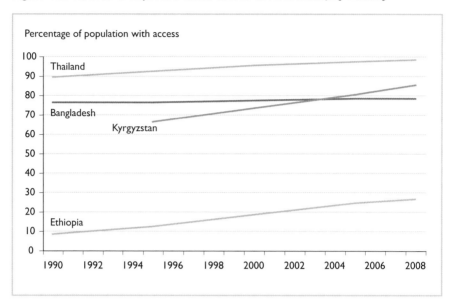

Source: Reference 47.

In 2003, there was a higher density of roads in Bangladesh than in the United Kingdom (166 km compared with 163 km per 100 km of land area). As Chapter 3 suggests, better road infrastructure may have contributed to improved access to emergency obstetric care in Bangladesh, which has reduced adverse outcomes despite the persisting high level of home-based and unattended delivery. With an improved transport infrastructure, the government was able to introduce financing innovations such as a voucher scheme to reimburse transport costs. As an indirect effect, health improved as better (and subsidized) transport made it easier for patients to access services provided at rural clinics.

The overall evidence for the importance of investment in water supply and effective sanitation for general health outcomes is well documented[44,45]. Although there has been a steady increase in access to water in rural areas of Ethiopia, Kyrgyzstan and Thailand (Figure 10.3), the health benefits are not always evident. In one study in Ethiopia, the expected improvement to women's health from access to clean water (assumed to lower the time taken to collect water and therefore to improve quality of life) was not seen. Instead fertility increased, increasing the demand for resources, which in turn, led to higher child malnutrition[46]. This is an example of the substantial complexity in this area. Improved sanitation is likely to have contributed to improvements in child mortality seen in these five countries, particularly in Kyrgyzstan (access to an improved water supply increased from 66% to 85% of the population in rural areas between 1990 and 2008) and Ethiopia (from 8% to 26%) (Figure 10.3). Improved access to sanitation may come about either through deliberate policy-making (whether around planning of settlements or building of new facilities), or because of migration into cities. All five countries have higher access to sanitation within urban areas than in rural areas, dramatically so in some cases such as in Ethiopia. This may also come about simply because increased family income allows families to build their own facilities. However, sanitation and improved access to water alone cannot account for the improvements seen in health in most of these countries.

Rapid expansion of communications technology is an important development in Bangladesh that has not been considered in many previous studies. With 80% access, television has become the primary mode for communicating health messages. For example, it was used most effectively to raise awareness about the efficacy of using zinc to treat childhood diarrhoea and about population control. A good example of the use of media is the Behavioral Change Communication campaign. As described Chapter 3, this intervention capitalized on opportunities provided by the rapidly expanding communication networks, putting emphasis on multimedia, multichannel and intersectoral approaches. Mobile phone technology – sending timely health messages directly to people's handsets – is one potential way to raise awareness of health issues but there are limited data to support the argument that it has led to better health[48,49]. However, family welfare assistants communicate with each other and with families mainly via mobile phones and this has facilitated the rapid scale up of the programme.

Equity of wealth distribution and health outcomes

Addressing the non-health factors that help to explain 'good health at low cost' inevitably raises the question: good health *for whom*? In 2010, the United Nations Development Programme's Human Development Report included a new inequality measure – the inequality-adjusted human development index. With renewed attention on the MDGs, the report stressed that it would be entirely possible to achieve MDG1, MDG4 and MDG6 without improving the lot of the poorest 20%[50]. Each of the five countries in our study performed better than expected in terms of child and maternal mortality outcomes compared with other countries with similar GDPs and each has implemented targeted policies that have benefited the health of the poor. However, as Figure 10.4 shows, some of these countries have performed better than others.

Figure 10.4 Trends in the Gini index

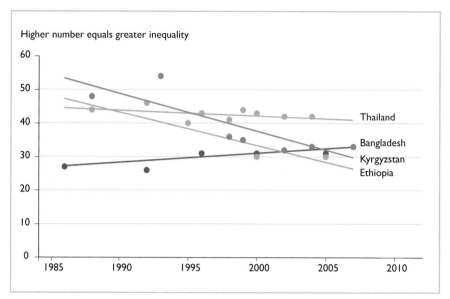

Source: Reference 47.

Figure 10.4 shows the Gini index – a standard economic measure of income inequality – for four of the five case studies (data were unavailable for Tamil Nadu). Ethiopia, Kyrgyzstan and Thailand show progress in terms of reducing inequality but inequality is increasing in Bangladesh due to a number of inter-linked factors. The last is a good example of a country in which improved health outcomes preceded economic growth – a country with "health without wealth"[12]. Microcredit provided by the Grameen Bank and other sources as well as an expanding garment industry are often cited as factors contributing to poverty reduction. However, the pathways from microcredit to good health are not always explicit, and microcredit may help only those who are already on the road to economic recovery[51]. Yet, other authors provide some evidence to suggest that some women have used microcredit schemes to enrich their lives and emancipate themselves from domestic violence[16]. Paradoxically, the health sector is becoming a generator of poverty through out-of-pocket expenditures. Although primary health care is free at the point of delivery, expenditures in the private sector are contributing to a medical poverty trap for the poorest sectors of society (see Chapter 3).

An important element of the inequality and health debate is the disparity in access to health services between urban and rural populations. Rural communi-

Figure 10.5 Urban population as percentage of total population

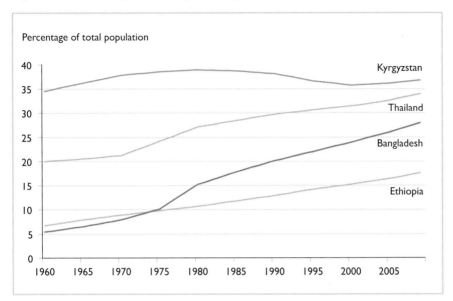

Source: Reference 47.

ties worldwide suffer from progressive underinvestment in infrastructure and amenities and experience disproportionate levels of poverty and poor living conditions[52]. These often lead to migration to urban centres (Figure 10.5). The five countries studied are predominately rural but it appears that governments have recognized the need to address urban–rural inequalities, including access to a range of basic health services. In Ethiopia and Thailand the fact that leaders come from, or have worked in, rural areas could help to explain their commitment to improving health in such areas. However, the rate of urbanization is accelerating and leading to improved access to health care – Tamil Nadu is one of the most urbanized states in India with 47% of the population living in urban areas.

Bangladesh has experienced extremely high growth in the urban population, estimated at more than 7% per year, and Dhaka is expected to have a population of 22 million by 2025. The complex impact of urbanization on health outcomes is of public concern. On one hand, people living in urban areas have better health outcomes and higher levels of utilization of services. On the other, there are concerns about the health of the urban hard-to-reach, although the gap is narrowing through concerted government action. Ensuring access to basic services (including health) is a challenge that the Bangladeshi Government must overcome in order to continue to improve health outcomes. Although Ethiopia is one of the least urbanized countries in east Africa, urbanization is identified as an increasing health problem as many people are now living in large peri-urban slums with little access to services. While there have been government efforts to improve access to primary health care services in rural and hard-to-reach areas, there is an acknowledgement that these have had limited success.

Challenges facing the rural poor in Kyrgyzstan are well documented in Chapter 5, but data suggest that the number of people not accessing services because they are either too far away or too expensive is decreasing. The chapter suggests that targeting these groups in terms of access to reproductive health services and contraceptives is vital if further progress is to be made. In Thailand, the focus on improving rural health appears to have been part of a concerted and long-term effort to improve the rural infrastructure and standards of living. This effort has focused on improving access to paved roads, electricity, piped water and health facilities. Thai health officials acknowledge that their policies have been pro-poor and pro-rural. Health disparities between rural and urban areas are decreasing and policies such as bonding doctors to rural areas and creating the Rural Doctors Society have helped to retain doctors in rural areas. The reduced inequalities in health identified in Thailand (similarly in Tamil Nadu) and elsewhere have been a result of long-term initiatives to improve the health of people living in rural areas[53].

In summary, it is worth reiterating the point that the focus countries have enjoyed better health outcomes than some other countries *despite* lower incomes and weaker economic growth. While not underplaying the relationship between health and wealth, there is clearly more to health development than a country's GDP. If there is an overarching theme to the economic pathways described above, it is the commitment that each country has shown to improving infrastructure. This has then improved *access* to health services through better roads and utilities, loans from microcredit schemes and access to knowledge via modern technologies. Health development is not necessarily about making people richer but also about making drugs and services cheaper and more widely available.

Summary points

- International donor funding has increased but the direct benefit of these funds for mother and child health is unclear; targeted support for specific policies has provided essential support during periods of political instability.

- Although the relationship between economic development and good mother and child health is complex and contested, improvements in infrastructure have helped to improve access to services and raised awareness through investment in communication technologies.

- Despite pro-poor policies and improvements in infrastructure, and despite some signs of improvement in reducing the equality gap, inequality continues to impede mother and child health in each of the five case study countries.

■ Social pathways to 'good health at low cost'

In each of the country studies, three social factors – empowering women, education and civil society – recur and were widely seen to have impacted positively on good health outcomes. While presented here as social factors, it is evident that these factors are complexly interrelated with clear political and economic dimensions.

Empowering women

There is a considerable literature that argues that the empowerment of women is a "neglected instrument for health"[54], and that "gender relations of power constitute the root causes of gender inequality, and are amongst the most influential of the social determinants of health"[55,56]. This has particular resonance for mother and child health[57]. It has been argued that MDG4 and MDG5 will not be achieved without more progress towards the achievement of MDG3 – which pertains to promoting gender equality and empowering women. The five case studies were, therefore, reviewed with a gender lens to see whether part of the explanation for achieving 'good health at low cost' (especially given the focus on mother and child health outcomes), was related to the status of gender equity and empowerment of women.

The answer to whether gender empowerment is important to achieving good health is complex and not clear-cut. However, it appears that some awareness of, and effort towards, gender equality forms part of a virtuous cycle in which decisions at individual and household levels concerning fertility and female schooling interact with income and health system changes to increase human development and health outcomes[58]. Thus, while gender empowerment does not seem to be a single causal factor that distinguishes the case studies (or explains the good outcomes described) it may be part of the context explaining why progress in terms of mother and child health outcomes has been possible at low cost. For example, research from the Indian subcontinent suggests that a range of gender-related non-health factors may help to explain why states in southern India have experienced better mother and child health outcomes and lower fertility rates than elsewhere in the region. Women's autonomy – in terms of decision-making; mobility; freedom from threatening relations with spouse; and access to, and control over, economic resources – was constrained in all three settings. However, women in Tamil Nadu fared considerably better than women from the northern portions of the subcontinent because patriarchal and gender-stratified structures were less constraining[59].

As acknowledged in Chapters 1 and 2, the relationship between the determinants of health, the role of health systems and health outcomes are "inherently complex" with "time lags between each determinant and its effect on health". Weaving gender into these relationships makes it yet more complex, partly because of the way that gender intersects with economic inequality, racial or ethnic hierarchy, caste domination, differences based on sexual orientation and a number of other social markers[56,60]. An additional challenge in assessing gender's role in achieving good health outcomes is how to measure and evaluate progress towards gender equality in health systems, especially in low- and middle-income countries. There are a number of standard indicators. For example, the Gender-related Development Index (GDI) introduced in the Human Development Report 1995 aims to assess whether men and women are making the same progress in terms of the Human Development Index (HDI). The Gender Empowerment Measure (GEM) looks at the degree to which women play an active role in political and economic life. Also, health outcome and health intervention data increasingly take gender into consideration – albeit only by disaggregating the data by sex.

None of the five case study countries is a consistently high performer across the standard indicators of gender/equality-related outcomes. Thailand drafted legislation in the late 1970s that sought to empower women by increasing their roles in the political process (see Chapter 7) and is also a high performer in terms of GDI, ranking 15th of the 155 countries in the world for which such a ranking is available. However, Thailand performs less well on the GEM score, ranking only 76th of the 109 countries for which there is a ranking. Women in the other four countries enjoy higher political profiles – Kyrgyzstan elected the first woman president in central Asia and has achieved considerable improvements in improving the status of women in comparison with its neighbours; Bangladesh has had a female prime minister and leader of the opposition for the last two decades and within the current 2011 cabinet both the home and the foreign minister are women; since 1991 a woman has been one of the two alternating chief ministers in Tamil Nadu; and in Ethiopia the Prime Minister's wife is also the Minister for Women).

However, as Bangladesh, Kyrgyzstan and Ethiopia (no data are available for Tamil Nadu) are all relatively poor performers in terms of both GDI and GEM ratings, it is questionable whether this has really led to significant shifts in attitudes towards, or improvements in opportunities for, women in these countries. While political leadership is lacking in this area, our case studies suggest considerable civil society commitment to empowering women and making progress towards gender equality in Tamil Nadu, Ethiopia, Bangladesh and Thailand. Kyrgyzstan is the exception, reflecting a regional trend, as the United Nations Development Programme concluded in a 2008 study[61]. While the former USSR has inherited a historical legacy of equality in access to education and to paid employment, it seems that the withdrawal of public services and periods of economic uncertainty have particularly burdened women.

Education

In addressing the question of why women die in childbirth, Kristof and Wudun argue that education is associated with decreased family size, increased use of contraception and increased use of hospitals[16]. However, the authors point out that correlation is not causation and provide a list of caveats to the claim that education necessarily leads to an individual's social and economic development. Establishing a link between education and improved health is equally – perhaps more – difficult. Chapter 3 suggests that a combination of factors contributed to the increases in adult female literacy rates in Bangladesh (from 18% in 1980 to 51% in 2008): government provision of free secondary schooling for girls; civil society, especially BRAC's involvement in the delivery of education; and microcredit. It remains unclear how this improvement has translated into better health status.

Furthermore, the relationship between education and better health remains ambiguous. On the one hand, while maternal and child mortality and morbidity is lower in (for example) Bangladesh than in neighbouring countries, the country has only outperformed Nepal regionally in terms of the increase in mean number of years of education for women aged 25–34[62]. On the other hand, when seeking to identify causal direction, it is not always possible to separate demand-side from supply-side factors. For example, was it the demand for education and women's autonomy that led to the dramatic reduction in fertility rates in Tamil Nadu or was this due to increased opportunities for improved education and women's autonomy? Breierova and Duflo found that increased school attendance in Indonesia resulted in women marrying later and having fewer children, while Osili and Long concluded that each additional year of primary education attended by a girl in Nigeria led to a reduction of 0.26

Figure 10.6 Thailand: adult literacy rate, by gender

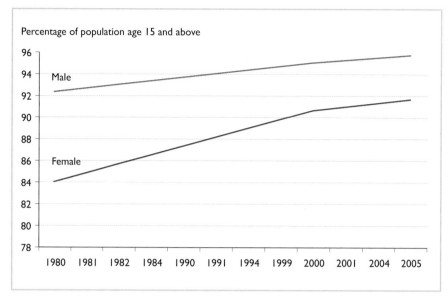

Percentage of population age 15 and above

Source: Reference 48.

children (both studies cited by Kristof & Wudun[16]). However, it is not clear whether demand or supply factors were more important. Looking at literacy levels, in Tamil Nadu, female literacy was important only to some extent[63] while other studies in southern Asia were unable to determine what level of female literacy would precipitate a sharp decline in fertility[64]. Indeed, one study[63] indicated that demand-side explanations of rapid drops in fertility – including education and female autonomy – "are unable to explain the full course of fertility transition taking place in many developing countries including some of the states in India and Bangladesh" (p. 1). Tamil Nadu's impressive reduction in fertility – reaching replacement level of 2.1 by 1990/1991 – also requires an understanding of supply-side factors such as "vigorous implementation of family planning services" *and* understanding the mechanism through which the know-ledge of services and practise was diffused through communities to individuals[63,65].

Thailand's experience of improved female literacy shows the importance of education as a social pathway to better health (Figure 10.6). The case study suggests that improved health outcomes were the result of improvements in youth and adult education and in reducing the gender education gap. As the country chapter reported, a one-year increment in a mother's education corresponded to a 7–9% decline in the under-5 mortality rate. Furthermore, education exercised a stronger influence in early and later childhood than during infancy. Although Thailand has a relatively low GEM ranking, women have had more opportunity to study and obtain employment. Female literacy rates among youths increased from 97% in 1980 to 99% in 2002. Thai gender-disaggregated statistics also showed that in 2006 enrolment rates for females were higher than for males, especially at the tertiary level. With better education, Thai women were more able to find employment. Data from 2002 to 2006 showed that women held a higher proportion of jobs than men, improving women's economic status.

Kyrgyzstan has benefited from the inherited model of near universal education for men and women operating during the Soviet regime, which is seen to benefit the development of the country, and to a large degree this has been sustained in the face of subsequent shortages.

Civil society

What emerges from the country chapters is that many of these countries have a vibrant NGO community working to empower women and interacting with the health sector in interesting and innovative ways. Previous studies have come to similar conclusions, noting the importance of civil society in addressing inequality in society[34]. For example, the *World Health Report* 2005 recognized that civil society in Bangladesh was crucial for changing health priorities and agendas, describing it as "the mass base" of support and impetus for forging broad political alliances – sowing the seeds for political reform[66].

Historically, the involvement of NGOs and civil society organizations has been very different across the five case studies. Ethiopia and Kyrgyzstan have relatively new but increasing nongovernment sectors (since the country gained independence, more than 2000 NGOs are now working in Kyrgyzstan's health sector, largely thanks to international donor support). Bangladesh and Thailand both have a long and lively history of indigenous (and international) civil society – Bangladesh is host to BRAC, the world's largest NGO. Another example from Bangladesh is the women's group Naripokkho, which has been strengthening gender awareness in subdistricts. One of its actions was to set up health advisory committees as part of the devolution of public services. It also mobilized journalists and local women's groups to lobby these committees to make gender-specific decisions. These included demands to increase the number of female gynaecologists and to decrease women's waiting times for medical services[67]. In Bangladesh, women's rights groups were asked to participate in formulating the government's Health and Population Sector Programme. Some ideas were apparently incorporated, but implementation and oversight has been weak[68].

In Tamil Nadu, the Campaign Against Sex Selective Abortion used the Right to Information Act 2005 to obtain district-wide data on sex ratio at birth from the Department of Health, enabling it to identify where problems existed. This organisation has waged a campaign to have doctors who disclose the sex of a fetus (which is illegal in India) deregistered from the Medical Council and have campaigned against problems in the relatively unregulated private sector, where the law is regularly flouted[68,69]. This group has encouraged pregnant women to go into private clinics and hospitals as mystery patients to see if doctors break the law. Where this has occurred, the group then attempts to have them prosecuted. The action of this and other groups working with the state health department and the media seems to offer at least part of the explanation why Tamil Nadu's sex ratio is now better than in many states in India.

In Ethiopia, the involvement of civil society in policy decisions is less well understood. Chapter 4 provides some positive examples of civil society participation but it is noted that the decentralization process was not inclusive and hence probably less effective than it could have been. However, positive advances in women's participation in the political process have been achieved through a Ministry of Women's Affairs, affirmative action and legal protection for women against early marriage.

In summary, this section has explored three social pathways to good health: empowering women, education and civil society. These pathways intersect at various points and have contributed to good health outcomes, as described in the country chapters. However, the directional arrows of causation between empowerment and education are not always clear: are women empowered because they are better educated, or does an empowered community demand better education? Gender adds a further dimension. None of the five countries performs particularly well against gender equality indicators and pointing to the presence of women in a country's government is surely too crude an indication of shifting cultural practices. A vibrant civil society is another recurring motif in some, though not all, of the country chapters. The role of civil society in good mother and child health outcomes remains weakly understood and warrants much closer scrutiny.

Summary points

- Women's empowerment is a likely factor contributing indirectly to advancements in mother and child health but the relationship is complex.

- Education is a strong explanatory non-health factor leading to better health in some of our country case studies but the relative importance of supply and demand factors is not always clear.

- Civil society played an important role in securing good mother and child health, through redressing inequality of access to services and, specifically, through working to empower women.

◾ Conclusions

Political, economic and social factors have contributed to the improvements in mother and child health seen in our five country case studies. Complex political, economic and social relations compound efforts to establish significant correlations between variables and outcomes. A working group set up to report on health inequalities in the United Kingdom expressed the problem well: "We are dealing with 'wicked problems', that is, problems that defy easy or single bullet solutions. They have complex causes and require complex solutions"[70]. That complexity is captured in this chapter and it illustrates the importance of context in understanding how interventions are derived and why they are effective.

Political commitment to improving maternal and child health outcomes is a common theme that emerges from each of the case studies. However, the devil is in the detail and it is essential to understand the political nuance. On the one hand, top-down hierarchies that get things done seem to be effective in increasing access to services and thus affecting health, especially where they work with civil society. On the other hand, bottom-up services provided by civil society may not be accurately captured through current health governance indicators, where 'voice' is only a crude indicator of engagement in the policy process. Further work is required to understand the role of civil society over time in achieving good mother and child health outcomes. Little is understood about the way relationships between government and civil society emerge or about processes of adaptation, accommodation and challenge.

Inequity lies at the heart of the country chapters, notably inequity between urban and rural areas and within regions and cities. Redressing the urban bias in infrastructure and services depends on investment in the rural sector to provide not just health care services but also education free at the point of use, reliable utilities, usable roads and accessible public transport. The demonstrable and positive effect of low cost communication technology on people's access to health care is one bright light at the end of a still too dark tunnel.

Although the pathway to good health is complex, gender equality appears to be an important part of a virtuous cycle. Changes linked to decisions at individual and household levels concerning fertility and female schooling interact with income and health system changes to increase human development and health outcomes. Exploring direct cultural pathways, this chapter suggests that health outcomes are improved where women are more engaged in decision-making, more mobile and relatively free from threatening relations.

Better-educated women and children lead healthier lives. The data on education from our focus countries do not establish a clear causal pathway to 'good health at low cost' but strongly support other evidence which links education to better health. Some of the case studies suggest that female empowerment is an important pathway to good health outcomes. Improved economic opportunities coupled with strong pressure by civil society in some countries have resulted in greater access to health services and rights.

Challenges remain. All of our countries face significant inequalities in income and health. Non-health factors that provide an initial boost to health – such as better employment opportunities, increased urban infrastructure, more disposable income – also lead to increases in chronic noncommunicable diseases and other health burdens for which our countries show varying levels of preparedness.

ACKNOWLEDGEMENTS

I would like to thank Loveday Penn-Kekana and Nicola Watt for their input to sections of early drafts of this chapter. The chapter as a whole was significantly restructured following an intensive workshop at the Rockefeller Bellagio Centre and I am very grateful to all the participants for their incisive feedback. Finally, the entire manuscript has benefited from the editorial guidance of a number of colleagues but in particular Dina Balabanova, Lesong Conteh, Mushtaq Khan, Martin McKee and Anne Mills.

REFERENCES

1. Rosenfield P. Social and political factors. In: Halsted SB, Walsh JA, Warren KS, eds. *Good health at low cost: proceedings of a conference held at the Bellagio Conference Centre.* New York: Rockefeller Foundation; 1985:173–80.

2. Cueto M. The origins of primary health care and selective primary health care. *American Journal of Public Health* 2004; 94(11):1864–74.

3. Bryant J. *Health and the developing world.* New York: Cornell University Press; 1969.

4. Buse K, Waxman A. Public–private partnerships: a strategy for WHO. *Bulletin of the World Health Organization* 2001; 79(8):748–54.

5. Ooms G et al. The diagonal approach to global fund financing: a cure for the broader malaise of health systems? *Globalization and Health* 2008; 4:6.

6. De Savigny D, Adam T. *Systems thinking for health systems.* Geneva: World Health Organization; 2009.

7. CSDH. *Closing the gap in a generation: health equity through action on the social determinants of health.* Geneva: World Health Organization, Commission on Social Determinants of Health; 2005.

8. Shiffman J. Generating political priorities for maternal mortality reduction in 5 developing countries. *American Journal of Public Health* 2007; 97(5):796–803.

9. Alvarez J et al. Factors associated with maternal mortality in sub-Saharan Africa: an ecological study. *BMC Public Health* 2009; 9:462.

10. Cleland J, van Ginneken JK. Maternal education and child survival in developing countries: the search for pathways of influence. *Social Science & Medicine* 1988; 27(12):1357–68.

11. Caldwell JC. Routes to low mortality in poor countries. *Population and Development Review* 1986; 12(2):171–220.

12. Reich M. The political economy of health transitions in the third world. In: Chen L, Kleinman A, Ware NC, eds. *Health and social change in international perspective.* Boston, MA: Harvard School of Public Health; 1994:413–51.

13. Bloom DE, Canning D. The health and wealth of nations. *Science* 2000; 287(5456):1207–9.

14. Croghan TW, Beatty A, Ron A. Routes to better health for children in four developing countries. *Millbank Quarterly* 2006; 84(2):333–58.

15. Lykens K et al. Social, economic, and political factors in progress towards improving child survival in developing nations. *Journal of Health Care for the Poor and Underserved* 2009; 20(4 Suppl):137–48.

16. Kristof N, Wudun S. *Half the sky: how to change the world.* London: Virago; 2010.

17. World Bank. *Worldwide governance indicators* [online database]. Washington, DC: World Bank; 2010 (http://info.worldbank.org/governance/wgi/index.asp, accessed 1 August 2011).

18. Kaufmann D, Kraay A, Mastruzzi M. *The worldwide governance indicators: methodology and analytical issues.* Washington, DC: World Bank; 2010 (Policy Research Working Paper 54).

19. Geneau R et al. Raising the priority of preventing chronic diseases: a political process. *Lancet* 2010; 376(9753):1689–98.

20. Greco G et al. Countdown to 2015: assessment of donor assistance to maternal newborn, and child health between 2003 and 2006. *Lancet* 2008; 371(9620):1268–75.

21. Reich M. Bangladesh pharmaceutical policy and politics. *Health Policy and Planning* 1994; 9(2):130–43.

22. Padmanaban P, Raman PS, Mavalankar D. Innovations and challenges in reducing maternal mortality in Tamil Nadu, India. *Journal of Health, Population and Nutrition* 2009; 27(2):202–19.

23. Finkelstein L. What is global governance? *Global Governance* 1995; 1:368.

24. Davis K, Kingsbury B, Merry S. *Indicators as a technology of global governance.* New York: New York University School of Law; 2010 (IILJ Working Paper 2010/2).

25. Attaran A. An immeasurable crisis? A criticism of the millennium development goals and why they cannot be measured. *PLoS Medicine* 2005; 2(10):e318.

26. Hill P. Understanding global health governance as a complex adaptive system. *Global Public Health* 2010; 28 April:1–13.

27. World Bank. *Worldwide governance indicators: documentation.* Paris: World Bank; 2010 (http://info.worldbank.org/governance/wgi/resources.htm, accessed 1 August 2011).

28. Devarajan S. Two comments on "Governance indicators: where are we, where should we be going?" by Daniel Kaufmann and Aart Kraay. *World Bank Research Observer* 2008; 23(1):31–6.

29. Langbein L, Knack S. The worldwide governance indicators: six, one, or none? *Journal of Development Studies* 2010; 46(2):350–70.

30. Kaufmann D, Kraay A, Mastruzzi M. Response to: "The worldwide governance indicators: six, one, or none?" Washington, DC: World Bank; 2010 (http://info.worldbank.org/governance/wgi/pdf/ResponseKL.pdf, accessed 27 July 2011).

31. Ensor T, Savelyeva L. Informal payments for health care in the former Soviet Union: some evidence from Kazakhstan. *Health Policy and Planning* 1998; 13(1):41–9.

32. UNICEF. *The state of the world's children: maternal and newborn health.* Geneva: United Nations Children's Fund; 2009.

33. Powell-Jackson T et al. Democracy and growth in divided societies: a health inequality trap? *Social Science & Medicine* 2011; (73(1):33–41.

34. Cattaneo A et al. Progress towards the achievement of MDG4 in the Commonwealth of Independent States: uncertain data, clear priorities. *Health Research Policy and Systems* 2010; 8:5.

35. Kenny C. *Getting better: why global development is succeeding.* New York: Basic Books; 2011.

36. Pitt C et al. Countdown to 2015: assessment of official development assistance to maternal, newborn, and child health, 2003–2008. *Lancet* 2010; 376(9751):1485–96.

37. Taskforce on Innovative International Financing for Health Systems. *More money for health, and more health for the money.* Geneva: International Health Partnership; 2009 (http://www.internationalhealthpartnership.net/CMS_files/documents/taskforce_report_EN.pdf, accessed 20 April 2011).

38. Lu C et al. Public financing of health in developing countries: a cross-national systematic analysis. *Lancet* 2010; 375(9723):1375–87.

39. Stuckler D, Basu S, McKee M. What causes aid displacement? International Monetary Fund and aid displacement. *International Journal of Health Services* 2011; 41(1):67–76.

40. Blas E, Kurup AS. *Equity, social determinants and public health programmes.* Geneva: World Health Organization; 2010.

41. Harbison S, Robinson W. Rural electrification and fertility change. *Population Research and Policy Review* 1985; 4(2):149–71.

42. Independent Evaluation Group. *The welfare impact of rural electrification: a reassessment of the costs and benefits.* Washington, DC: World Bank; 2008.

43. Fan S, Yu B, Jitsuchon S. Does allocation of public spending matter in poverty reduction? Evidence from Thailand. *Asian Economic Journal* 2008; 22(4):411–30.

44. Genser B et al. Impact of a city-wide sanitation intervention in a large urban centre on social, environmental and behavioural determinants of childhood diarrhoea: analysis of two cohort studies. *International Journal of Epidemiology* 2008; 37(4):831–40.

45. Fewtrell L et al. Water, sanitation, and hygiene interventions to reduce diarrhoea in less developed countries: a systematic review and meta-analysis. *Lancet Infectious Diseases* 2004; 5(1):42–52.

46. Gibson M, Mace R. An energy-saving development initiative increases birth rate and childhood malnutrition in rural Ethiopia. *PLoS Medicine* 2006; 3(4):e87.

47. World Bank. *World Development Indicators* [online database]. Washington, DC: World Bank (http://data.worldbank.org/data-catalog/world-development-indicators, accessed 1 August 2011).

48. Etzo S, Collender G. The mobile phone revolution in Africa: rhetoric or reality? *African Affairs* 2010; 109(437):659–68.

49. Lester RT et al. Effects of a mobile phone short message service on antiretroviral treatment adherence in Kenya (WelTel Kenya1): a randomized trial. *Lancet* 2010; 376(9755):1838–45.

50. Barros F et al. Health and nutrition of children: equity and social determinants. In: Blas E, Kurup A, eds. *Equity, social determinants and public health programmes.* Geneva: World Health Organization; 2010:49–75.

51. Schurmann A, Johnston H. The group-lending model and social closure: microcredit, exclusion, and health in Bangladesh. *Journal of Health, Population and Nutrition* 2009; 27(4):518–27.

52. Ooi G, Phua K. Urbanization and slum formation. *Journal of Urban Health* 2007; 84(Suppl 1):27–34.

53. Gravel N, Mukhopadhyay A. Is India better off today than 15 years ago? A robust multidimensional answer. *Journal of Economic Inequality* 2010; 8(2):173–95.

54. Editorial. Gender equity is the key to maternal and child health. *Lancet* 2010; 375(9730):1939.

55. Marmot M, on behalf of the Commission on Social Determinants of Health. Achieving health equity: from root causes to fair outcomes. *Lancet* 2007; 370(9593):1153–63.

56. Sen G, Ostlin P. *Unequal, unfair, ineffective and inefficient. Gender inequality in health: why it exists and how we can change it: Final Report to the WHO Commission on Social Determinants of Health, Women and Gender Equity Knowledge Network.* Stockholm: Karolinska Institute; 2007.

57. Bhutta Z et al. Delivering interventions to reduce the global burden of stillbirths: improving service supply and community demand. *BMC Pregnancy and Childbirth* 2009; 9(Suppl 1):S7.

58. Molina G, Purser M. *Human development trends since 1970: a social convergence story.* Geneva: United Nations Development Programme; 2010 (Human Development Research Paper 2010/2).

59. Jejeebhoy J, Sathar Z. Women's autonomy in India and Pakistan: the influence of religion and region. *Population and Development Review* 2001; 27(4):687–712.

60. WHO. Women and health. *Today's evidence, tomorrow's agenda.* Geneva: World Health Organization; 2009.

61. UNDP. *Regional gender equality strategy, 2008–2011.* New York: United Nations Development Programme Regional Bureau for Europe and the Commonwealth of Independent States; 2008 (http://europeandcis.undp.org/uploads/public1/files/RBEC%20%20Gender%20Equality%20Strategy%20%202008%20-%202011%20revised%20FINAL.doc, accessed 20 April 2011).

62. Gakidou E et al. Increased educational attainment and its effect on child mortality in 175 countries between 1970 and 2009: a systematic analysis. *Lancet* 2010; 376(9745):959–74.

63. Dev SM, James KS, Sen B. *Causes of fertility decline in India and Bangladesh: an investigation.* New Delhi: South Asia Network of Economic Research Institutes. SANEI; 2002:27.

64. Visaria P, Visaria L. Demographic transition: accelerating fertility decline in 1980s. *Economic and Political Weekly* 1994; 29(51–52):3281–92.

65. Guilmoto CZ, Irudaya Rajan S, eds. *Fertility transition in south India.* London: Sage; 2005.

66. WHO. *The world health report 2005 – make every mother and child count.* Geneva: World Health Organization; 2005: 166.

67. Naripokkho. Women's health and rights advocacy partnership completion report: 2003–2006. Dhaka: Naripokkho; 2006 (Internal document).

68. Murthy RK. Strengthening accountability to citizens on gender and health. *Global Public Health* 2008; 3(Suppl 1):104–20.

69. Joseph J. *Reflections on the campaign against sex selection and exploring ways forward.* New Delhi: Centre for Youth Development Activities; 2007 (india.unfpa.org/drive/Reflections.pdf, accessed 20 April 2011) (Report commissioned by the UN Population Fund).

70. Hunter DJ et al. *Learning lessons from the past: shaping a different future.* Durham: University of Durham; 2009:9 (http://www.dur.ac.uk/resources/public.health/news/FinalSynthesisedReporttoMarmotReview-WC3subNov09.pdf, accessed 28 July 2011) (Marmot Review Working Committee 3, Cross-cutting Sub-Group Report).

Chapter 11

CONCLUSIONS

Good Health at Low Cost research team

This book has explored the experiences of five countries. Each was selected because it had made consistent progress in improving the health of its population and had improved access to key services. Some of these countries have fared better than many others at similar levels of economic development. And each has made progress in designing and implementing imaginative and innovative reforms to its health care system. Each has done so despite having limited resources. Some of these achievements have been sustained over long periods of time. Yet the countries are all quite different from one another. They have different political systems. They inherited different levels of resources, whether expressed in terms of money or in terms of people and physical infrastructure. And they have pursued different combinations of policies in developing their health systems. Our question is how have they achieved what they have? Are there lessons that we can draw that will be of relevance to other countries seeking to improve their health systems?

'Good health at low cost' remains an attractive slogan but confusing phrase. The original 1985 report *Good health at low cost* captured the aspirations of the moment: to ensure access to key low cost interventions, particularly within primary health care. The phrase highlights the achievements given low levels of resources. 'Low cost' was understood broadly, in terms of total financial cost, but also in terms of resources available (Halstead S. Personal communication at *Good health at low cost* meeting in Bellagio, August 2010). In our study, 'good health at low cost' was viewed as the achievement of good health in countries with a relatively low level of income. Our countries spend quite different amounts of money, whether viewed in terms of total or only government health expenditure. Although health expenditure has increased somewhat in absolute terms, it has not changed substantially as a share of GDP over the years in all five countries. Nonetheless, it appears that substantial health improvements have been made, without a substantial increase in the share of national resources spent on health. In this respect, our five countries do indeed appear to have achieved 'good health at low cost'. Our question is, how?

An obvious starting point is the original *Good health at low cost* report. Now 25 years old, its findings have stood the test of time. The case studies in this book, and the subsequent experiences of the original countries included in that report, confirm the importance of sustained investment in health systems, especially in primary care, with an emphasis on sustainable funding and the development of a skilled health workforce, strong political commitment to good health for the whole population, a high degree of community involvement, measures to ensure equity of access and use, and health-promoting policies that go beyond the health system. Indeed, some of these are more important than ever. This is clearly the case for a skilled workforce. The technology available 25 years ago limited what could be done in low resource settings. This has changed dramatically and there are now many low cost interventions that can be life saving, but only if administered by skilled health workers. Each of the countries examined in this book provides examples of innovative strategies to increase the size and skills of the health workforce, especially in traditionally underserved rural areas.

However, it is now possible to step back and ask what are the factors that enable some countries to adopt these measures while others do not? It cannot simply be a lack of knowledge. The arguments in favour of primary health care have been well-rehearsed[1], with the most recent evidence being assembled in the 2008 *World Health Report*[2]. The evidence for intersectoral action to promote health is also well established[3], having also been updated recently, in the *Report of the Commission on Social Determinants of Health*[4]. There is a wealth of scientific literature on how best to improve access to care. The answer must lie somewhere else than lack of evidence.

Work over the past decade has demonstrated that health systems are complex and require a systems thinking approach[5] that understands the relationships between different health systems components, the context in which the systems exist, and the sequencing of actions. Health system strengthening is much more than a mechanistic implementation of a series of essential interventions and there is great scope for unintended consequences[6].

Gathering the information in this book has involved each of us going on a journey. This journey involved more than crossing national borders to gather the information needed to assemble the case studies. Much more importantly, it involved crossing disciplinary and cognitive borders, requiring each of us to look at our own health system through the eyes of others, taking nothing for granted and asking fundamental questions about why things are as they are, how they got there and why they changed.

Four interlinked factors necessary for a health system to succeed emerged from this process (Figure 11.1). Conveniently, each can be expressed as a word beginning with C. They are *capacity* (the individuals and, especially, institutions necessary to design and implement reform), *continuity* (the stability required for reforms to be seen through to completion, coupled with the institutional memory that prevents the same mistakes being made each time), *catalysts* (meaning the ability to seize windows of opportunity) and *context* (or more precisely, the ability to take context into account when developing policies that are relevant and appropriate to the given circumstances). We will now consider each of these in turn.

Figure 11.1 Key themes emerging from the research

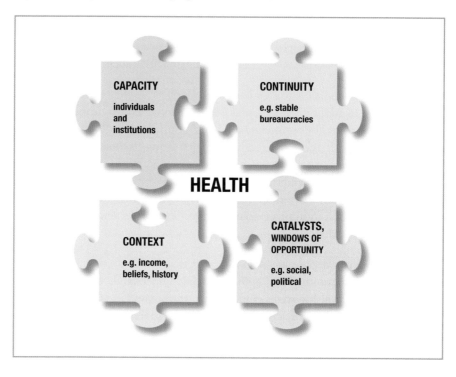

Capacity

Individuals matter. Our case studies contain many examples of individuals who have had a vision of where they wanted to be and have inspired those around them to get there. Some, but not all, have worked in the health sector. They include heads of governments, such as the current Ethiopian Prime Minister and the first Kyrgyz President after independence from the USSR, who simply wanted to make their country a better place to live. In both cases, achievements in health care have been accompanied by enhancements in education, transport links, safe water supplies and other areas that improve the lives of ordinary people while, in addition, alleviating the burden of disease and improving access to care. They also include health ministers, such as Tedros Adhanom Ghebreyesus, who articulated his four-step plan to achieve the health Millennium Development Goals (MDGs) in the *Lancet*[7]. We are, of course, aware that, despite their achievements, some of these individuals have attracted controversy as they sought to implement wide-ranging changes and we recognize that some have questioned whether the ends always justified the means. We simply conclude that addressing some of the challenges they inherited required very difficult decisions.

We also found many examples of individuals who, while they might not aspire to be leaders, also played a key role in making things happen. These are the bureaucrats, a term that is often seen in negative terms as a consequence of sustained attacks by political commentators looking to score easy points. Yet bureaucrats are essential if things are to change. Often poorly paid, always undervalued, many work tirelessly for little reward to improve the lives of their fellow citizens. Of course we realize that not all do so, and there are still many who exploit their positions for personal gain, with profound consequences for those often-voiceless people who depend on the services they administer. But in the countries we studied there was clear evidence that good practices were being encouraged while bad practices were being dealt with.

Individuals working alone can, however, only achieve so much. A second aspect of capacity that emerged strongly was that of strong institutions. Where these were most successful they provided a degree of stability that transcended the careers of individuals, ensuring institutional memory. The best are also learning institutions, drawing lessons from their own experiences but also from those of others working in similar situations elsewhere. They have access to emerging research and have systems in place to ensure that it is absorbed, adapted and implemented, something encouraged by the presence of long-term technical experts based within health ministries[8]. They also have a degree of autonomy, giving them the ability to think outside the box in order to arrive at innovative solutions to difficult problems. However, such institutions also have strong incentives to collaborate where they recognize that improving health is everyone's business and a common reason for failure is the inability to emerge from one's own sectoral silo[9]. In Tamil Nadu, district-level health managers and effective management systems have enabled expansion of access to primary care workers and essential drugs. We have also seen how a lack of institutional capacity can limit the success of reforms, as in the neighbouring state of Kerala following decentralization of social welfare provision, where local health planners were insufficiently prepared to manage scarce decentralized funds.

Individual institutions exist within a broader institutional framework. This can provide the basis for a set of formal and informal rules that facilitate the translation of evidence into practice, avoiding high transaction costs associated with a market-based approach[10]. The institutional framework interfaces with what is termed governance, which includes issues such as the rule of law, the ability to raise taxes and transparency. In their absence, it is very difficult to deliver effective and responsive health care for all. In most of the study countries we can see evidence of wider processes of state and institution-building that have created a framework for reform of health systems. Notable examples include Thailand and Kyrgyzstan, where health systems development has benefited from strengthening systems of accountability. This is also apparent in China, one of the original *Good health at low cost* countries[11].

Yet the countries studied suffered from a severe inherited lack of health system capacity. Recognizing the gaps, they have been open to innovation in seeking to use these resources more effectively. For example, all face shortages of health workers, especially in rural and remote areas. In response, they sought to create a new community-based cadre of health workers (Bangladesh, Tamil Nadu, Thailand) or launched mass retraining of existing physicians as family practitioners (Kyrgyzstan), recognizing the need to be flexible in finding ways to respond to the needs of their populations given the scarce resources. The most successful health systems have also seized on existing capacities outside the health sector, such as exploiting improved road and communications infrastructure. For example, in Bangladesh, health assistants' use of mobile phones to communicate with clients and each other, and manage workload in isolated rural areas, has improved deployment and programme efficiency, and also responsiveness.

Finally, there is the issue of capacity to monitor what is happening. Even in the richest countries, there are often major gaps in the information to track progress towards the goals of reform. Our case studies included several examples of systems that had established effective monitoring mechanisms linked to the policy process, such as those in Thailand and Kyrgyzstan. Similarly, in Tamil Nadu, there is a process of learning from local innovation, ensuring that the lessons are incorporated into policy.

■ Continuity

Although there is a school of thought that welcomes turmoil, seeing opportunities in what is termed creative destruction, a key finding to emerge from our case studies is the importance of continuity. This is linked to the development of a vision that can be articulated and communicated to those who must implement it, something only possible with inspirational leaders and receptive institutions.

Health systems are complex adaptive systems. They require resources that take time to produce, and contain institutions that take time to change and people who take time to learn. What can be achieved – and how quickly – is constrained by where they started from, a phenomenon known as path dependency[12]. Health systems cannot be changed overnight and those who believe that they can do so with some kind of "big bang" are deluding themselves.

Many of the successes described in this book incorporated careful sequencing. Change was seen as requiring a sequence of steps, each interlinked and mutually interdependent. For example, the Thai road to universal coverage took place in several stages, each based on ever more ambitious national plans. Expansion of access to key reproductive health interventions in Bangladesh and Tamil Nadu was incremental, learning lessons from previous experience every step of the way.

One way to ensure continuity is to create stable, professional bureaucracies. This will often require considerable investment in training to ensure that there are individuals with the requisite skills, as happened with the dedicated public health cadre unique in India to Tamil Nadu. This is easiest in countries which have stable governments, such as Costa Rica, one of the original *Good health at low cost* countries. However, it is possible, and indeed desirable, to develop mechanisms by which national plans and actions can transcend political and economic transition. Perhaps the best example is in Kyrgyzstan, where the key elements of the two consecutive reform plans (*Manas* and *Manas Taalimi*) survived intact despite several violent changes of government. However, the core elements of the Thai reforms also survived unscathed from the Asian financial crisis of the 1990s. In Costa Rica, the expansion of primary care in the early 1990s, regarded as the completion of the unfinished agenda to universalize access to primary care in the 1970s, was able to proceed despite a change in political administration. These health systems demonstrate a high degree of resilience, as do the systems in Ethiopia and Bangladesh that have established mechanisms to sustain health care delivery in the face of repeated natural disasters. Yet there is still much to be learned about how a health system can develop and maintain such resilience.

Several of the countries we studied were major recipients of development assistance. For them, continuity involves more than just their domestic institutions. It also involves managing what can be a remarkably complex collection of donor agencies. We found a range of examples of success in creating mechanisms to ensure synergies among donors and consistency of policies over time, for example the well regarded Sector–wide Approaches (SWAps) in Kyrgyzstan and Ethiopia.

Continuity was often evident in the effective engagement of the nongovernmental and private sectors, recognizing the important role of the private and voluntary sectors in delivering care in many countries. Successful reforms have pursued greater integration of public and private sectors, often building on private sector capacity, for example scaling up access to essential maternal and child services by underserved populations in Bangladesh and strengthening HIV/AIDS and tuberculosis prevention in Tamil Nadu.

Despite pluralistic health care provision in Bangladesh, Thailand and Tamil Nadu, government leadership is evident in formulating policies, initiating mutually beneficial collaborations and seeking to protect public interest. The mechanisms that promote trends for closer engagement also promote continuity by negotiating shared goals and establishing ways of monitoring progress towards them.

◼ Catalysts

There are many examples throughout history of health system reforms that have been implemented in the aftermath of a crisis. This has required individuals with the vision and ability to seize windows of opportunity. Examples of crises from our case studies include the achievement of independence by Bangladesh in 1971, and Kyrgyzstan in 1991. In Ethiopia, the opening up of the country and increasing donor involvement since 1994 has led to more intensive reforms in the health and other sectors. China's various experiences in health financing reform since the introduction of economic liberalization in the 1970s have provided important lessons on both the potential hazards of rapid economic growth for health and promising ways of reinvesting its new wealth to address them. Success is greatly assisted by having responsive, flexible institutions that can support the process, although in practice it has often been necessary to create them as part of the reform process, as was done in Kyrgyzstan.

Economic shocks can also catalyse health systems developments. After the collapse of the Soviet Union, the loss of subsidies from Moscow and regional trade links triggered a severe economic crisis in Kyrgyzstan, and brought the health system to a standstill. This situation helped to foster consensus about the urgent need to reform the health system and the enactment of the radical *Manas* programme in 1996, the most radical of its kind in central Asia.

Natural disasters have also acted as catalysts for strengthening health systems resilience through developing health systems preparedness to respond to external threats. This includes ability to plan early warning mechanisms and implement multifaceted strategies. The competencies associated with these efforts have led to improvements in overall service delivery in communities at risk in Bangladesh, Ethiopia and Thailand.

◼ Context

Health systems are embedded in larger social systems, at national and international levels. They are influenced by their history and the histories of the countries in which they exist. They shape and, in turn are shaped, by policies in many other sectors. Most obviously, there is a synergistic relationship with the national economy whereby economic growth can, if fairly distributed, support effective health systems, while effective health systems, by promoting a healthy workforce, can boost economic growth[13]. Similarly, investment in education creates a skilled health workforce and empowered, informed patients, while the promise of a longer and healthier life provides a stimulus for people to secure education for themselves[14]. It is these types of virtuous cycle that were established early in the original *Good health at low cost* countries and that underlie their continued health improvement.

Financial resources are only a part of the answer. The economic growth in some of the countries, such as Thailand and China, may have helped to create a momentum and population demand for expanding coverage and encouraged sophisticated reform initiatives in the health systems and in other sectors. However, the overall level of resources in the health system did not emerge as a key determinant of success across the countries, although reforms to enhance financial protection (Thailand, Kyrgyzstan, China) have played an important role in expanding access to essential services. Interestingly, health systems have not benefited disproportionately from increased national income. There is scope to spend more, improve financial protection, reduce out-of-pocket payments and address needs, and Thailand is moving in this direction.

Another element of the context involves cultural norms and national identity. Work undertaken to inform the development of this project identified the role played by ethnic and linguistic fragmentation in slowing progress in child health[15]. Essentially, it can be argued that countries where the ruling groups retain separate identities from others in the same country are less willing to invest in systems that redistribute resources, such as those to deliver health care. In this respect, the achievement of Ethiopia is notable. Despite the extreme degree of ethnic and linguistic diversity that characterizes the country, strenuous efforts have been made to carve out a coherent national identity supported by measures to achieve equitable allocation of resources. Another example of seeking a fit between health system strategies and population preferences is the emphasis on home-based maternal and reproductive care aimed at isolated and marginalized groups (Bangladesh, Tamil Nadu).

A third aspect of context relates to geography. Countries with widely dispersed rural populations, such as Ethiopia, or with particularly isolated groups, such as Bangladesh and Thailand, have had to find ways of deploying health workers with at least basic skills where they are needed most. Yet challenges remain as the Ethiopian Government embarks on the next stage, which is to reach out to the smallest villages and to the nomadic population[16].

Socioeconomic, regional and ethnic inequalities and the expansion of the private sector have led to widening health inequalities in several countries, despite considerable successes in improving average figures, and this problem is exemplified by China. The importance of providing a basic package of health care to those in need has been a driving principle in many of the countries included in both this and the original set of countries. This supports Amartya Sen's belief that "If a significant proportion of people are left out of ongoing health facilities for one reason or another, the health of the people will clearly suffer"[17]. While in some countries such as Thailand and Costa Rica, health sector developments have been underpinned by concerns to uphold equity, this remains rare. Reforms have promoted aggregate health gain, rather than achieving equitable health gain; the needs of specific population groups may not have been sufficiently addressed. This raises serious questions for the future and whether seeking both aggregate and relative health gains are possible.

■ In conclusion

Box 11.1 summarizes the pathways to improving health and access to care that have emerged from our research. The key message of this book is that success in improving health and delivering health care is facilitated by capacity, both individual and institutional, continuity, or the ability to maintain a course even when all around is changing, catalysts, or the ability to seize windows of opportunity, and sensitivity to context, so that policies that are adopted take account of the circumstances in which they will be implemented.

Although we have been able to chart many successes, it is clear that considerable challenges remain. It cannot be assumed that the countries in this study will sustain their achievements in the face of emerging challenges. Of the original four countries, only two (Sri Lanka and Costa Rica) have done so, although the achievements in Sri Lanka have continued despite a divisive, damaging and brutal civil war. In China, some of the earlier achievements have been reversed, due to growing income inequalities hampering access and to the dismantling of many community-based services during the reform process.

Each of the new countries included in this book still has some way to go to provide accessible and affordable services to the whole population, especially in remote rural areas and in the emerging pockets of deprivation in urban settings, and to achieve protection from catastrophic expenditure in the event of family illness. In some of them there are concerns about political stability. In each, the achievement of equity remains a long-term goal, although this is something shared with much wealthier countries. Thailand and Kyrgyzstan are, however,

Box 11.1 Pathways to improving health and access to care

- *Political commitment* to improve health outcomes, and effective leadership and willingness by governments to prioritize health, innovate and embed reform in systems, giving space for front-line workers to make a difference.

- Commitment by governments to *more equitable and pro-poor policies and female empowerment*.

- *Effective and stable street-level bureaucrats* that have institutional memory.

- *Collaboration* by different sectors, actors and programmes involving communities, grassroots groups and the media in order to increase the awareness of entitlements and rights and coverage of underserved populations.

- *Flexible use of health workers* to ensure that those with the most appropriate skills deliver care, particularly to women and children.

- *Building health system resilience*, to allow it to withstand shocks and emerging threats, combined with innovative use of scarce resources, and the capacity to incorporate bottom-up innovation.

- *Economic factors*, including strengthened infrastructure, economic growth, increased external funding, communication technology and the ability to draw on resources beyond the public sector.

- *Social development*, including government commitment to more equitable and pro-poor policies (e.g. empowering women, education).

- The presence of *individuals and political elites*, along with strong institutions implementing policies adapted to context, who choose to lead change, seizing windows of opportunity for developing viable and affordable health systems.

making significant progress in this direction. Progress is, perhaps inevitably, uneven; while Tamil Nadu has achieved a substantial decline in maternal and child mortality, it still faces widespread undernutrition, in large part as a consequence of its inability to tackle deeply rooted inequalities.

Looking ahead, a major concern must be the changing nature of the diseases that health systems must respond to. In this respect, they can be seen as victims of their own success. Having picked the low-hanging fruit that make up the common causes of childhood death, they must develop the capacity to move to the next stage of the epidemiological transition in which urbanization, and its accompanying lifestyles, fuel an epidemic of noncommunicable diseases. Some, such as Costa Rica, Thailand and Kyrgyzstan, have already had to do this and have made notable progress; others, such as Kerala and China, continue to struggle. Yet others, such as Ethiopia and Bangladesh, are at a much earlier stage in the process. This will require interventions with an entirely different degree of complexity to those required now. We hope that the systems that have been put in place in the countries we have studied will help them to prepare for this challenge. By the time another 25 years has passed, we will know, one way or the other.

REFERENCES

1. Starfield B. *Primary care: balancing health needs, services, and technology.* New York: Oxford University Press; 1998.

2. WHO. *The world health report 2008. Primary health care – now more than ever.* Geneva: World Health Organization; 2008.

3. Sindall C. Intersectoral collaboration: the best of times, the worst of times. *Health Promotion International* 1997; 12(1):5–6.

4. CSDH. Closing the gap in a generation: health equity through action on the social determinants of health. In: *Final report of the Commission on Social Determinants of Health.* Geneva: World Health Organization; 2008.

5. de Savigny D, Adam T, eds. *Systems thinking for health systems strengthening in English.* Geneva: Alliance for Health Policy and Systems Research, World Health Organization; 2009.

6. WHO. *Everybody's business: strengthening health systems to improve health outcomes.* [WHO's framework for action.] Geneva: World Health Organization; 2009.

7. Ghebreyesus TA. Achieving the health MDGs: country ownership in four steps. *Lancet* 2010; 376(9747):1127–8.

8. Wisman R, Heller J, Clark P. A blueprint for country-driven development. *Lancet* 2011; 377(9781):1902–3.

9. Chernichovsky D, Martinez G, Aguilera N. Reforming "developing" health systems: Tanzania, Mexico, and the United States. *Advances in Health Economics and Health Service Research* 2009; 21:313–38.

10. Bloom G, Standing H, Lloyd R. Markets, information asymmetry and health care: towards new social contracts. *Social Science & Medicine* 2008; 66(10):2076–87.

11. Bloom G. Building institutions for an effective health system: lessons from China's experience with rural health reform. *Social Science & Medicine* 2011; 72(8):1302–9.

12. Altenstetter C, Busse R. Health care reform in Germany: patchwork change within established governance structures. *Journal of Health Politics, Policy and Law* 2005; 30(1–2):121–42.

13. McKee M et al. Health systems, health, and wealth: a European perspective. *Lancet* 2009; 373(9660):349–51.

14. Strauss J, Thomas D. Health, nutrition and economic development. *Journal of Economic Literature* 1998; 36:766–817.

15. Powell-Jackson T et al. Democracy and growth in divided societies: a health-inequality trap? *Social Science & Medicine* 2011; 73(1):33–41.

16. Donnelly J. Ethiopia gears up for more major health reforms. *Lancet* 2011; 377:1907–8.

17. Sen A. Learning from others. *Lancet* 2011; 377(9761):200–1.

Annex

METHODOLOGY

■ Bangladesh

Quantitative and qualitative methods were employed in generating this case study. The work was carried out in two streams which informed each other: first, an extensive review of secondary data was conducted in conjunction with a review of the grey and published literature; second, in-depth interviews and focus group discussions were conducted, some at subdistrict level.

Quantitative methods

Data sources

In Stage 1, an extensive review of secondary grey and published literature was conducted (from national surveys and routine data) in order to track changes in selected health outcomes and health system related factors influencing these outcomes. These were supplemented using international data sources and an extensive literature review using the search methodology described below. A data inventory was created that summarized findings and described the local sources (Table A.1).

Table A.1 Key local data sources, Bangladesh (examples)

Sources	Time periods
Bangladesh Demographic and Health Survey (BDHS)	1993–1994, 1996–1999, 1999–2000, 2004, 2007
Urban Health Survey	2006
Bangladesh Maternal Health Services and Maternal Mortality Survey	2001
Bangladesh Adult Literacy Assessment Survey	2008
National Health Accounts	1996–2002
Bangladesh Health Watch Report	2007–2009
Social sector performance surveys: health and family planning	2004–2005
Human Resources Development Data Sheets,	2002–2010
Sample Vital Registration System, Bangladesh Bureau of Statistics	
First – Fifth Five Year Plans in Health and Population Sector,	
Annual programme reviews of HPSP and HNPSP	
The Constitution of Bangladesh	
Draft National Health Policy, Health Services Report	

Figure A.1 Search results for PubMed and EconLit, Bangladesh

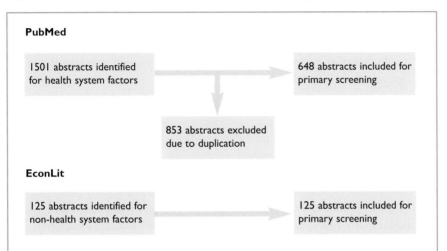

Qualitative methods

Literature review

Literature searches were conducted focusing on both health and non-health factors affecting health (Figure A.1). PubMed was searched for health- and health systems-related factors. Eighteen different searches were implemented in three major outcome areas. Specifically, a country-specific core was used and then intermediary outcomes or final outcomes were searched within the six health systems building blocks, for example Bangladesh *and* immunization *and* service delivery. For non-health systems-related factors, a search was conducted in EconLit. The review also involved manual reference tracing. Ultimately, a total of 773 titles and/or abstracts were identified for inclusion. Further, a comprehensive review of the grey literature was undertaken, including books on the development of the nation that have been published in Bangladesh.

Key informant interviews and focus group discussions

The conceptual model underlying the study (see Chapter 2, Figure 2.3) was used to draw on the Stage 1 findings, including the health system and the wider policy context in which it operates. The model on health systems adopted by the WHO[1] was employed to explore the key changes over time relating to the six building blocks of the health system.

Based on past or present engagement in our areas of interest, 18 key informants were selected for interview: policy-makers, programme managers at both national and *upazila* (subdistrict) level and public sector programme specialists (12); politicians and activists from NGOs and the private sector (2); international and development partners (2); academics (1); researchers (1). A pre-tested, open-ended questionnaire adapted for the Bangladesh context was used in the interviews. All interview participants gave written informed consent prior to participating in the interview.

In addition, 20 focus group discussions were conducted with government field workers (health assistants, family welfare assistants/skilled birth attendants, family welfare visitors), private providers (traditional birth attendants and informal providers) and NGO-sponsored community health workers (urban birth attendants, health workers/paramedics, health volunteers and health educators/counsellors) in selected rural and urban areas (including ICDDR,B's rural health system observatories in Abhoynagar and Mirsarai subdistricts and Dhaka city slums having BRAC's maternal, neonatal and child health programme). The gender breakdown of the focus groups was 79 men and 60 women.

Transcripts of the key informant interviews and focus group discussions were developed in Bangla and summarized in English. Reviews of local research/evaluation findings and/or policy briefs on relevant non-health sectors such as education, employment, food security, climate change, water–sanitation, social safety nets, poverty reduction, disaster management were undertaken to supplement the health-sector information. Finally, triangulation of evidence from multiple sources was conducted.

Data analysis

Findings were integrated in order to explain the improved health outcomes observed in Bangladesh with reference to the conceptual model and timeframe. Thematic analysis of qualitative information was employed to identify themes, subthemes relating to the framework, as well as emergent issues, with a particular emphasis on context. Efforts were made to validate qualitative information through triangulation of information derived from multiple sources.

Finally, an iterative feedback process was ongoing with our key informants and other stakeholders within Bangladesh, enabling the inclusion in the chapter of up-to-date material as it was released. Preliminary findings were presented at conferences and enriched by additional insights.

REFERENCE

1. WHO. *Everybody's business: strengthening health systems to improve health outcomes. WHO's framework for action.* Geneva: World Health Organization; 2007.

■ Ethiopia

Both quantitative and qualitative data were reviewed and analyzed from government, nongovernment and private published documents and key informant interviews. The following represents the main data sources for the study.

Quantitative methods

Data sources

A review and time-series analysis of available documents was undertaken, covering the critical period between 1974 (the time when a communist military junta took power) and 2010. The analysis used secondary data and materials mostly on health indicators that focused on child and maternal mortality. Additional data on human, commodity and financial resources were also included. Table A.2 shows the sources, time period and indicators used in the study.

Qualitative methods

Literature review

This included review and analysis of health policies, reforms and innovations as well as health research conducted in the country between 1994 (when the Imperial era ended with a military coup) and 2010. The main ones are shown in Table A.3.

Key informant interviews

Eighteen interviews were conducted with key informants, involving health policy-makers, implementers and health driving forces and stakeholders. Specifically representatives were interviewed from Ethiopian Health and Nutrition Research Institute (EHNRI); Tulane University, Ethiopia; the Federal Ministry of Health, CCM-GF Secretariat, Ethiopia; National HAPCO; Health Bureau, Affar Region; Columbia University, Ethiopia; MSH; USAID; UNICEF; Health Bureau, Amhara Region Referral Hospital, Amhara Region; and World Bank, Ethiopia.

Data analysis

In general, as indicated above, data collection involved in-depth interviews with policy-makers, document review on health and related policy issues, and secondary data collection mostly on appropriate health and household indicators/outcomes. As far as possible, the data collection covered the following three

Table A.2   Key data sources, Ethiopia (examples)

Type of database	Time periods	Variables of interest
Household surveys (Ethiopia Demographic and Health Survey, 2000 and 2005)		
Central Statistical Agency	2000, 2005	Change in under-5 mortality by region, Ethiopia
Administrative reports (Federal Ministry of Health, 2009)		
Health and Health Indicators, Ethiopia	2004, 2008	Selected indicators in maternal, child health
	2007, 2008	Per capita expenditure for health by region
	2002/03–2007/08	Access to safe water
	2002/03–2007/08	Human resources – ratio of physicians to population,
International databases (data for selected East African countries)		
World Development Indicators, World Bank	1990–2008	GDP per capita (constant 2000 US$)
	1990–2008	Under-5 mortality
	2006–2009	% children aged <5 sleeping under insecticide-treated nets
	2004–2007	Physicians per million population
	2003–2007	Per capita expenditure on health (current US$)
	2003–2007	Share of out-of-pocket health expenditure
	2003–2007	Share of health expenditure from external sources
WHOSIS, 2009	2001–2007	Median availability of generic essential medicines

timeframes, in chronological order: (i) 1974–1991: to provide general *historical context* and the constraints that may have prevailed at the time including major socioeconomic, policy, political, natural and man-made events; (ii) 1992–2000: the *time of transition*, including major health and political policy formations; implementations and possible outcomes; along with infrastructural develop-ments; and (iii) 2001– present: the *time of policy innovation and implementation*, (including donor involvement) and specific health and related outcomes.

Table A.3   Health policies, reforms, innovations and research, 1994–2010

Source/year	Document
TGE, 1993	The Health Policy of the Transitional Government of Ethiopia. Addis Ababa, Ethiopia
FMOH, 2009	Annual Performance Report of HSDP III (2008/9). Addis Ababa, Ethiopia
FMOH, 1998	The HIV/AIDS Policy of the Federal Democratic Government of Ethiopia. Addis Ababa, Ethiopia
FMOH, 2009	Results of Baseline Survey on Alignment and Harmonization for IHP Compact. Addis Ababa, Ethiopia
FMOH, 2008	Appraisal of MDG Performance Fund: The Programming Component. Addis Ababa, Ethiopia
FMOH, 2008	Scaling up aid for better health in Ethiopia, the IHP Road Map. Addis Ababa, Ethiopia
FMOH, 2010	4th National Health Accounts 2007/8. Addis Ababa, Ethiopia
MOFED, 2006	Ethiopia: Building on Progress A plan for Accelerated and Sustained Development to End Poverty (PASDEP), 2006/6–2009/10
MOFED, 2008	Joint financial arrangement between the Federal Democratic Republic of Ethiopia and development partners on support to the MDG-Fund. Addis Ababa, Ethiopia
WHO, 2009	Health-related millennium development goals. World Health Statistics 2006 and 2009 (WHOSIS). ITS Statistical Information system. Geneva
WHOSIS, 2006; 2009	Health-related millennium development goals
Miz-Hasab Research Centre, 2010	The System Wide Effects of the Scale Up of HIV/AIDs, Tuberculosis, and Malaria Services in Ethiopia
Miz-Hasab Research Centre, 2006	Hospital-based ART [antiretrovral therapy] scale-up in Ethiopia

In-depth interview transcripts and notes were coded by salient themes using NUD*IST as necessary. Secondary data were analysed by looking at trends (when possible, for instance with DHS and MOH indicators); and by overview when data were not consistently available. Health system elements were correlated with health outcomes. Health outcomes data were analysed in relation to policy, political and health systems – demonstrating how favourable political, policy and health systems yielded better health outcomes with lower investment in health.

■ Kyrgyzstan

Quantitative methods

Data sources

Information was drawn from secondary sources that are regularly used for the monitoring and evaluation of health systems in Kyrgyzstan. A data inventory was created, providing a detailed snapshot of data available on each indicator, data reliability and variations in data by source (Table A.4).

Data analysis

The primary approach was time-series analysis, tracking the progress in health systems inputs, outputs and outcomes during the period 1997–2009.

Qualitative methods

Literature review

Reviews were done of relevant local (both published and unpublished) and international literature on determinants of health improvement, wider economic and social changes that might have improved health, the historical evolution of the Kyrgyz health system, achievements and challenges, and evidence on how policy-makers had managed to promote the health reforms and improve health system outcomes. Other sources of documentary evidence included relevant local reports and regulations.

Key informant interviews and focus group discussions

In-depth interviews and focus groups were carried out at the national and regional levels. The in-depth interviews were administered to the policy-makers at the different levels and not limited to only the health sector. Focus groups with doctors (general practitioners) were conducted. Interview guidelines developed by the team at the London School of Hygiene & Tropical Medicine were adapted to the Kyrgyz context and piloted with two policy-makers. The questionnaire was semi-structured and included additional probes under each health system building block. The interviews allowed some variation of the sequence of topic areas was possible, but covered key areas of the framework of the *Good health at low cost* project (see Figure 2.3).

Twenty-eight in-depth interviews and five focus groups (three to five people per group) were carried out across the country. There were no refusals. On average,

Table A.4   Key data sources, Kyrgyzstan (examples)

Types of databases	Time periods	Variables of interest
Household surveys		
UNICEF Multiple Indicator Cluster Surveys	2006	Maternal mortality ratio Infant mortality rate Under-5 mortality rate
DHS	1997	Maternal mortality ratio Infant mortality rate Under-5 mortality rate
Health module of the Kyrgyz Integrated Household Survey	2001, 2004, 2007, 2010	Financing burden (OOPs) Equity Access to health care Effectiveness of health system
Discharged patient survey	02/2001, 07/2001, 04/2003, 04/2004, 10/2006	Financing burden (OOPs) Equity Access to health care
Administrative reports		
Republican Medical Information Centre		Cardiovascular disease Tuberculosis HIV/AIDS Human resource indicators
National Statistic Committee (non-health system indicators)	1990–2009	Macroeconomic indicators (GDP, poverty rate, etc.) Education Gender Governance
Millennium Development Goals revised report	2010	Maternal mortality ratio Infant mortality rate Under-5 mortality rate
National Health Accounts	2010	Total health expenditure OOPs
International databases		
WHO Health for All database	01/2011	Cardiovascular disease Tuberculosis Life expectancy Financing indicators (total health expenditure, OOPs)

Note: OOP: out-of-pocket expenditure

Table A.5   Characteristics of key informants, Kyrgyzstan

Key informant types	Total number	Mean age (years)	Gender		Professional background					
			M	F	Medical doctor	Nurse	Public health	Econo-mist	Acade-mic	Other
National level	9	45	4	4	4			3		2
Oblast level	11	55	7	4		4		3		4
District level	15ª	55		15	8	5				2
International organizations and projects	5	45	5		3			1	1	
Former government policy-makers	3	65	3	1	1					2
Total	43	54.2	19	24	16	9		7	1	10

Notes:

National level: Central Agency of Development, Investment and Innovations; Ministry of Health; State Agency of Social provision; State Mandatory Health Insurance Fund; NGOs; etc.

Oblast level: Territorial hospitals, family medical centres, *oblast* social departments within the local authorities, territorial departments of the Mandatory Health Insurance Fund.

District level: Family group practices, feldsher–midwifery posts, village health committees.

International organizations and projects: WHO, World Bank, UNICEF, Medicines Transparency Alliance.

Former policy-makers: A few key informants who used to work in the government.

ª Five focus groups at *rayon* level with doctors with 3–5 people.

interviews lasted between 1.5 and 3 hours and were tape-recorded. Sampling was purposive, seeking to identify people who had played key roles in the policy process and health system development during the previous 20 years. Respondents were selected from four *oblasts* (districts), to represent regional variation; exposure to, and experience of, reforms; and a mixture of resource constraints. Table A.5 presents the characteristics of all key informants.

Data analysis

Interview guidelines developed by the team at the London School of Hygiene & Tropical Medicine were adapted to the Kyrgyz context and piloted. The semi-structured questionnaire was developed in Russian and included additional probes under each health system building blocks. As well as the themes identified under the remit of health, the Kyrgyz team reviewed different local reports and policy briefs on non-health sectors themes, such as gender, education, employment and poverty reduction, to supplement the health-sector information. As a result, triangulation of evidence from multiple sources was conducted.

■ Tamil Nadu

Quantitative methods

Data sources

Information was drawn primarily from secondary sources both at national and state levels to make a comparison between Tamil Nadu and the rest of India. Certain indicators, such as out-of-pocket expenditure and equity, were estimated using National Sample Survey Organisation (NSSO) data. Table A.6 summarizes data sources, time periods and variables used.

Data analysis

The primary approach was time-series analysis, tracking the progress in health systems inputs, outputs and outcomes over a period of approximately four decades.

Qualitative methods

Literature review

Review of literature included both published and unpublished academic as well as administrative documents on determinants of health improvements, economic and social factors that might have affected health, the historical evolution of the Tamil Nadu and the Indian health system, achievements and challenges, and evidence on how policy-makers and implementers managed to improve health outcomes. The databases PubMed, EconLit, EBSCO and ScienceDirect were used to collect literature on both health and non-health system factors. Other sources of documentary evidence included Five-Year Plan documents, health policy reports, policy documents of the Tamil Nadu State Government, performance reports of the Department of Health and Family Welfare (Government of Tamil Nadu), surveys undertaken by central and state government agencies such as the NSSO, the International Institute of Population Sciences and publications relating to India by international organizations such as World Bank, WHO and UNICEF.

Table A.6   Description of key data sources for analysis, Tamil Nadu

Types of databases	Time periods	Variables of interest
Household surveys		
Morbidity and Health Care (NSSO)	1995–1996 2004	Non-hospitalized and hospitalized illnesses Health care choices and quantity of service used Sociodemographic characteristics
National Family Health Survey (NFHS)	1992 1998 2005	Family welfare and health indicators by background characteristics at the national and state levels Perinatal mortality, adolescent reproductive health, high-risk sexual behaviour, tuberculosis, malaria
Census of India	1991 2001	Literacy, sex ratio
Sample Registration System (SRS) Bulletin	1985 1990 1995 2000 2005	Vital events such as birth rate, death rate, infant mortality rate, maternal mortality ratio, under-5 mortality
Administrative reports		
Vital statistics	1971–2007	Population and vital statistics (life expectancy, infant, child and maternal mortality, and crude birth rate)
Policy Note, Department of Health and Family Welfare, Tamil Nadu Government	1985–2006	Budget, number and type of hospitals, beds, doctors, nurses, and others; child immunization coverage of various basic vaccines
National Health Accounts, India	2001/2002 2004/2005	Health spending by functions, financing agents, and health care providers
Statistical Handbook of Tamil Nadu	1996–2008	State GPD
International databases		
University of Washington Institute of Health Metrics and Evaluation	1970–2007	Under-5 mortality Vaccination for diphtheria, pertussis, tetanus coverage 1982–2006

Table A.7   Characteristics of key informants, Tamil Nadu

Key informant types	Total number	Mean age (years)	Gender		Professional background					
			M	F	Medical doctors	Nurse	Public health	Economist statistician	Acade-mic	Other
Policy makers at the federal/state level										
Serving	5	53	3	2	3					2
Retired	15	67	11	4	13					2
Implementers, MOPH (in 3 provinces)	10	35	6	4	5	3	1	1		
Research institutes	4	55	2	2	2			2		
Outside MOPH	5	51	3	2	2			1	1	1
Total	39	55	25	14	25	3	1	4	1	5

Key informant interviews

In-depth interviews were carried out with four groups of key informants in 2010: policy makers in the Ministry of Health and Family Planning (both of the Government of India and of the Government of Tamil Nadu), retired health administrators (directors) who were at the helm of the affairs during the 1980s and 1990s, and administrators (technocrats) in service, researchers and respondents in other sectors. Details are provided in the Table A.7.

Fifteen retired health administrators, who had seen the evolution of the health system and were in key positions in the 1980s and 1990s, were identified from the list provided by the Directorate of Medical Services and snowball sampling used to identify further respondents in the Department of Health and other sectors until a consensus has reached about the evolution and factors responsible for the development of the sector. Semi-structured questionnaires were used as a guideline and most of the interviews were recorded with their oral consent. On average, interviews lasted 2.5 hours.

Data analysis

Using content analysis, a descriptive narrative was prepared, and information was triangulated in several ways including with published literature.

■ Thailand

The country chapter drew on series of quantitative and qualitative analyses that supplemented each other and sought to identify factors promoting health and access to services over time.

Quantitative methods

Data sources

Information was drawn from both primary and secondary sources used regularly for the monitoring and evaluation of health systems in Thailand[1,2], and a number of national household survey datasets were re-analysed. Table A.8 summarizes data sources, with time periods and variables used.

Data analysis

The primary approach was time-series analysis, tracking the progress in health systems inputs, outputs and outcomes over a period of approximately four decades.

Changes in health infrastructures and human resources over time were normalized to population density ratios using the Ministry of Interior Department of Public Administration's reports on the mid-year population.

Average annual changes in important outcome/output and input indicators were determined for each major event period using interrupted, time-series analysis. Serial correlation between the current value and its lags was controlled for using an appropriate auto-regressive model.

Qualitative methods

Literature review

The authors carried out reviews of relevant published and unpublished literature on determinants of health improvement, wider economic and social changes that might have improved health, the historical evolution of the Thai health system, achievements and challenges, and evidence on how policy-makers and policy implementers had managed to improve health outcomes. Other sources of documentary evidence included a long series of national Five-Year Health Development Plans, published literature relevant to maternal and child health in Thailand, and publications relating to Thailand by international organizations such as WHO and UNICEF.

Table A.8   Description of key data sources for analysis, Thailand

Types of databases	Time periods	Variables of interest
Household surveys		
Health and welfare surveys	1974–1978 (q 1 yr) 1981–2001 (q 5 yr) 2003–2007 (q 1 yr) 2009 onward (q 2 yr)	Non-hospitalized and hospitalized illnesses Health care choices and quantity of service used Sociodemographic characteristics
Socioeconomic surveys	1957–1986 (q 5 yr) 1988–2006 (q 2 yr) 2007 onward (q 1 yr)	Consumption and non-consumption expenditures including for health care Earned/unearned money and in-kind incomes Socioeconomic status variables
Surveys of population change	1942–1952 1965–2005 (Inter-census, q 10 yr)	Births, deaths and migration
Population and housing census	1909–1929 1937–1947 1960–2010 (q 10 yr)	Births, deaths and migration
Administrative reports		
Vital statistics	1957–2007	Population and vital statistics from national civil registration systems (life expectancy, infant, child and maternal mortality, and crude birth rate)
Health Resource Surveys	1962–2007	Number and type of hospitals, beds, doctors, nurses and others
National Health Accounts	1994–2008	Health spending by functions, financing agents and health care providers
Thailand health profiles	1996–2008	Child immunization coverage of various basic vaccines
International databases[3]		
	1970–2007	Under-5 mortality Vaccination for diphtheria, pertussis, tetanus coverage 1982–2006[4]

Table A.9   Characteristics of key informants, Thailand

Key informant group	Total number	Mean age (years)	Gender		Professional background					
			M	F	Medical doctor	Nurse	Public health	Econo-mist	Acade-mic	Other
Policy-makers, MOPH at national level	4	61	4		4					
Implementers, MOPH (in 3 provinces)	11	53	5	6	5	5	1			
Research institutes	2	55	2		2					
Outside MOPH	5	52	3	2	2			1	1	1
Total	22	55	14	8	13	5	1	1	1	1

Key informant interviews

In-depth interviews were carried out with four groups of key informants during the first half of 2010: policy-makers in the Ministry of Public Health (MOPH), implementers (technocrats) in the MOPH, researchers, and respondents in other sectors (Table A.9). Two eminent key informants (policy-makers) were identified initially, and the snowball sampling was used to identify further respondents in the MOPH and other sectors until no new information emerged. Semi-structured questionnaires were used and there were no refusals. On average, interviews lasted 1.5–3 hours and were tape-recorded (with permission).

Data analysis

Content analysis was applied, a descriptive narrative prepared, and information was triangulated in several ways including with published literature. A member of the research team was also interviewed as an eyewitness of district health systems development.

REFERENCES

1. Tangcharoensathien V, Limwattananon S, Prakongsai P. Improving health-related information systems to monitor equity in health: lessons from Thailand. In: McIntyre D, Mooney G, eds. *The economics of health equity.* Cambridge: Cambridge University Press; 2007:222–45..

2. Limwattananon S et al. *Reviews of existing databases for monitoring and evaluation of equity in health in Thailand.* Nonthaburi: ASEM Trust Fund; 2006.

3. Murray CJL et al. Can we achieve Millennium Development Goal 4? New analysis of country trends and forecasts of under-5 mortality to 2015. *Lancet* 2007; 370:1040–54.

4. Lim SS et al. Tracking progress towards universal childhood immunisation and the impact of global initiatives: a systematic analysis of three-dose diphtheria, tetanus, and pertussis immunisation coverage. *Lancet* 2008; 372:2031–46.